Objective Assessment of Hearing

Core Clinical Concepts in Audiology

Series Editors
James W. Hall III, PhD
Virginia Ramachandran, AuD

Basic Audiometry
Pure-Tone Audiometry and Masking
By Maureen Valente

Electrodiagnostic Audiology
Objective Assessment of Hearing
James W. Hall III, PhD
De Wet Swanepoel, PhD

Objective Assessment of Hearing

James W. Hall III, PhD
De Wet Swanepoel, PhD

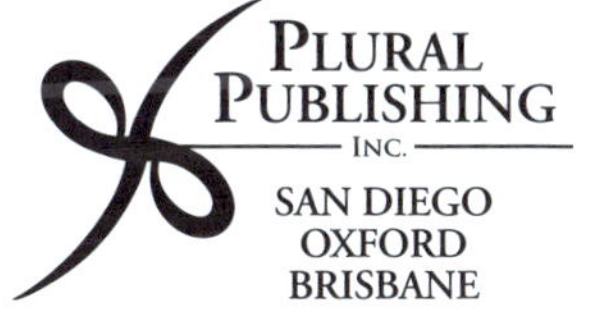

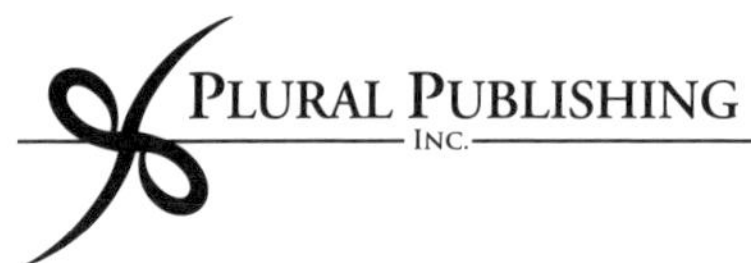

5521 Ruffin Road
San Diego, CA 92123

e-mail: info@pluralpublishing.com
Web site: http://www.pluralpublishing.com

49 Bath Street
Abingdon, Oxfordshire OX14 1EA
United Kingdom

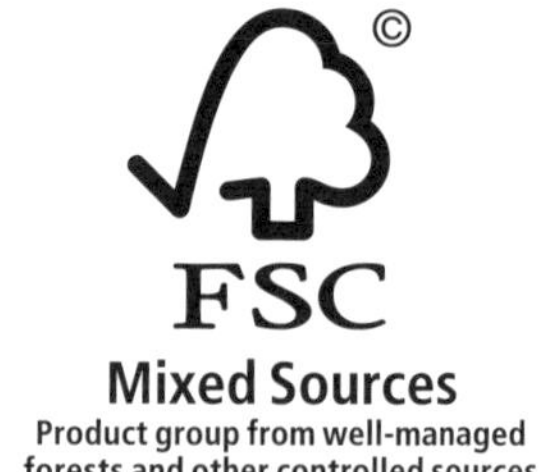

Typeset in 11/13 Palatino by Flanagan's Publishing Services, Inc.
Printed in the United States of America by McNaughton and Gunn, Inc.

Library of Congress Cataloging-in-Publication Data

Hall, James W. (James Wilbur), 1948-
Objective assessment of hearing / James W. Hall III and De Wet Swanepoel.
p. ; cm. — (Core clinical concepts in audiology)
Includes bibliographical references.
ISBN-13: 978-1-59756-353-6 (alk. paper)
ISBN-10: 1-59756-353-6 (alk. paper)
1. Audiometry. 2. Hearing disorders—Diagnosis. I. Swanepoel, De Wet. II. Title. III. Series: Core clinical concepts in audiology.
[DNLM: 1. Hearing Disorders—diagnosis. 2. Hearing Tests—methods. WV 272 H177o 2010]
RF294.H323 2010
617.8'075—dc22

2009036441

Contents

Foreword

How can we make learning in audiology more effective? This is the question that we began with in designing the Core Clinical Concepts in Audiology series. Our answer is revealed in the construction of the books of the series in which we seek to provide palatable and useful information to students and practitioners to develop and refine clinical skills for audiology practice.

By and large, texts available for our field provide exhaustive examination of broad topic areas. Although these texts are useful and necessary for advanced scholarship, we currently lack pedagogic materials that focus on basic clinical methods and knowledge. The books in this series are designed for teaching and learning.

These books are written for the student. The scope of practice for audiology has expanded dramatically since the inception of our field. Today's students must acquire a tremendous arsenal of clinical skills and knowledge in a very short period of time. The books of the CCC series are meant to be clear and comprehensible to students, focusing on the content necessary to achieve knowledge and skills for clinical practice. Furthermore, the books are designed to be economical, both financially and in time spent in learning.

These books are written for the clinician. With expansion of the scope of audiology practice, currently practicing clinicians must acquire new skill sets while continuing to serve their patients. Not a small feat. Hard-working practitioners deserve educational materials compatible with the real-world demands of fast-paced and time-limited clinical practice. In response to these needs, the books of the CCC series are designed to be concise. The succinct construction of the series is meant to allow readers to efficiently acquire the essential concepts and skills described in the books.

These books are written for the instructor. Most instructors of audiology courses are familiar with the frustration of searching for materials that cover the topics which reflect the learning outcomes of their courses. Especially lacking are materials designed to promote clinical learning. The books of the CCC series are designed to focus on specific areas of clinical practice. They are targeted toward the learning outcomes commonly found in audiology curricula. Due to the economical nature of the books, instructors can feel comfortable in creatively combining different Core Clinical Concepts in Audiology books to support the unique and diverse learning demands of specific courses.

These books are written for the user. The needs of the reader are our primary concerns. These books are written to help readers learn to be outstanding clinical audiologists. To be sure, these are lofty goals. The authors of the CCC series books have put forth their best effort to accomplish these goals.

Objective Assessment of Hearing by James W. Hall III and DeWet Swanepoel was written to provide a practical guide to the use of objective measures for prediction of hearing sensitivity. Some of the measures described in the text have been around for a long time. Electrocochleography (ECochG), for example, predates the beginnings of audiology. Other objective procedures, including acoustic immittance measures, have for many years proven their worth in clinical audiology. Yet, we've witnessed in recent years innovative applications for these time-tested procedures, such as high frequency probe tone tympanometry in neonates or acoustic reflexes in the diagnosis of auditory neuropathy spectrum disorder. Several measures included in the book are relatively new additions to the clinical test battery, among them otoacoustic emissions (OAEs) and the auditory steady-state response (ASSR).

Even seasoned clinicians will appreciate the up-to-date and evidence-based recommendations for practice included in the text. The book was written by two audiologists who indeed "clinically practice what they preach." Newer clinicians and students will appreciate the simply stated broad perspective on application of objective tests, and the common sense tips on how to strategically apply objective tests for quantifying hearing ability. As with the other books of the CCC series, the organization and construction of the book works to provide important and necessary information in a manner consistent with the needs of readers.

James W. Hall III, PhD
Virginia Ramachandran, AuD
Series Editors

Preface

The Core Clinical Concepts Series is designed to present a series of textbooks, each of which addresses a topic in an in-depth and comprehensive manner. *Objective Assessment of Hearing* is the first offering within the Electrophysiology component of the CCC series. In this text, the use of objective audiologic measures available to audiologists is explored in an effort to expand daily application of the measures in the timely and accurate measurement of hearing in infants, children, and adults.

Chapter 1 provides the context for the use of objective measures in audiometric assessment. Chapter 2 is an up-to-date review the varied clinical applications of aural immittance measures, including tympanometry and acoustic reflexes. The inclusion of case studies in this chapter demonstrates the valuable contribution of immittance measures in interpretation of patterns of audiometric findings. In Chapter 3, another electroacoustic procedure—otoacoustic emissions—is explored concisely, with specific reference to the rather unique applications of OAEs in screening for and diagnosis of auditory dysfunction. Chapter 4 introduces the reader to electrophysiologic measures by describing the invaluable use of electrocochleography in diagnostic audiologic assessment of infants and young children. In Chapter 5, the varied roles of the auditory brainstem response (ABR) are reviewed including applications in hearing screening, frequency-specific estimation of hearing sensitivity, and neurodiagnosis. Bone-conduction and tone burst ABR protocols are outlined, as well as practical strategies and methods for analysis of findings. The auditory steady-state response is covered in Chapter 6, with a simple but complete description of how the ASSR can contribute importantly to estimation of hearing sensitivity. Chapter 7 reviews current evidence-based recommendations for use of objective measures for screening, identification, and quantification and of hearing loss. The final chapter (8) consists of case studies illustrating the multiple clinical uses and advantages of objective measures for diagnostic auditory assessment of infants and young children.

We gratefully dedicate this book to those innovative audiologists and hearing scientists who initially published research evidence in support of the valuable diagnostic application of objective measures of auditory function, including:

James Jerger: Aural immittance (impedance) measures
Robert Galambos: Auditory brainstem response
David Kemp and Brenda Lonsbury-Martin: Otoacoustic emissions
Gary Rance and Terence Picton: Auditory steady-state response

1

Rationale for Objective Hearing Assessment

A WORD ABOUT TERMINOLOGY

Important Terms and Concepts

At the very outset of the book, we should define four terms that will be repeatedly cited throughout:

- Auditory function (dysfunction)
- Auditory sensitivity
- Hearing sensitivity
- Hearing

Each of these terms refers to a distinctly different concept. Consequently, misuse of the terms can lead to inaccuracy in reports of test findings and, potentially, misdiagnosis and mismanagement. Unfortunately, the terms are sometimes inappropriately used interchangeably or even synonymously in clinical audiology. *Auditory dysfunction* is, as the term clearly implies, abnormal auditory function somewhere in the auditory system, from the external ear to the auditory cortex. Auditory dysfunction is often best detected with electroacoustic and/or electrophysiologic measures that have proven sensitivity to dysfunction at each level of the auditory system (e.g., middle ear, cochlea, eighth [auditory] cranial nerve, etc.). Importantly, auditory dysfunction is not necessarily associated with a decrease in hearing sensitivity or a hearing loss. There are many common clinical examples of this independence between auditory dysfunction and hearing loss. Abnormal otoacoustic emissions confirming cochlear (outer hair cell) auditory dysfunction are often found in persons with completely normal hearing sensitivity (no hearing loss). And even marked central auditory nervous system dysfunction may be present and confirmed with either electrophysiological measures and/or diagnostic measures of auditory processing in patients with perfectly normal hearing sensitivity (again, no hearing loss).

Auditory sensitivity refers to the threshold for some type of auditory response, but not necessarily a behavioral response. Of course, auditory sensitivity and *hearing sensitivity* may be the same in a given person, particularly an adult. However, it is not uncommon in pediatric patients for auditory sensitivity to be better than or worse than behavioral measures of hearing threshold. An example of the latter is an infant who has behavioral hearing thresholds outside the adult normal range due to normal immaturity of the sensory nervous system and motor response to sound, yet auditory brainstem response (ABR) thresholds are at 0 dB nHL or even lower (better). Conversely, for adult subjects auditory thresholds as indicated by the single lowest intensity level eliciting the ABR are usually 5 to 10 dB worse (greater) than behavioral hearing threshold for the same stimulus.

One of the most important distinctions in clinical audiology, and one that is not always appreciated by clinical audiologists, is the difference between hearing sensitivity and *hearing*. Hearing sensitivity is usually measured with pure-tone audiometry. It's common to read in the report of a basic hearing assessment a statement such as, "Pure-tone thresholds were within normal limits consistent with normal hearing," or even more misleading and inaccurate, "The presence of otoacoustic emissions (OAEs) is consistent with normal hearing." Persons with normal pure-tone audiometry may have normal hearing sensitivity, but not necessarily normal hearing. And about all we can say about a person with even totally normal OAEs is that the outer hair cells are probably intact. Normal hearing requires entirely normal auditory processing at all levels of the auditory system from the cochlea to the cortex, for even complex and demanding auditory tasks. The important point here is that "we hear with our brain." The pure-tone audiogram measures only one of the most basic of auditory processes—detection of a very simple and rather long duration sinusoidal sound—under ideal conditions. OAEs are not, of course, a test of hearing. Persons with normal hearing sensitivity and with normal cochlear function can, and sometimes do, have major hearing problems associated with very poor speech perception that produce serious hearing handicap and disability. It is critical in analyzing and interpreting auditory findings, and describing them in clinical reports, to keep in mind these distinctions in terminology, striving always for precision and accuracy in terminology.

Several other terms that are related but with different meanings are:

- Hearing loss
- Hearing impairment
- Hearing handicap
- Hearing disability

A *hearing loss* is usually described as a loss or deficit in hearing sensitivity resulting from auditory dysfunction anywhere within the peripheral and/or central auditory system. Clinically, hearing loss often suggests a problem that warrants at the least the consideration of intervention, either medical (drug therapy or surgery) or nonmedical (some type of assistive device or rehabilitation). One could argue that from a statistical perspective hearing loss begins when hearing thresholds exceed 15 dB HL. With the typical 5 dB step size in signal intensity used in clinical assessment of hearing, the standard deviation for hearing thresholds is 5 dB. Therefore, a hearing threshold level of, for example, 20 dB is four standard deviations greater than normal (audiometric zero or 0 dB HL). The cutoff for normal versus abnormal hearing sensitivity, that is, for defining what constitutes a hearing loss, may vary depending on the age of the patient. Hearing threshold levels greater than 20 or 25 dB may be considered a hearing loss for adults, whereas with children thresholds exceeding 15 dB HL are generally viewed as a hearing loss. The term *hearing loss* may be qualified with adjectives (e.g., mild hearing loss or severe hearing loss) or even with a specific reference to hearing threshold levels in dB and/or frequencies in Hz (e.g., a 45 dB hearing loss at 1000 Hz) to describe the degree or magnitude of the deficit.

The term *hearing impairment* is often used interchangeably with hearing loss and, in fact, the distinction between the two terms is modest. Usually, a hearing impairment is considered a deficit in hearing function that is based on dysfunction with the auditory system or is psychological in nature. The term *hearing handicap* refers to the impact of the hearing loss on a person's goals and on their personal and professional roles and responsibilities (e.g., as an employee, spouse, etc.). Finally, *hearing disability* describes the impact of a hearing loss on a person's social functions and activities. Importantly, a person with a clear hearing loss or hearing impairment documented with audiologic data does not necessarily have a hearing handicap. Similarly, a person with a hearing handicap doesn't invariably have a hearing disability. Determining the extent a hearing loss negatively impacts on quality of life and on social and vocational daily activities goes far beyond a simple audiogram and other diagnostic audiologic measures.

Detection versus Diagnosis

In each chapter of this book, we first discuss detection of auditory dysfunction or hearing loss (carefully using the two terms appropriately!) and then we discuss the diagnosis of auditory dysfunction or hearing loss. We use the term *detection* synonymously with *identification*. These terms define the overall goal of screening for any type of auditory dysfunction. The criteria for the disorder to be detected with the screening must be defined in advance (a priori). That is, is our goal to differentiate those persons with normal auditory function from those with any auditory dysfunction, or is our goal to identify persons with hearing loss meeting some preestablished criteria? Criteria might include hearing loss exceeding a certain degree, such as 25 dB HL, hearing loss exceeding a certain degree for specific frequencies or within a specific frequency region, or perhaps, hearing loss sufficient to adversely affect communication. In turn, we manipulate the screening protocol and also the criteria for a Pass versus a Refer (e.g., Fail) screening outcome to meet the preestablished criteria. Electroacoustic and electrophysiologic procedures (specifically OAEs and ABR) are, of course, the most well-accepted approaches for "hearing" screening. Any discussion of the detection of auditory dysfunction or hearing loss must also take into account the test performance of the screening measure, that is, the sensitivity, specificity, positive predictive value, and negative predictive value. Terms important in the discussion of test performance are defined briefly in Table 1–1. These terms will be further defined and illustrated in subsequent discussions of different electroacoustic and electrophysiologic auditory measures in other chapters of the book.

The phrase *diagnosis of hearing loss* probably has different meanings for different people. To paraphrase the conventional medical use of the term *diagnosis* and adapt it to audiology, diagnosis is the use of scientific and skillful methods to establish the cause and nature of a hearing loss. At the very least, the overall objective in diagnosis of hearing loss is estimation of, as accurately as possible, the degree and configuration of hearing loss for each ear. There are four requirements to meet this diagnostic objective:

- Auditory procedures that are valid and reliable in persons of all ages
- Frequency-specific auditory or hearing thresholds in some dimension of dB (e.g., dB HL, dB nHL)
- Ear-specific (right and left ear) auditory or hearing thresholds and, as indicated by the other findings
- Auditory thresholds for air- versus bone-conduction stimulation

Table 1–1. Definition of terms related to the performance of screening methods

Term	
Target disorder or hearing loss	Specified disorder or hearing loss for detection by screening method
Sensitivity	Ability of screening method to correctly identify the target disorder (reported as % value)
Specificity	Ability of screening method to correctly identify individuals without the target disorder (reported as % value)
Positive predictive value	Chance that an individual who fails the screening test will have the target disorder (reported as % value)
Negative predictive value	Chance that an individual who passes the screening test will not have the target disorder or hearing loss (reported as % value)
False-positive	Incorrect fail result on screen for an individual without the target disorder
False-negative	Incorrect "pass" result on screen for an individual with the target disorder

With this information, it is possible to describe multiple important dimensions of hearing loss. Dimensions contributing to accurate definition of hearing loss are summarized in Table 1–2. It's possible, for example, to estimate with reasonable accuracy the degree of hearing loss at different frequencies for both ears. In addition, audiologists almost always seek to define in all patients (children and adults) the type of hearing loss, that is, sensory, conductive, mixed, neural including auditory neuropathy, or central, attributing the hearing loss to auditory dysfunction in one or more regions of the auditory system. Finally, with comprehensive diagnostic auditory findings, typically including those for both electroacoustic and electrophysiologic measures, evaluated in the context of a thorough medical history and perhaps other diagnostic findings (e.g., laboratory or neuroradiological studies), it is sometimes possible for the audiologist to further specify a likely etiology or underlying pathology for the hearing loss.

Table 1–2. Dimensions of hearing loss diagnosis

Type	Nature of loss (conductive, sensory, neural, i.e., auditory neuropathy, mixed, central)
Degree	Severity of loss across frequencies (e.g., mild, moderate, severe, profound)
Configuration	Frequency-specific pattern of loss (e.g., steeply sloping high frequency loss, low frequency loss, high frequency notch)
Symmetry	Ear affected (bilateral or unilateral)
Cause	Etiology of loss related to many factors (e.g., genetic, environmental, medical treatment, disease processes, aging, etc.)
Onset	Time when loss started (congenital, progressive, childhood-onset, adult-onset, etc.)
Impact	Effect of loss on functioning (e.g., speech perception in quiet and in noise)

CLINICAL LIMITATIONS OF BEHAVIORAL AUDIOMETRY

Clinical limitations of behavioral audiometry form the rationale for electroacoustic and electrophysiologic auditory measures in all patients, but particularly in infants and young children. Very simply, we need electroacoustic and electrophysiologic auditory measures because behavioral audiometry does not always provide valid and reliable information on auditory function (the four requirements listed above) necessary for timely diagnosis and intervention (Table 1–3). Perhaps the most obvious limitation of behavioral audiometry techniques is the inability to obtain valid and reliable information in infants and young children. This is not to imply that electroacoustic and electrophysiologic auditory measures are independent of age or maturation. Although the functional anatomy of the ear is reasonably intact by about 30 weeks gestational age, developmental trends and chronological age must regularly be taken into account for all electroacoustic and electrophysiologic auditory measures. Findings must be analyzed with age-corrected normative data as indicated by the maturational gradient of the auditory measure that is being applied in a child. A variety of *listener variables* potentially have an important influence on behavioral auditory responses, among them:

- Age and development
- Neurological immaturity (sensory and motor)
- Cognitive factors
- Language
- Attention and state of arousal
- Motivation

Electroacoustic and electrophysiologic auditory measures are clinically very useful also in patients whose sickness precludes valid behavioral audiometry, and in persons who cannot or will not cooperate and voluntarily respond to the demands of the task. Selected electroacoustic and electrophysiologic auditory measures can be recorded in patients who are asleep, sedated, or anesthetized. And there are automated electroacoustic and electrophysiologic auditory measures permitting data

Table 1-3. A summary of the general clinical strengths and weaknesses of electroacoustical and electrophysiological auditory measures available to clinical audiologists

Strengths
• Do not require a behavioral response from the patient
• Results are not influenced by motivation
• Results are not influenced by cognitive status
• Results generally are not influenced by state of arousal
• Measurements can be made with patient sedated or anesthetized
• Results are not influenced by native language
• Patient is not required to follow detailed verbal instructions
• Results not influenced by motor status
• Measures provide information on regions of the auditory system from the middle ear to the cerebral cortex
• Generally high degree of sensitivity to auditory dysfunction
• Generally provide site-specific information on auditory dysfunction
• Valid measures are possible from infants and young children
• Reasonable test time
Weaknesses
• Do not measure "hearing"
• Limited or no information on cortical auditory dysfunction
• Abnormal finding does not invariably indicate hearing loss
• Single measure generally provides limited information on hearing status
• No information on speech perception or understanding

Note. Specific advantages associated with each measure are detailed in the chapter devoted to the measure.

collection and analysis by nonaudiologic personnel. Finally, as noted throughout this book, even when behavioral audiometry is feasible clinically, electroacoustic and electrophysiologic auditory measures may offer the advantage of enhanced sensitivity and site-specificity for peripheral and central auditory dysfunction. Even after itemizing the limitations of behavioral audiometry and emphasizing the strengths of electroacoustic and electrophysiologic auditory measures, we must stress a basic axiom of diagnostic audiometry . . . only behavioral measures provide a true measure of hearing. Our initial diagnostic information may be derived from electroacoustic and electrophysiologic auditory measures, and we almost certainly will initiate referrals to other professionals, and audiologic intervention, based on these initial findings. However, whenever possible the diagnostic process should continue until auditory function is thoroughly assessed and the effectiveness of intervention confirmed with behavioral measures.

CROSS-CHECK PRINCIPLE REVISITED

Over 30 years ago, James Jerger and Deborah Hayes published a paper that is as timely today as it was then. In "The Cross-Check Principle in

Pediatric Audiology" (Jerger & Hayes, 1976), the authors summarize the limitations and pitfalls associated with exclusive reliance on behavioral test results. They then make a strong case for the use of aural immittance (then impedance) measures and/or auditory brainstem response (then brainstem-evoked response) to verify or "cross-check" the behavioral test results. After presenting four case reports to illustrate the often disastrous diagnostic and management outcomes that can result from stubborn reliance on behavioral tests alone, Jerger and Hayes conclude:

> In summary, we believe that the unique limitations of conventional behavioral audiometry dictate the need for a "test battery" approach. The key concept governing our assessment strategy is the cross-check principle. The basic operation of this principle is that no result be accepted until it is confirmed by an independent measure. (Jerger & Hayes, 1976, p. 620)

The *cross-check principle* remains unchanged 30 years later, but the test battery has expanded considerably. Augmenting the original test battery of behavioral audiometry, immittance measures, and the ABR are clinically-resurrected and better understood diagnostic procedures, such as electrocochleagraphy (ECochG) and some cortical auditory evoked responses, otoacoustic emissions, and a procedure that is relatively new to the clinical scene . . . the auditory steady state response (ASSR). As we will demonstrate often in this book, the rationale and clinical application of the additions to the diagnostic test battery is evidence based. Consistent with existing guidelines and developing guidelines for best practice in audiology today, clinical application of auditory procedures should be based on research findings or, minimally, accumulated clinical findings published in peer-reviewed journals. Ample data now exist in support of the clinical applications of the electroacoustic and electrophysiologic auditory measures reviewed in this book. As stated so eloquently by Leonardo da Vinci (1452–1519) about 500 years ago: "Those who fall in love with practice without science are like a sailor who steers a ship without a rudder or compass, and who can never be certain whither he is going."

2

Aural Immittance Measurements

INTRODUCTION

Terminology

Aural immittance measurements are proven tools for hearing screening and they are a valuable component of the diagnostic audiologic test battery. Measurement of aural immittance is the original electroacoustic technique to be incorporated into the diagnostic test battery. The term *immittance* is really a hybrid word for middle ear measurements combining portions of the terms *im*pedance and ad*mittance*. Impedance (Z_a) is the opposition to acoustic energy flow through the middle ear system (in acoustic ohms). The subscript *a* refers to acoustical. The two forms of impedance are mechanical and electrical. The reciprocal of Z_a, admittance (Y_a), is the ease of acoustic energy flow through the middle ear system. It is described in *acoustic millimhos*, or mmhos (ohms spelled backwards). As noted in Chapter 1, all electroacoustical and electrophysiological measures offer major clinical advantages for auditory assessment. The specific, and rather compelling, clinical advantages or rationale for routinely performing aural immittance measurements in the diagnostic test battery, particularly in pediatric patient populations, are summarized in Table 2–1. Immittance measurements are quick, are technically simple, and can be recorded in persons of all ages without regard to developmental or cognitive status. The sensitivity of tympanometry and acoustic reflexes to middle ear dysfunction is well established. Moreover, immittance measures are useful diagnostically in patients with a wide assortment of audiologic, otologic, and neurologic diseases and disorders.

Historical Perspective

Initial investigations of tympanometry and acoustic reflexes date back over 60 years, although British physicists (e.g., Sir Charles Wheatstone) conducted more general studies with acoustical, mechanical, and electrical impedance bridges as early as the early 1800s The person credited with the development and earliest clinical applications of impedance measurements is Otto Metz (1905–1993), a German otolaryngologist and scientist who fled from Nazi Germany to Denmark in 1938 just before Hitler led the country into World War II (Figure 2–1A). Using a cumbersome mechano-acoustic device, an impedance bridge, Metz collaborated with Danish auditory researchers in a Copenhagen hospital in further clinical studies of the new technique. As an aside, in 1943 Dr. Metz again was forced to flee from Nazi capture in Denmark to safety in an auditory research laboratory at the University Hospital in Lund, Sweden. Returning to Denmark after the end of the war,

Table 2–1. Summary of clinical strengths versus weaknesses of aural immittance measures

Strengths
• Equipment is widely accessible
• Clinically proven with over 30 years of clinical experience and research
• Normative data are available
• Anatomy and physiology relatively well defined
• Relatively unaffected by developmental age or status
• Brief test time
• Relatively simple techniques
• Useful as a screening technique
• Measurement does not require sedation or anesthesia
• High degree of sensitivity to middle ear dysfunction
• Provides information on middle ear mechanics (tympanometry)
• Detects and confirms perforation of the tympanic membrane
• Detects and confirms patent ventilation tubes
• Provides information on afferent auditory pathways (acoustic reflex)
• Sensitive to retrocochlear auditory dysfunction (acoustic reflex)
• Provides information on caudal (lower) brainstem auditory pathways (acoustic reflex)
• Provides information on seventh cranial (facial) nerve (acoustic reflex)
• Estimation of the degree of hearing loss (acoustic reflex)
Weaknesses
• Not a measure of "hearing"
• Measurement requires an airtight (hermetic) seal within external ear canal
• Only provides information on middle ear status (tympanometry)
• No information on rostral (higher) brainstem auditory function
• No information on cortical auditory function
• No information on speech perception or understanding
• Does not provide precise index of the degree of hearing loss
• Findings are limited in patients with middle ear dysfunction (acoustic reflex)

Note. All electroacoustic and electrophysiologic measures share a number of clinical advantages, as summarized in Chapter 1 and described in detail throughout the text.

Metz published in 1946 a classic paper entitled, "The Acoustic Impedance Measured on Normal and Pathological Ears" (Metz, 1946) and, in the 1950s, important papers on the acoustic reflex.

In the early 1960s, James Jerger (Figure 2–1B) visited Denmark, ironically after attending an audiology conference in Bonn, Germany, and observed measurement of middle ear impedance with a new and improved electroacoustic impedance bridge (Madsen ZO 61) developed by other Danes, including Knud Terkildsen (1918–1984), K. A. Thomsen, and an engineer, Dr. Scott-Nielson. Soon one of

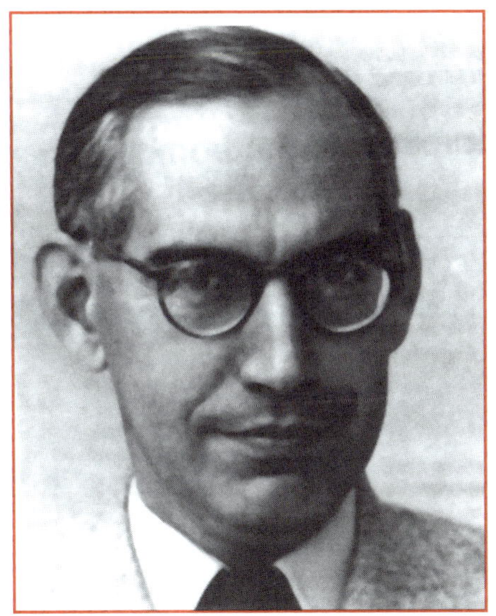

A

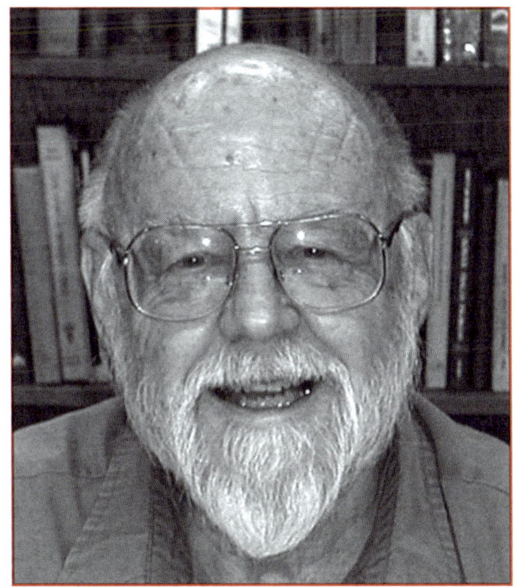

B

FIGURE 2–1. **A.** Otto Metz, a German scientist who developed an electromechanical impedance bridge that was a very early forerunner of modern immittance devices. **B.** James Jerger, also known as "the father of diagnostic audiology," who introduced impedance measurements to clinical audiologists in the United States and then around the world.

the new impedance devices was shipped to Dr. Jerger. With his move to Baylor College of Medicine in Houston, Dr. Jerger began to consistently collect data from large series of children and adults with a wide variety of pathologies. By 1970, he published the first of a lengthy series of clinical trials of the new clinical technique (with a newer Madsen ZO 70 device). Immittance measurement (then still called *impedance audiometry*) was immediately a hot research topic. In addition, many big-name audiologists, among them James Jerger, Chuck Berlin, and Jerry Northern in the United States, traveled extensively throughout the 1970s giving practical workshops on the new technique, and generating considerable clinical interest in impedance audiometry. An entire textbook entitled *Clinical Impedance Audiometry* appeared in 1975, followed by a second edition in 1980. Understandably, with the discovery of the auditory brainstem response (ABR) in 1971, and its rapid growth as a clinical technique in the early 1980s, most of the excitement in audiology about impedance/immittance measures rather suddenly diminished. However, immittance measurements are no less valuable today than they were 30 years ago.

Current Status of Immittance Measures

Without question, immittance measures are even now the most sensitive and clinically feasible technique for evaluating middle ear function. Measurement of the acoustic reflex quickly provides clinically useful information on a substantial portion of the auditory system, as well as a nonauditory structure (the seventh cranial nerve). Given the many and varied advantages of immittance measurement (see Table 2–1), it is safe to claim that no other widely accessible procedure in audiology provides as much diagnostic information with such a modest investment of time and effort. Instrumentation for immittance measurements is widely accessible. Tympanometers are found in virtually all audiology clinics and private practices, and even in the offices of pediatricians and other health professionals. However, according to a recent survey, only 45% of audiologists routinely perform tympanometry in audiologic assessments and only one in five audiologists (20%) record acoustic reflexes.

The following review focuses on the applications of tympanometry and the acoustic reflex for detecting and diagnosing auditory dysfunction. The primary purpose of this chapter is not to provide a novel and highly scientific review of immittance measurements. We also do not pretend to present a thorough treatise on a topic that has been extensively treated in many previous books, monographs, book chapters, and journal articles. Rather, our main objective is to encourage audiologists to fully exploit immittance measurements on a daily basis in their clinical practice, and to view measurement of aural immittance as an essential technique for the identification and diagnosis of auditory dysfunction.

FUNCTIONAL ANATOMY

Introduction

Immittance measurement involves multiple auditory structures, ranging laterally from the external ear canal centrally to the caudal portion (pons) of the auditory brainstem. A detailed discussion of the rather complex anatomical bases of each immittance measure and each component of aural immittance (e.g., reactance, susceptance, conductance, and phase), as well as the common clinical measures tympanometry and acoustic reflexes, is far beyond the scope of this book. What follows herein is a brief overview of the major anatomic structures that underlie the most commonly applied immittance measures, tympanometry and acoustic reflexes, with an emphasis on how anatomic abnormalities and disorders affect these measures. A logical, and clinically practical, starting point is to consider the well-known formulae for acoustic impedance (Z_a) and acoustic admittance (Y_a):

$$Z_a = R_a^2 + X_a^2$$

where R_a = acoustic resistance (i.e., impedance due to friction), $X_a = 2\pi f M (-k/2p\pi f)$, and X_a = acoustic reactance (i.e., impedance due to mass [M] and to stiffness [elastic or compliance] components).

$$Y_a = G_a^2 + B_a^2$$

where Y phase angle = arctan (B_a / G_a), G_a = acoustic conductance (admittance due to friction), and B_a = acoustic susceptance, that is, admittance due to mass and stiffness (or compliance) components. Conventional aural immittance measurements are made with a low frequency probe tone of 220 or 226 Hz and, therefore, with a long wavelength (about 5 feet or 160 cm). With the low frequency probe tone, immittance measurements reflect mostly stiffness (i.e., compliance or elastic reactance). In the normal adult ear, anatomic structures contributing to mass and stiffness include the tympanic membrane and the ossicular chain. Most resistance in immittance measurements is created by the influence of the friction on stapes footplate movement created by cochlear fluid pressure. Tympanometry is less straightforward in infants under the age of 6 months. A higher frequency probe tone is necessary for valid measurement of middle ear status. This clinically important topic is discussed further in a following section on high probe tone immittance measurement.

External Auditory Canal

The first step in immittance measurement is insertion of a soft probe tip into the outer portion of the external ear canal until an airtight (hermetic) seal is formed. Immittance measurement does not contribute to the diagnosis of external ear canal pathology. Quite the contrary, there is always a slight chance that insertion of a nonsterile probe during immittance measurement could interfere with, or even exacerbate, external ear canal pathology. Therefore, prior to the beginning of immittance measurement the external ear canal should routinely be carefully inspected with an otoscope to rule out pathology or other disorders or aberrations. Examples of external ear canal pathology include cysts, fibromas, external otitis, benign tumors (e.g., exostosis), and malignant tumors (e.g., melanoma). Among the nonpathologic conditions in the external ear canal are cerumen and a wide variety of foreign bodies (e.g., pebbles, insects, toys). The latter are, of course, most often discovered in the ear canals of young children. Criteria for medical referral based on history and otoscopic examination are summarized in Table 2–2.

An almost incidental but useful clinical finding in immittance measurement is a rough estimation of the ear canal volume enclosed in the space between the medial edge of the probe tip and the tympanic membrane. At high (e.g., +200 daPa [decapascals]) or low (e.g., –200 to –400 daPa) pressures, the middle ear is essentially decoupled from the immittance measurement permitting estimation of the compliance of the air within the external ear canal (medial to the probe tip). If there is a perforation in the tympanic membrane or if there is a patent (open) ventilation tube within the tympanic membrane, an abnormally large ear canal volume will be measured. Of course, ear canal volumes are directly related to age and to body size, and usually affected also by gender. That is, ear canal volumes increase with age from infants through adolescence and with body size across the age span. Ear canal volumes are generally larger for males than for females. Also, assuming consistent technique for inserting the probe tip in the right and left ears, ear canal volumes are reasonably symmetrical. Meaningful interpretation of immittance findings requires an appreciation of normal expectations for ear canal volume and factors influencing ear canal volume (Table 2–3).

Table 2–2. Hearing and tympanometric criteria for audiologic and/or medical referral

History
• Otalgia
• Otorrhea
Visual inspection of the ear
• Structural defect of the ear, head, or neck
• Ear canal abnormalities
– Blood or effusion
– Occlusion
– Inflammation
Excessive cerumen, tumor, or foreign materials
• Eardrum abnormalities
• Abnormal color
• Bulging eardrum
• Fluid line or bubbles
Perforation

Source. From "Guidelines for Screening for Hearing Impairment and Middle-Ear Disorders," by American Speech-Language-Hearing Association, 1990, *ASHA*, *32*(Suppl. 2), p. 17–24. Reprinted with permission.

Middle Ear

As evident from the formulae for acoustic impedance, particularly the symbol *f*, mass reactance increases directly in relation to frequency, whereas the stiffness (elastic reactance) component of impedance decreases as frequency is increased. Resistance (the friction component) of impedance is independent of frequency. The clinical implications of these relations between frequency and impedance components are well known. The majority of disorders and diseases affecting the middle ear increase stiffness of the middle ear system. The middle ear abnormalities that increase stiffness reduce the transmission of energy in the low frequency region and, therefore, are associated

Table 2–3. Factors influencing ear canal volume in immittance measurement

Factor	*Ear Canal Volume (in cc or ml)*
Age	
Infants	<0.5
Children	0.3 to 1.0
Adults	0.65 to 1.75
Gender	males > females
Symmetry	+/– 20%

Note. Single component (e.g., impedance or admittance) tympanometry recorded with low (220 or 226 Hz) probe tone.

with a low frequency conductive hearing loss. Clinical entities producing a low frequency hearing loss include, of course, fixation of the ossicular chain (e.g., otosclerosis). Conversely, when the mass component of aural impedance is affected, the result is a high frequency conductive hearing loss. Two clinical entities producing a high frequency hearing loss include disarticulation (discontinuity) of the ossicular chain and sometimes a cholesteatoma. The audiogram patterns related to these two impedance abnormalities are sometimes referred to as the *stiffness tilt* and the *mass tilt*. Because mass and stiffness are separate components within the impedance formula, it is possible for a middle ear abnormality to affect both of them in the same patient. Suppurative otitis media, for example, produces a low frequency stiffness-related hearing loss and a high frequency hearing loss, with relatively better hearing in the intermediate frequency region (around 1500 Hz).

Immittance measurements reflect mechanical properties of the middle ear and abnormalities in middle ear anatomy, in turn, can affect mechanical properties. The relation between middle ear abnormalities and tympanometry is imprecise and, interpreted in isolation, of limited clinical value. For example, a normal tympanogram can certainly be recorded in persons with middle ear pathology. The most obvious example of this finding is fixation of the ossicular chain. The classic finding in this clinical entity is a shallow tympanogram, but many other findings are certainly possible and encountered clinically when anatomic abnormalities occur in combination. A person with fixation of the ossicular chain and also a scarred tympanic membrane may yield a very deep tympanogram consistent with a compliant middle ear system. Multiple etiologies can be associated with a shallow, normally-shaped tympanogram, among them otosclerosis, congenital fixation of the ossicular chain, and fibrous adhesions subsequent to middle ear disease that involve the ossicles. A shallow tympanogram may, in fact, be a normal finding in an older adult with otherwise entirely normal auditory function. A variety of pathologies can be reflected in a flat tympanogram, ranging from some form of otitis media, to hemotympanum (blood within the middle ear space), to a cholesteatoma involving the ossicular chain. In short, the sensitivity of tympanometry to middle ear dysfunction is reasonably good but the specificity of tympanometry in differentiating among anatomic abnormalities is poor.

Cochlear and Retrocochlear Pathways

The acoustic reflex is a *sonomotor* response, that is, a muscle response to sound. The acoustic reflex, therefore, falls in the same general category as the postauricular muscle response, the eye blink response, and the startle response. Careful measurement of stapedial acoustic reflexes, especially under four test conditions—ipsilateral and contralateral stimulation of the right and left ears—yields considerable information on the anatomical status of the auditory system. The major pathways in the acoustic reflex arc are illustrated in Figure 2–2. The acoustic reflex pathways can be divided anatomically into four general portions: (a) the afferent pathways consisting of the cochlea and the eighth (auditory) cranial nerve, (b) brainstem neurons within the cochlear nuclei and, for contralateral pathways, the trapezoid body and medial superior olivary complex, (c) the efferent pathway involving motor fibers within the seventh cranial nerve, and (d) for contralateral acoustic reflexes polysynaptic pathways including neurons within the reticular formation (reticular activating system). The presence of acoustic reflexes is, of course, dependant on essentially normal middle ear function. Most middle ear abnormalities obscure confident detection of acoustic reflexes, even without markedly abnormal tympanograms and in the presence of a modest (5 to 10 dB) gap between air- and bone-conduction pure tone thresholds. Also relevant to acoustic reflex measurement in young children, drugs affecting consciousness by suppressing the reticular activating system will influence, and may even totally suppress, acoustic reflexes. For more detailed information on the anatomical and physiological bases of the acoustic reflex, the reader is referred to Hall (1985).

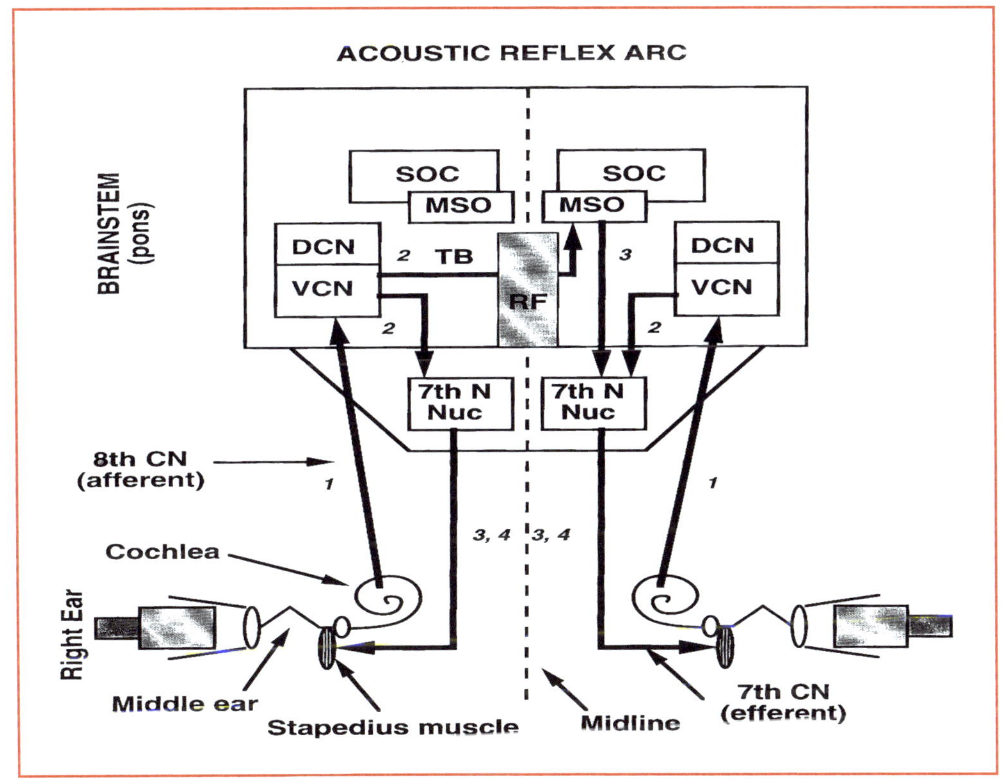

FIGURE 2–2. Diagram of the acoustic reflex pathways. SOC = Superior Olivary Complex; MSO = Medial Superior Olivary; RF = Reticular Formation; TB = Trapezoid Body; DCN = Dorsal Cochlear Nucleus; VCN = Ventral Cochlear Nucleus; 7th Nerve Nucleus; CN = Cochlear Nerve.

IDENTIFICATION (SCREENING) OF AUDITORY DYSFUNCTION

Tympanometry

Introduction

Tympanometry is a fundamental and essential procedure for detection of auditory dysfunction. Clinical acceptance and application of any audiologic procedure is enhanced by technical simplicity in performing the procedure and simplicity in analysis and interpretation of the findings. Of course, the clinical acceptance and appeal of a procedure is also highly dependent on its clinical value and contribution to the diagnosis of auditory dysfunction. Tympanometry unquestionably meets both of these criteria for a clinical technique. To a large extent, clinical audiologists readily accepted, and routinely applied, tympanometry because there was a simple and easily remembered system for categorizing normal versus abnormal findings. The familiar approach for classifying tympanograms according to the initial letters of the alphabet (A, B, C) was first suggested in 1962 at an audiology conference by Gunnar Lidén (1918–2003), a Swedish pediatrician who, reportedly because he didn't like the smell of dirty diapers, turned first to otology and then became very well known for his clinical research in audiology. However, it was James Jerger who in the early 1970s further developed and clinically validated a system for classifying tympanogram types. Reported in a series of journal articles and books, and presented at many workshop and professional conferences, the *Jerger tympanogram system* soon became, and remains to this day, the most common approach for analysis and interpretation of tympanometry.

Jerger Tympanogram Classification System

Examples of the three basic tympanogram types in the Jerger classification system are shown in Figure 2–3. Definitions for Type A, B, and C tympanograms from the original paper by Dr. Jerger are summarized in Table 2–4. It is important clinically to note that the original tympanogram types were based on measurements made with a change in ear canal pressure from +200 mmH_2O downward to –200 mmH_2O (a descending change). Tympanogram height and pressure peak, and even classification, may be altered when tympanograms are recorded instead with pressure increasing (ascending) from a negative value (e.g., –200 daPA) to a positive extreme. Hall and Chandler (1994) reported tympanogram findings as a function of the direction of pressure change in a series of 182 adult subjects. The peak of the tympanogram was different for descending versus ascending pressure change in 84% of the subjects. A total of 62% of subjects yielded lower peak amplitude in the descending direction than in the ascending, whereas the reverse trend (lower amplitude in the ascending direction) was observed in 21% of the subjects. The pressure where the peak was recorded also was markedly affected by the direction of air pressure change by as much as +/–170 daPA. Furthermore, these authors found that for 13% of the subjects changing the direction of the air pressure change within the external ear canal altered the Jerger tympanogram type.

Although the three original tympanogram types account for most middle ear conditions, variations of the types have been introduced to better describe and differentiate selected middle ear disorders. Severely restricted mobility of the ossicular chain results in a very shallow (Type As) version of the Type A tympanogram, characterized by a distinct tympanogram peak, but with a height of <0.30 mL. At the other extreme, the Ad (*d* for deep) tympanogram has excessive height (>1.5 mL). The use of higher frequency probe tones (e.g., 600 or 1000 Hz) during tympanometry will sometimes result in what are known as *W-shaped* tympanograms, sometimes in persons with entirely normal hearing sensitivity.

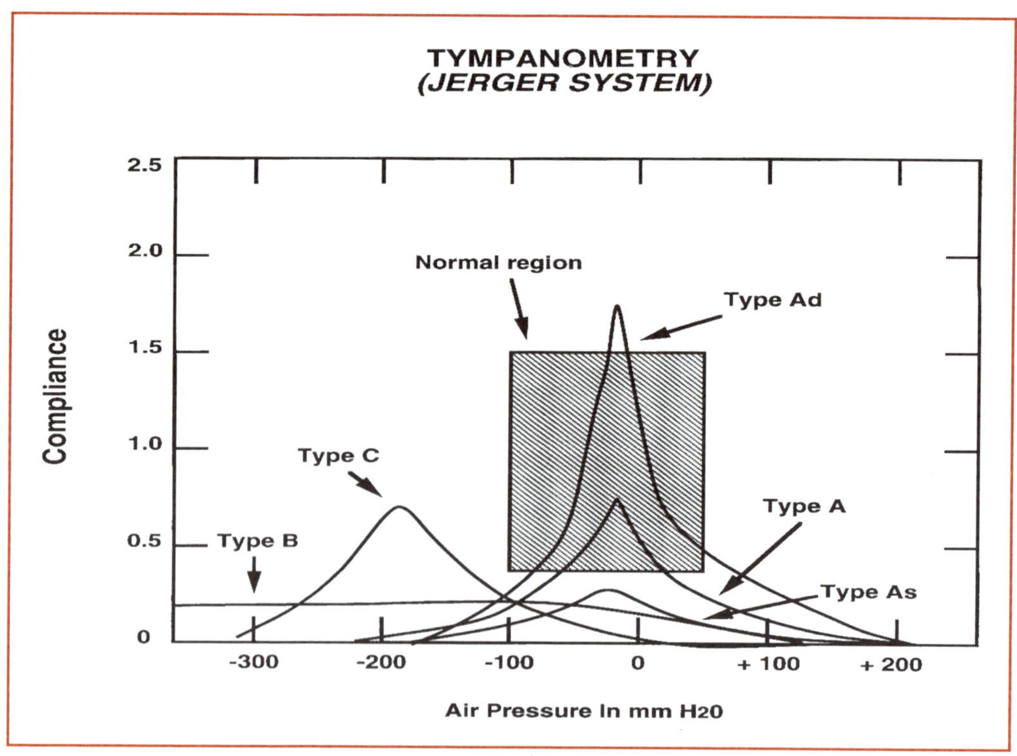

FIGURE 2–3. Traditional Jerger system for categorizing tympanograms.

Table 2–4. Impedance (immittance) protocol used in the pioneering studies by Dr. James Jerger and colleagues at Baylor College of Medicine that resulted in the categories for tympanograms

Parameter	Selection
Instrumentation Device	Madsen Z0–70
Probe tone frequency	220 Hz
Air pressure direction	+200 to −200 or −400 daPa
Rate of pressure change	Not specified
Tympanogram type definitions	
Type A	Characterized by a relatively sharp maximum at or near 0 mm. Type A is found in normal and otosclerotic ears.
Type B	Little or no maximum. Compliance remains essentially unchanged over a large range of pressure variation. Type B is found in ears with serous or adhesive otitis media.
Type C	The maximum is shifted to the left of zero by negative pressure in the middle ear. Slight negative pressure is quite common in many otherwise normal ears, but when the maximum equals or exceeds approximately −100 daPa, significant negative pressure in the middle ear may be presumed.

Source. From "Clinical Experience with Impedance Audiometry," by J. Jerger, 1970, *Archives of Otolarygology*, *92*, pp. 311–324. Reprinted with permission.

Gradient

Coined by Brooks (1968), *gradient* is the term used for a computation of tympanogram admittance relative to a pressure range. First reported in the early 1980s (e.g., Cooper, Hearne, & Gates, 1982; de Jonge, 1986; Koebsell & Margolis, 1986), gradient is defined by identifying the half-amplitude admittance (Y) point on the positive and negative side of the tympanogram, and then dividing the total amplitude on each side by two. The main steps in manual calculation of tympanogram gradient are illustrated in Figure 2–4. The difference in air pressure between each of these points on the slope of the tympanogram is referred to as delta (difference) pressure (dP) and expressed in daPa. The gradient measure, therefore, takes into account two tympanogram response parameters —height and width. The objective in using the gradient clinically, rather than the conventional tympanogram peak or the pressure at which the peak occurs, is to more effectively detect middle ear disorders, especially middle ear effusion. Some aural immittance meters automatically calculate and display the tympanogram gradient. Table 2–5 shows published normative values (children and adults) for analysis of tympanogram gradient, and for distinguishing normal versus abnormal gradient findings clinically. The theory behind the gradient is clinically attractive, that is, enhancing sensitivity and specificity of tympanometry in the detection of middle ear dysfunction. However, in a study of 80 children with normal middle ear status and 80 children with otologically confirmed otitis media, Tompkins and Hall (1990) found no clinically important difference in the detection of children with otitis media when the gradient measure (automatically calculated with a GSI 33 Middle Ear Analyzer) was compared with conventional tympanogram analysis (i.e., using Types A, B, and C). Mean gradient values in this study were 0.53 for the normal group and 0.20 for the otitis media subject group. Unfortunately, for about one third of the children with otitis media and very flat tympanograms, the immittance device did not automatically calculate a gradient.

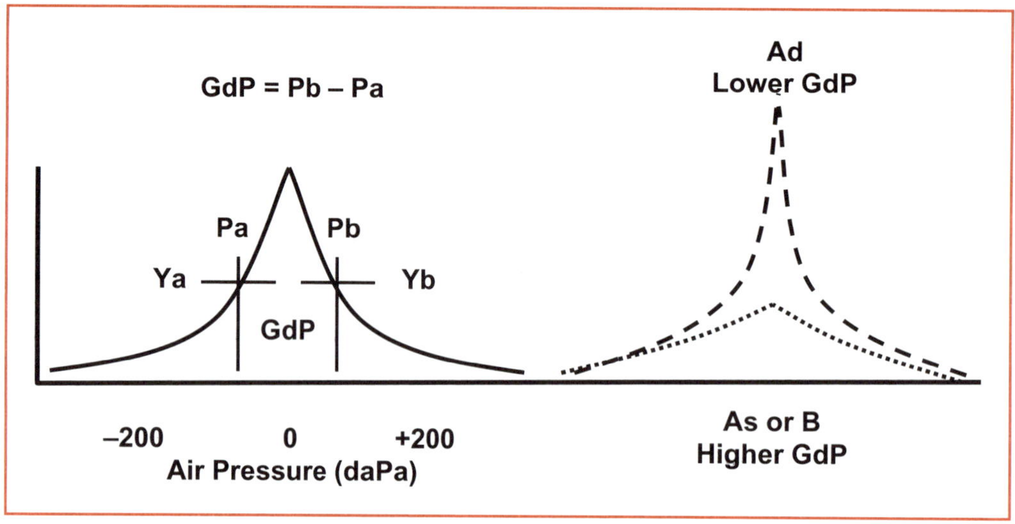

FIGURE 2–4. Important steps in calculating the gradient measure of tympanogram properties.

Table 2–5. Normal data for the tympanometric gradient (GdP) measured from children and adults

Population	*Index*	*GdP (daPa)*
Children*	Mean	133
	10th percentile	80
	90th percentile	200
Adults**	50th percentile	110
	5th percentile	63
	95th percentile	162

Note. GdP is defined as the difference in pressure between the half-amplitude points on an admittance tympanogram. Data were collected with a 226-Hz probe tone and an air pump speed of 50 daPa/sec.

*Data for 88 ears of 46 children between the ages of 3.7 and 5.8 years, as reported in "Tympanometric Gradient Measured from Normal Preschool Children," by K. A. Koebsell & R. H. Margolis, 1986, *Audiology*, *25*, pp. 149–157. Reprinted with permission.

**Data for right ears of 83 college students with an average age of 22 years, as reported in "Normal Tympanometric Gradient: A Comparison of Three Methods," by R. de Jonge, 1986, *Audiology*, 25, pp. 299–308. Reprinted with permission.

The gradient measure may have some role in the quantification of tympanogram status by nonaudiologists, but it doesn't appear to offer any compelling advantage in comparison to conventional and manual analysis of tympanogram types.

Guidelines for Screening with Tympanometry

Most states within the United States have official guidelines for hearing screening that include middle ear immittance measurements. A representative example of these typically rather simple guidelines is the Ohio State Licensure Board definition of screening with tympanometry: "Tympanometry screening" means "a pass/fail dynamic measure of middle ear compliance of no less than 0.2 ml of H_20, within the pressure range of +150 to –150 daPa." The American Speech-Language-Hearing Association produced guidelines (ASHA, 1997) that were an outgrowth of the work of a task force, and that were based on one published study by Roush et al. (1995) and two studies by Nozza and colleagues (Nozza, Bluestone, Kardatzke, & Bachman, 1992, 1994). Roush et al. (1995) reported data for 88 mostly African American children aged 6 to 30 months who attended day care centers. Children in the studies reported by Nozza and colleagues were aged 1 to 16 years with histories of chronic or recurrent otitis media who were receiving medical care for their middle ear disorders in a university hospital. Confirmation of middle ear effusion was available from either otoscopy (Roush et al.) or otoscopy plus findings at surgery. The 1996 ASHA Guidelines require calculation of tympanogram peak and width, and provide criteria for pass versus fail outcomes in two age groups. Tympanogram peak is measured in mL from the base of the tympanogram (at +200 or −400 daPa) to the peak on the tympanogram. Tympanogram width is defined as the pressure interval in daPa where a horizontal line intersects the tympanogram at 50% of the peak height. Calculation of tympanogram height and width is illustrated in Figure 2–4. For children between the ages of 7 and 12 months, the tympanogram meets pass criteria when the height static admittance is ≥0.2 mL, and the tympanogram height fail outcome is <0.2 mL. The pass/fail criterion for tympanogram height for children 13 to 35 months is ≥0.3 mL and <0.3 mL. For children between the ages of 7 and 12 months, the tympanogram width criteria is ≤235 daPa for a pass outcome, and <235 daPa for a fail outcome. The pass/fail criterion for tympanogram width for children 13 to 35 months is ≤200 daPa and >200 daPa.

Smith et al. (2006) recently investigated in a series of 3686 children under the age of 3 years the probability of predicting the presence or absence of middle ear effusion (MEE) using tympanometry. The authors described three tympanogram measurements in their study that can be derived from the printouts of any commercially available immittance device:

- The height of the tympanogram peak was measured in mL, which is equivalent to millimhos (mmhos).
- The pressure of the tympanometric peak was calculated as the location of the peak deflection on the *x*-axis in relation to atmospheric pressure. It was measured in decapascals (daPa).
- Tympanogram width was defined as the pressure interval in daPa where a horizontal line intersects the tympanogram at 50% of the tympanic peak height.

Smith et al. (2006) make the point that

> ... most tympanograms are associated with either a relatively low probability (<30%) or a relatively high probability (>70%) of MEE and, accordingly, can be helpful in either reassuring the clinician that MEE probably is not present or raising the clinician's index of suspicion that MEE is present. Thus, the types of tympanograms found most commonly among healthy, asymptomatic children >6 months of age, namely, tympanograms with height ≥0.3 mL and width ≤200 daPa, have such a low probability of associated MEE . . . that they might serve to obviate the necessity of otoscopic examination in evaluating such children clinically. (p. 12)

The findings of Smith et al. (2006) can be put into context by referring back to Figure 2–3. The probability of MEE associated with each of the tympanograms in the figure is very low (1%) for the normally shaped tympanogram (A), moderate (42%) for the rounded tympanogram (C), and relatively high (80%) for the flat tympanogram (B). Screening with tympanometry, as with any screening technique, may yield false negative and false positive outcomes. In addition, the sensitivity, specificity, and both positive and negative predictive values differ substantially depending on the criteria for a pass versus fail outcome. Increased sensitivity is invariably purchased with decreased specificity, and vice versa.

Single versus Multifrequency and Multicomponent Tympanometry

Studies of multifrequency and multicomponent tympanometry were first reported in the mid-1970s (e.g., Colletti, 1975; Vanhuyse, Creten, & Van Camp, 1975). Since then, many researchers have conducted in normal and abnormal ears investigations of tympanometry with precise measurement of the individual components of acoustic admittance (resistance and reactance [conductance and susceptance]) and phase angle (ϕ). As a number of authors, working groups, panels, and committees have accurately noted over the past 30 years, multifrequency and multicomponent tympanogram techniques are more sensitive to low impedance pathologies (e.g., tympanic membrane and ossicular chain abnormalities) than simple admittance tympanograms recorded with a single low frequency probe tone. However, audiologists rely almost exclusively on single component/single frequency tympanometry for detection and diagnosis of auditory dysfunction. According to a survey reported by Hanks and Kinder at the 2007 Early Hearing Detection and Intervention (EHDI) Conference, the majority of audiologist respondents reported using a single-component admittance tympanometry technique, rather than a multicomponent technique. Two factors—simplicity and clinical yield—probably explain the longstanding clinical reliance on this approach. Tympanometry and analysis of tympanogram findings are clearly simpler when one component is recorded for one probe tone frequency. Multicomponent tympanometry yields a wide variety of different "types", including multiple normal variations. In addition, in pediatric populations most middle ear pathology is detected and adequately described with single-component and single-frequency tympanometry. There appears to be a common perception among audiologists that the simple tympanometry approach is adequate for diagnosis and management of children with middle ear pathology.

There are clear clinical indications for the use of high frequency (1000 Hz) versus low frequency (226 Hz) tympanometry in infants, up to the age of at least 4 months. Aural immittance characteristics differ substantially for infants versus older children and adults. Specifically, in comparison to older persons the middle ears of infants have a higher resistance component for a low frequency probe tone (e.g., 226 Hz) and admittance phase angle near 0°, rather than –70°. Beginning in the 1970s, published reports described multipeaked tympanograms in infants with apparently normal middle ear function and normal appearing tympanograms with a low frequency probe tone in neonates with middle ear pathology (Holte, Margolis, & Cavanaugh, 1991; Margolis & Popelka, 1975; Paradise, Smith, & Bluestone, 1976). Exact explanations are lacking for the developmental changes observed in tympanometry, and for the presence of false negative tympanogram findings in neonates. Factors likely to contribute to these findings are residual mesenchyme within the middle ear space, immature status of the middle ear system and possibly immature development, and associated increased compliance of the osseous portion of the of ear canal walls in young infants. In any event, as infants reach 4 to 6 months of age tympanogram characteristics become more adult-like and low frequency probe tone tympanometry yields a valid measure of middle ear status. A probe tone frequency of 1000 Hz is recommended for tympanometry in neonates and older infants, and normative data are now available (Kei et al., 2003; Margolis, Bass-Ringdahl, Hanks, Holte & Zapala, 2003). Ear canal volume measurements in infants, however, should be conducted for a low frequency (e.g., 226 Hz) probe tone. Most audiologists involved in pediatric auditory assessment appear to appreciate the importance of utilizing a high frequency probe tone with tympanometry in infants. Hanks and Kinder (2007) found that almost all audiologists surveyed employed a 1000 Hz (versus 226, 678, or 800 Hz) probe tone in performing tympanometry in children under 6 months.

Wideband Reflectance

Another approach for middle ear assessment, measurement of wideband middle ear power (WMEP), offers potential advantages over conventional tympanometry, particularly for detection of pathology in neonates and young children (Hunter, Tubaugh, Jackson, & Prospes, 2008). Also known as *wideband reflectance* and *wideband middle ear impedance*, WMEP was until recently only a research technique performed with rather complex instrumentation in a laboratory setting (e.g., Allen, 1986; Keefe, 1992). Clinical equipment for WMEP measurement, coupled with otoacoustic emission (OAE; transient evoked and distortion product OAE) instrumentation, is now available commercially from Mimosa Acoustics. The WMEP involves essentially simultaneous measurement of power reflectance, impedance, and admittance using either a broadband (chirp) stimulus or multiple sinusoidal stimuli over a relatively wide frequency range. Experimental instrumentation permits WMEP measure for frequencies of less than 100 Hz to over 10,000 Hz. Clinical equipment permits WMEP measurement over a frequency range of 258 to 6000 Hz. WMEP measurements are made in six domains:

- Power reflectance (%)
- | R | 2 Power absorption (%)
- 1 – | R | 2 Transmittance (dB)
- 0 × log10[1 –(| R | 2)] Normalized resistance (real (Re) component)
- [Re(Z) / Zc] Normalized reactance (imaginary [Im] component)
- [Im(Z) / Zc] Normalized impedance magnitude (| Z /Zc |)

As the stimulus is presented to the external ear canal, it is partially reflected from the tympanic membrane. Power reflectance is the energy reflected back into the ear canal, and not absorbed by the middle ear system. Test time is appropriately brief (consistently less than 1 minute). Figure 2–5 illustrates representative WMEP printouts for normal and sensorineural ears (top panel) and, for comparison, an ear with otitis media. Importantly for clinical measurement in infants and young children, WMEP is measured at ambient pressure or without induced ear canal pressure. A hermetic (airtight) seal between the probe and the ear canal wall is not required. However, the quality of the seal and the insertion depth of the probe tip do influence test findings. With a loose seal, low frequency energy may escape from the ear canal and significantly reduce reflectance in the low frequency region. Also, the marked increase in the cross section of the external ear canal in infants as they mature is a potential factor affecting WMEP measurement. However, in a comprehensive study of 97 infants ranging in age from 3 days to 47 months utilizing the Mimosa Acoustics device, Hunter et al. (2008) reported no significant age effect. There was also in this study good test-retest reliability, and no ear or gender effect on WMEP parameters. These authors did find a statistically significant difference in WMEP measures (reflectance, absorption, and transmittance) within the 1000 to 4000 Hz region for infants with clinical evidence of otitis media with effusion versus infants with normal middle ear status. One possible limitation of WMEP measures, cited by Hunter et al. (2008), was a high degree of normal variability. In summary, WMEP has considerable potential value for detection of auditory dysfunction in infants and older children. WMEP measured in combination with

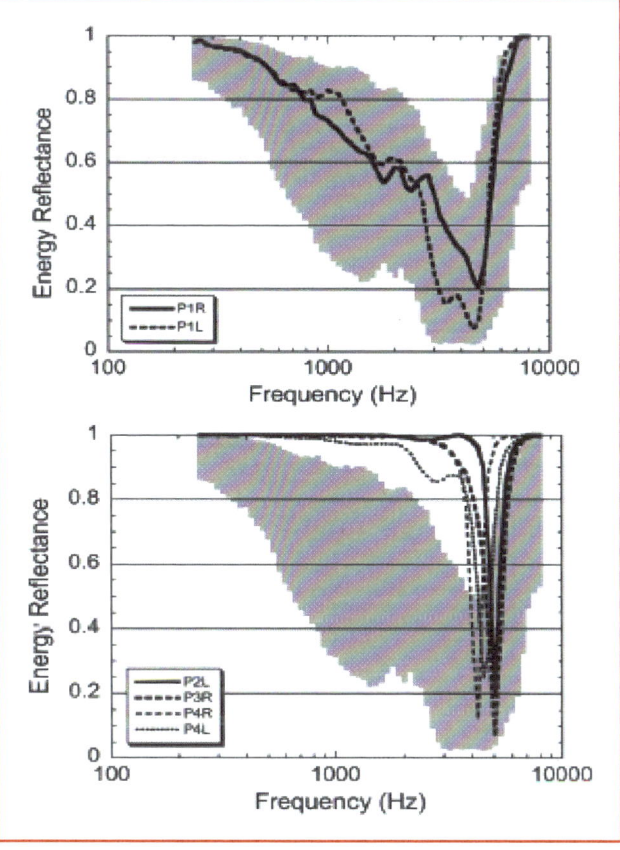

FIGURE 2–5. Normal range (*shaded area*) for wideband power reflectance (WBR) and findings for right and left ear for a patient with sensory hearing loss and normal middle ear function (*top*) and multiple patients with the diagnosis of otitis media and abnormal middle ear function (*bottom*).

OAEs, with both techniques recorded using the same instrumentation including a single probe, may result in the unusual merger of high sensitivity and high specificity for detection of middle ear disorders.

Acoustic Reflex Thresholds for Broadband Noise Signals

Tympanometry has unquestionable value as a screening tool for the detection of middle ear abnormalities. WMEP also shows promise for this clinical objective. However, as we emphasized at the outset of this chapter, hearing requires integrity of much more than the middle ear. The application of hearing loss estimation with acoustic reflex thresholds was first reported in the early 1970s (Jerger, Burney, Mauldin, & Crump, 1974; Niemeyer & Sesterhenn, 1972). An obvious and clinically real limitation of the acoustic reflex as a screening or diagnostic test is the adverse impact of middle ear dysfunction. Presuming normal middle ear function, acoustic reflexes permit quick and objective differentiation of normal versus abnormal cochlear function. We will review techniques for estimating the degree of sensory hearing loss in the next section of the chapter. First, we'll describe a very simple acoustic reflex technique for distinguishing between normal and disordered hearing that relies only on an acoustic reflex threshold for a single signal.

As clinical experience with acoustic reflex measurement accumulated, a direct relation was observed for hearing loss and the acoustic reflex for noise signals. In particular, the acoustic reflex threshold for broadband noise (BBN) increased rather systematically with hearing thresholds. In contrast, acoustic reflexes elicited with pure tone signals showed little change in threshold from normal hearing sensitivity through 50 or even 60 dB HL. Cursory inspection of Figure 2–6 reveals the differential effect of sensory hearing loss on acoustic reflex thresholds elicited with tonal versus BBN signals. In a study of 326 adult subjects with varying degrees of sensory hearing loss, Hall, Berry, and Olson (1982) evaluated the acoustic reflex threshold for a BBN signal (contralateral condition) in differentiating normal hearing (pure tone average <35 dB HL) from disordered (pure tone average ≥35 dB HL) ears, and offered guidelines for the clinical use of the strategy. The distributions of acoustic reflex thresholds for two groups of subjects (normal versus hearing loss) displayed in Figure 2–6 reveal that 76% of the 204 subjects with hearing thresholds in the 0 to 34 dB HL range yielded BBN elicited acoustic reflex thresholds of 90 dB SPL or less. In contrast, almost three fourths (72%) of the 122 subjects with serious hearing loss had BBN acoustic reflex thresholds exceeding 90 dB SPL. Importantly, no subject with hearing loss (pure tone average >35 dB HL) had an acoustic reflex threshold for BBN of less than 85 dB SPL.

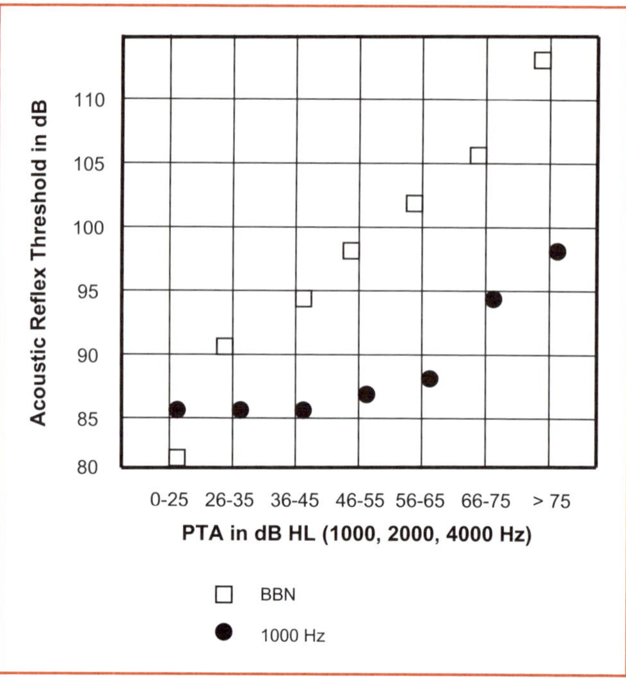

FIGURE 2–6. Relation of hearing thresholds and acoustic reflex thresholds for tonal and broadband noise signals (Hall, Berry & Olson, 1982).

The relationship between acoustic reflex threshold and hearing level is displayed in more detail in Table 2–6. Acoustic reflex thresholds of 65 through 80 dB SPL invariably ruled out the likelihood of serious sensory hearing loss, whereas acoustic reflex thresholds of 110 or 115 dB SPL identified serious hearing loss with 100% accuracy, and the majority of patients with reflex thresholds of 100 and 105 dB SPL also had hearing loss. Although these acoustic reflex data were collected in the contralateral signal condition (not the ipsilateral condition) and from adults (not children), the BBN acoustic reflex technique for hearing loss detection seems promising. The very simple measurement of a single acoustic reflex threshold for a BBN signal, or even "screening" for the acoustic reflex threshold at a fixed 80 dB SPL signal level, appears to have value for detection of hearing loss. In combination with other hearing detection techniques, such as otoacoustic emissions or speech awareness thresholds in the sound field, the acoustic reflex measurement for a BBN signal

Table 2–6. The proportion of subjects with no serious hearing loss versus those with serious hearing loss shown as a function of the level of the acoustic reflex threshold for a broadband noise (BBN) signal

Acoustic Reflex Threshold for BBN in dB SPL	(N)	Pure-Tone Average (500 to 4000 Hz)	
		<35 dB HL	>35 dB HL
65	(2)	100%	0%
70	(6)	100%	0%
75	(20)	100%	0%
80	(32)	100%	0%
85	(51)	69%	31%
90	(76)	76%	24%
95	(66)	55%	45%
100	(39)	28%	72%
105	(25)	16%	84%
110	(4)	0%	100%
115	(5)	0%	100%

Source. From "Identification of Serious Hearing Loss with Acoustic Reflex Data," by J. W. Hall, III, G. A. Berry, & K Olson, 1982, *Scandinavian Audiology*, *11*, pp. 251–255. Reprinted with permission.

provides a readily available, quick, and objective method for ear-specific identification of hearing loss in infants and young children.

DIAGNOSIS OF AUDITORY DYSFUNCTION

Introduction

The foregoing review confirms the evidenced-based documentation of immittance measures for detection of auditory dysfunction. However, as noted at the outset of this chapter, immittance measures analyzed and interpreted in isolation have relatively limited diagnostic value. In combination findings from other audiologic procedures, such as pure tone audiometry, otoacoustic emissions, and/or auditory brainstem response, immittance measures make an important, even critical, contribution to the diagnostic audiology test battery. This concept is, of course, now well appreciated and was articulated effectively over 30 years ago in the classic paper by Jerger and Hayes entitled "The Cross-Check Principle in Pediatric Audiometry" (1976)

Nonetheless, acoustic reflex findings are useful diagnostically for estimating degree of sensory hearing loss in patients who cannot volunteer valid pure tone findings, and for differentiating among sensory, neural, and some brainstem auditory abnormalities. Acoustic reflex measurements also play a small but very important role in the diagnosis of auditory neuropathy. The diagnostic contribution of acoustic reflexes in pediatric audiology is particularly noteworthy with patients for whom electrophysiological auditory measurements, such as ECochG, ABR, and ASSR, are contraindicated or for a variety of reasons cannot be completed. Two not uncommon explanations for the lack of auditory electrophysiology findings are the lack of access to auditory evoked response instrumentation and the requirement in many children for performing auditory evoked response assessment under sedation or anesthesia. In such cases, the modest diagnostic findings available from acoustic reflex measurements can provide enough information on the site of auditory dysfunction and the degree of hearing loss (or confirmation of normal hearing sensitivity) to allow the audiologist to promptly provide appropriate intervention. Furthermore, combining test results for tympanometry, acoustic reflex measurement, and even partial results for pure tone audiometry produces patterns of findings that, when carefully analyzed, yield an amazing amount of diagnostic information for patients of all ages and types of auditory dysfunction.

In this section, we review strategies for applying acoustic reflexes in estimating degree of sensory hearing loss. We also will highlight the diagnostic value inherent in patterns of findings for immittance measures and air conduction pure tone audiometry. A discussion of how test findings for all electroacoustical and electrophysiological measures can be fully exploited diagnostically is reserved for Chapter 7. Case reports illustrating multiple diagnostic patterns and outcomes following assessment with a comprehensive electroacoustical and electrophysiological test battery are presented in Chapter 8.

Tympanometry Findings in Auditory Dysfunction

As already pointed out, tympanometry findings taken alone are far more useful in detecting middle ear abnormality than contributing to the diagnosis. It is certainly not possible to predict the degree of hearing loss with tympanometry. Some authors have argued that inclusion of multiple probe tone frequencies and multicomponent analysis increases the diagnostic value of tympanometry. For example, Lilly (2005) stated:

> MFT [multifrequency tympanometry] seemed to record changes in the middle ear after acute otitis media that 226-Hz tympanometry was unable to detect, implying persistence of pathology. . . . With tympanometry, as with static acoustic-immittance measurements, the differential diagnosis of some middle-ear problems often is more accurate when both components of Za or Ya are available for analysis. . . . Clinically, unless one is working only with neonates, the need for multiple-component, multiple-frequency tympanometry exists for fewer than 20% of all patients evaluated. Still, these techniques are invaluable for the differential diagnosis of: 1) fixation of the lateral ossicular chain from fixation of the stapes; 2) profound mixed hearing losses; 3) clinical otosclerosis from disruption of the ossicular chain; 4) hypermobility of the incudostapedial joint; and 5) congenital ossicular fixation in children. (p. 6)

We would certainly agree that audiologists should take advantage of all of the techniques that are available to enhance diagnostic accuracy. However, considering the relatively low proportion of children with the pathologies just listed, diagnosis of hearing loss in the vast majority of children will not be markedly diminished by the exclusion of multicomponent tympanometry from the test battery.

Toynbee and Valsava Techniques

Two other longstanding and underutilized tympanometric measures of eustachian tube dysfunction warrant brief mention in our discussion of diagnosis of auditory dysfunction. Both tests are conducted with the patient in a sitting position using a conventional immittance device. The Toynbee test is named for Joseph Toynbee (1815–1866), an English otologist who dedicated his life to research of the anatomy and pathology of the ear. As an aside, Toynbee is given credit for recognizing the connection between stapes fixation and hearing loss. Also, according to most reports, Toynbee died when he inadvertently inhaled substances he was investigating as possible treatments for tinnitus (a combination of prussic acid and chloroform). With the Toynbee test tympanometry is first performed in the typical fashion. Then the patient is instructed to swallow (with mouth closed) while the patient's nose is compressed, preventing air from passing in or out. If the eustachian tube opens (a normal finding), middle ear pressure (and pressure in the nasopharynx) will decrease as documented by a shift in the pressure peak of the tympanometry before versus after the Toynbee maneuver). That is, the tympanogram peak moves toward the negative pressure region.

The Valsava Technique was named after a famous Italian philosopher, practicing physician (surgeon), and anatomist Antonio Maria Valsalva (1666–1723) who in his amazingly diverse and productive career established a name in medicine, public health, mental health, and especially for his detailed studies and classic textbooks on the anatomy of the ear. Dr. Valsalva actually devised the technique that now is named after him. Again, tympanometry is first recorded as usual. Then, with the patient's nose pinched together by the thumb and forefinger, the patient is instructed to inflate the mouth with air and try to exhale. The Valsalva maneuver is most useful to determine whether the eustachian tube can be forced open and negative middle ear pressure relieved by creating positive pressure within the mouth and nasopharynx. This is, of course, the same technique we often use to "clear our ears" while flying on an airplane that is descending.

Sensitivity Prediction by the Acoustic Reflex (SPAR)

German auditory researchers Niemeyer and Sesterhenn in 1972 introduced at an audiology congress the concept of hearing loss prediction from the acoustic reflex and published their findings 2 years later (Niemeyer & Sesterhenn, 1974). Data were limited to persons with normal hearing. Soon after, Jerger and colleagues (Jerger, Burney, Mauldin & Crump, 1974) at the Baylor College of Medicine investigated in a series of 1156 patients with varying degrees of sensory auditory dysfunction a clinical adaptation of this concept for hearing loss prediction based on acoustic reflex thresholds (ARTs) for pure tone versus noise signals. Briefly, the acoustic reflex threshold for a BBN signal was subtracted from the averaged reflex thresholds for pure tone signals of 500, 1000, and 2000 Hz. Then a correction factor, determined biologically for each impedance device, is added to the result. The calculation, summarized in the following equation, yielded a *noise tone difference* (NTD). Jerger and colleagues named the new procedure sensitivity prediction by the acoustic reflex, with the nautical sounding acronym SPAR.

$$\text{NTD} = \frac{[\text{ART 500 Hz HL} + \text{ART 1000 Hz HL} + \text{2000 Hz HL}]}{3} - \text{ART BBN SPL} + \text{correction}$$

Two years later, based on observations of inaccuracies for some patients in hearing loss prediction with the original SPAR, Jerger and colleagues refined the 1974 criteria for predicting hearing. Because of concerns about the overall low accuracy rate (<75%) along with troublesome false-positive predictive errors (e.g., prediction of a moderate hearing loss in a normal hearing person) even with revised 1976 SPAR criteria, Hall (1978) published findings for a further revised SPAR technique, referred to as the 1977 SPAR. Criteria employed in the simplified and improved 1977 SPAR technique are summarized in Table 2–7. The objective was to categorize hearing status as normal hearing, mild-moderate hearing loss, or severe hearing loss.

Other Acoustic Reflex Predictive Techniques

Also during the 1970s, David Lilly developed a method for hearing threshold prediction based on statistical regression techniques (Lilly, 1977). The original regression equation required acoustic reflex threshold data for octave frequencies from 500 Hz through 4000 Hz, as well as BBN. Due to the absence of valid data for the 4000 Hz test frequency in a substantial proportion of patients, Lilly soon reported a modified regression equation (Lilly, 1977). Other researchers (e.g., Rizzo & Greenberg, 1979) further refined the regression

Table 2–7. Criteria for the 1977 version of the sensitivity prediction by acoustic reflex (SPAR) technique

Noise-Tone Difference (NTD)	*Broadband Noise*	*Hearing Sensitivity Prediction*
≥20 dB and 1000 Hz ART ≤95 dB HL	Anywhere	Normal hearing sensitivity
<20 dB or 1000 Hz ART >95 dB HL	≤95 dB SPL	Mild-moderate hearing loss
<20 dB or 1000 Hz ART >95 dB HL	>95 dB SPL	Severe hearing loss

Note. ART = acoustic reflex threshold; HL = hearing level; SPL = sound pressure level.

Source. From "Predicting Hearing Loss from the Acoustic Reflex: A Comparison of Three Methods," by J. W. Hall, III, 1978, *Archives of Otolaryngology*, *104*, pp. 601–605. Reprinted with permission.

equation technique for hearing loss estimation with acoustic reflex data. Unfortunately, accuracy of all of the regression equation approaches was compromised by an unacceptable high rate of false positive errors in normal hearers but also underestimation of severe hearing loss even resulting in false negative errors (patients with hearing loss predicted to have normal hearing).

Recognizing the limitations of the regression equation approach for predicting hearing loss, and the importance of taking into account signal bandwidth in hearing loss prediction, Popelka, Margolis, and Wiley (1976) developed another novel technique for identifying hearing loss known as the *bivariate plot coordinate system*. Unique among predictive methods, the bivariate plot coordinate system took into account acoustic reflex thresholds for pure tone signals and both low and high pass noise bands, and it attempted to predict hearing status for three separate frequencies (500, 1000, and 2000 Hz). Acoustic reflex threshold data were literally plotted on a set of three graphs that were designed to simply and accurately separate persons with normal hearing versus "significant" hearing impairment. Subsequent clinical research confirmed that the bivariate plot coordinate system was characterized by a high rate of false negative errors with normal hearing predicted especially for patients with mild and/or high frequency sensory hearing loss (Hall, 1978).

Contraindications to Acoustic Reflex Measurement

The signals used to elicit the acoustic reflex are necessarily rather high in intensity, approaching the loudness discomfort level of some persons. Measurement of the acoustic reflex in patients complaining of hyperacusis and/or tinnitus is not advised. In most cases, the information gained from recording acoustic reflexes will not contribute to the diagnosis of their auditory dysfunction. Often concerns about possible retrocochlear auditory pathology are ruled out with neuroradiological imaging (e.g., CT or MRI). Conversely, the likelihood of doing harm to the patient, and exacerbating their hyperacusis and perception of tinnitus, is unacceptably high with acoustic reflex measurement. There are reported medico-legal cases of persons who have filed lawsuits against audiologists and others following acoustic reflex measurement, claiming that permanent noise-induced hearing loss resulted from the high intensity stimulus sounds. Also, acoustic reflex measurement is contraindicated for patients with a history of vertigo or other vestibular symptoms with exposure to high intensity sounds (Tullio phenomenon). It is wise clinical practice to first describe the acoustic reflex measurement process to the patient, and to inform the patient that she may request at any time that the test be discontinued. Any concerns the patient may express during or after acoustic reflex measurement should be documented in writing. Finally, there is little to be gained by exceeding stimulus intensity levels of 110 dB during acoustic reflex measurement.

Diagnosis Value of Patterns of Aural Immittance Findings

Introduction

Considerable diagnostic information is available from the administration of aural immittance measurements in combination with pure tone audiometry. More than 30 years ago, Susan Jerger and Jim Jerger (1977) first reported on the diagnostic application and value of acoustic reflex patterns. Some practice is required for pattern recognition skills to develop, but time spent in reviewing different patterns of findings for immittance measurement and pure tone audiometry is time well spent. We've reviewed tympanometry already in this chapter, and we will assume that the reader has a good grasp of pure tone audiometry. [*Note:* An entire textbook on pure tone audiometry is also available within the Plural Publishing Core Clinical Concepts Series.]

A brief explanation of acoustic reflex conditions and patterns is warranted. The reader may wish to first review the diagrammatic figure of acoustic reflex pathways presented earlier (see Figure 2–2). In discussing acoustic reflex patterns, it's important to make the distinction between *probe ear* and *stimulus ear*. The probe ear is, obviously, the ear on which tympanometry is performed. For ipsilateral reflexes, the probe ear and stimulus ear are the same. That is, the acoustic immittance change indicating the presence of an acoustic reflex occurs ipsilateral to (in the same ear as) the stimulation. The term *uncrossed* is also used for ipsilateral, as the acoustic reflex pathways do not cross the midline of the brainstem. For contralateral acoustic reflexes, stimulus is presented to the ear opposite the probe ear. That is, the acoustic immittance change indicating the presence of an acoustic reflex occurs contralateral to (in the same ear as) the stimulation. The term *crossed* is interchangeable with contralateral, as the acoustic reflex pathways cross the midline of the brainstem (via the trapezoid body) before coursing to the region of the motor nucleus of the seventh cranial (facial) nerve and then to the stapedius muscle via motor fibers within the seventh cranial nerve.

There is, then, the possibility of four distinct and different measurement conditions in acoustic reflex measurement: (a) right ear ipsilateral, (b) left ear ipsilateral, (c) contralateral reflexes with the probe in the right ear and sound in the left ear, and (d) contralateral reflexes with the probe in the left ear and sound in the right ear. These four measurement conditions, and normal findings for each, are often shown graphically in a "faces" figure (Figure 2–7). An open box in the figure indicates the presence of normal acoustic reflexes (thresholds of <90 dB HL). A shaded box indicates abnormal (elevated) acoustic reflexes, whereas a filled in (black) box indicates that no acoustic reflex activity was detected.

Combinations or patterns of findings for pure tone audiometry, tympanometry, and acoustic reflex recordings are related to likely clinical etiologies or diagnoses. In the figures and the explanation that follow, we refer to each of the six illustrative patterns of findings as cases (Case A, Case B, etc.). In viewing these figures and real world clinical findings, the reader is advised to first examine the tympanogram to confirm or rule out middle ear disorder. Then inspect the audiogram to determine whether there is evidence of conductive hearing loss. Finally, take a few moments to analyze the actual acoustic reflex pattern produced by findings for each of the four measurement conditions.

Case A: Vertical Acoustic Reflex Pattern (Mild Conductive)

The vertical pattern is often encountered clinically, particularly in pediatric populations where middle ear disorders are commonplace. As shown in Figure 2–8, the tympanogram on the right ear is clearly abnormal, immediately alerting the clinician to the likelihood of a conductive hearing loss. The suspicion is confirmed by a mild conductive hearing loss for the right ear, with an air-bone gap at all audiometric frequencies. Referring to the faces portion of the figure, acoustic reflexes are absent whenever the probe is in the right (conductive) ear. Detection of a normal contralateral acoustic reflex with sound in the right ear and probe in the normal left ear confirms (even without reference to pure tone findings) that the conductive hearing loss is mild at most. Greater conductive hearing loss for the right ear would result in elevation of the contralateral acoustic reflex (sound right and probe left). A conductive hearing loss essentially reduces the effectiveness of the acoustic reflex stimulation by the magnitude of air-bone gap. Because the acoustic reflex is normally activated with an intensity level of 85 dB HL, a conductive loss of 25 to 30 dB will raise the contralateral acoustic reflex threshold (sound in the conductive ear) to about 110 to 115 dB HL.

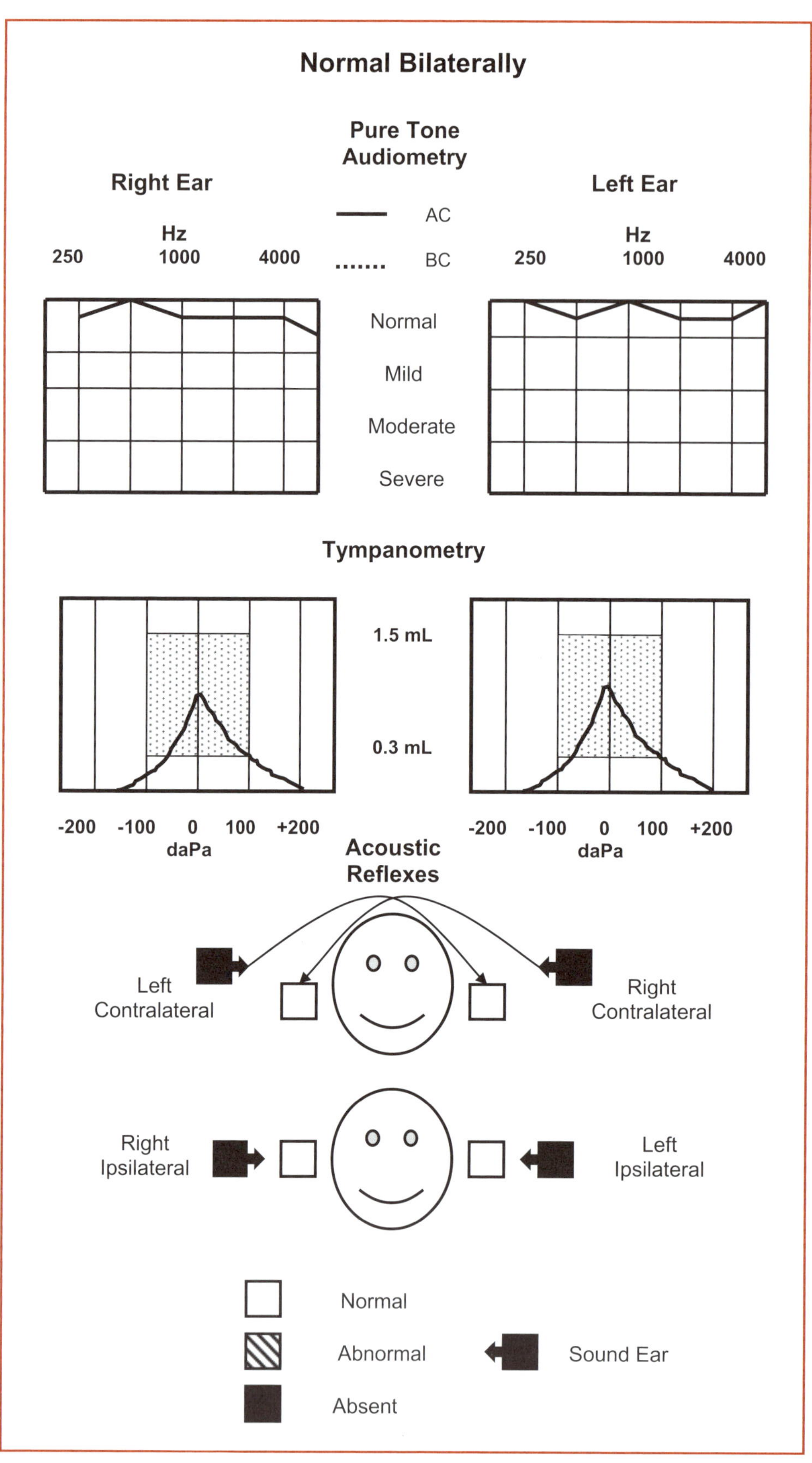

FIGURE 2–7. Relation among findings for the audiogram, tympanogram, and acoustic reflex findings for a person with normal hearing sensitivity.

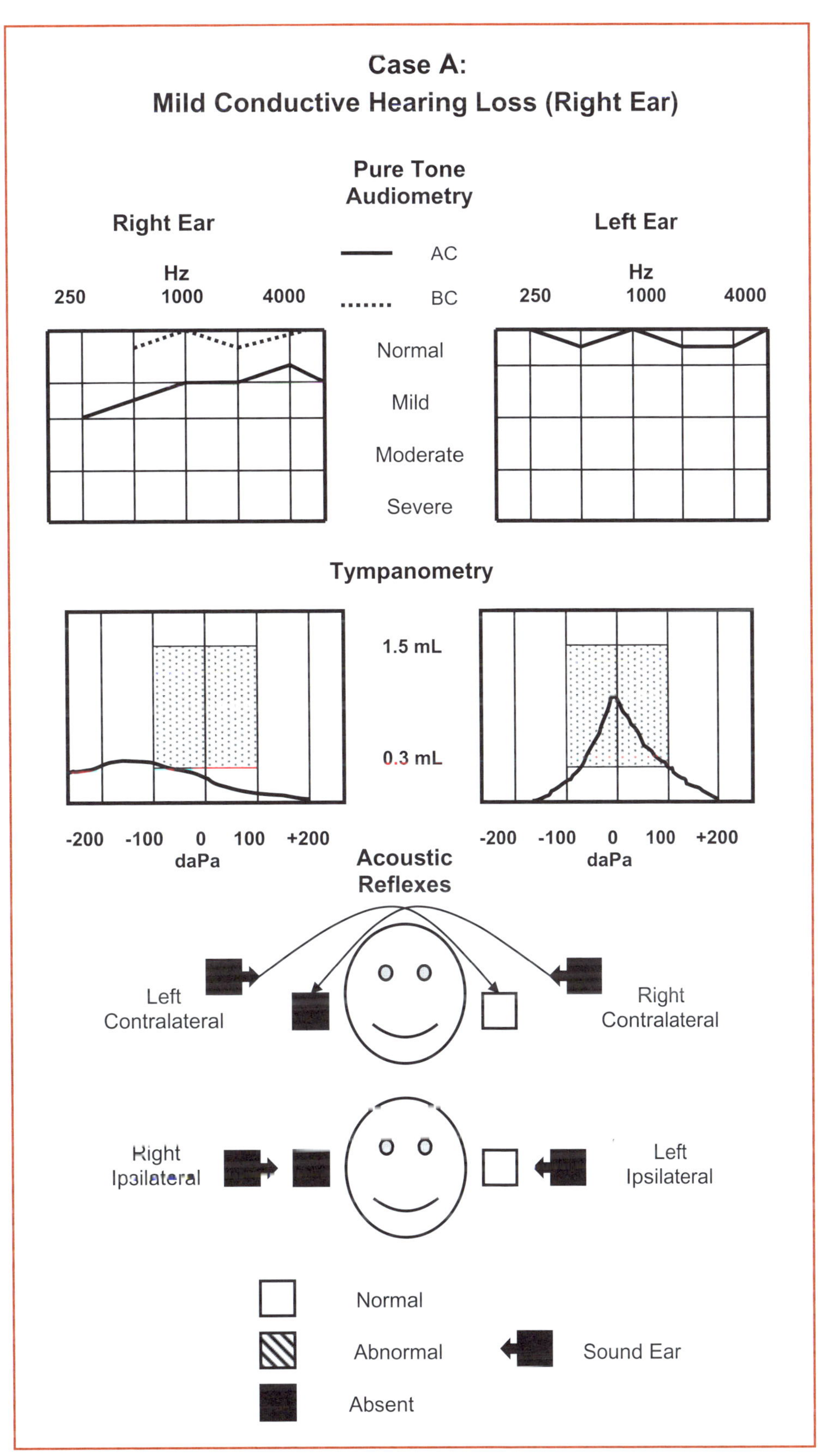

FIGURE 2–8. Relation among findings for the audiogram, tympanogram, and acoustic reflex findings for a child with a mild conductive hearing loss on the right ear.

Of course, the ipsilateral reflex, or any acoustic reflex measured with the probe in the ear with a middle ear disorder, is not observed even with a very modest (5 to 10 dB) air-bone gap. Prediction of degree of conductive hearing loss from the acoustic reflex pattern is especially useful in infants and young children for whom pure tone audiometry is not yet possible.

Case B: "Inverted L" Acoustic Reflex Pattern (Moderate Conductive)

The so-called "inverted L" pattern (Jerger & Jerger, 1977) for acoustic reflexes is really a vertical pattern with the addition of an abnormality in the contralateral acoustic reflex with sound in the conductive ear (probe in a normal ear) due to the degree of conductive hearing loss (Figure 2–9). Almost any degree of conductive loss will produce some elevation of the contralateral acoustic reflex with sound stimulation in the conductive loss. Greater degrees of conductive loss, or air-bone gaps, are associated with progressive elevations of the acoustic reflex.

Case C: Vertical Acoustic Reflex Pattern (Facial Nerve Disorder)

The facial nerve is the final efferent pathway to the stapedius muscle. Facial nerve disorder is a second explanation for the vertical pattern of acoustic reflex abnormality. Acoustic reflexes are abnormal (usually absent) whenever the probe is in the affected ear, as illustrated in Figure 2–10. Two factors clearly distinguish this vertical pattern from the acoustic reflex pattern typical of mild conductive hearing loss (illustrated by Case A). The most obvious factor is normal tympanometry in facial nerve disorder, consistent with normal middle ear function. The absence of middle ear disorder is confirmed by a normal audiogram or, in any event, no difference between air and bone conduction pure tone thresholds. Speech audiometry, specifically rollover on performance-intensity functions for PB words (PI-PB functions), may also reveal another clue for facial nerve disorder. At high intensity levels, word recognition may actually deteriorate in persons with facial nerve paralysis who lack the protective function of the acoustic reflex. Careful measurement of acoustic reflexes in the four possible conditions permits identification of facial nerve disorder in patients of all ages, even infants and young children with syndromes or diseases that include as a sign facial nerve pathology and paralysis.

Case D: Diagonal Acoustic Reflex Pattern (Sensory)

When acoustic reflexes are abnormal (e.g., elevated in threshold) or absent with sound in the suspect ear, the most likely explanation is a sensory hearing loss (Figure 2–11). Of course, the chances of detecting any acoustic reflex activity decline as the degree of sensory hearing loss increases. Normal acoustic reflex findings are anticipated in mild sensory hearing loss. Generally, acoustic reflexes for pure tone signals will be recorded, although at elevated thresholds, for moderate sensory hearing loss and until the degree of loss exceeds about 60 dB HL. Normal middle ear function in both ears is confirmed by the presence of normal acoustic reflexes with the probe in each ear under at least one condition.

Case E: Diagonal Acoustic Reflex Pattern (Neural)

At first glance the diagnostic pattern seen in Case E (Figure 2–12) may appear similar to, perhaps indistinguishable from, the diagnostic pattern just noted for Case D. Close inspection of all available findings clearly differentiates the two patterns. The big difference is the degree of hearing loss. With neural auditory dysfunction (e.g., an acoustic tumor or, more properly, vestibular schwannoma) the diagonal acoustic reflex abnormality is associated with even mild hearing loss, whereas a moderate-to-severe sensory loss is required to produce the same pattern. The neural pattern may also result from acoustic reflex decay, and not only elevation of the acoustic reflex thresholds.

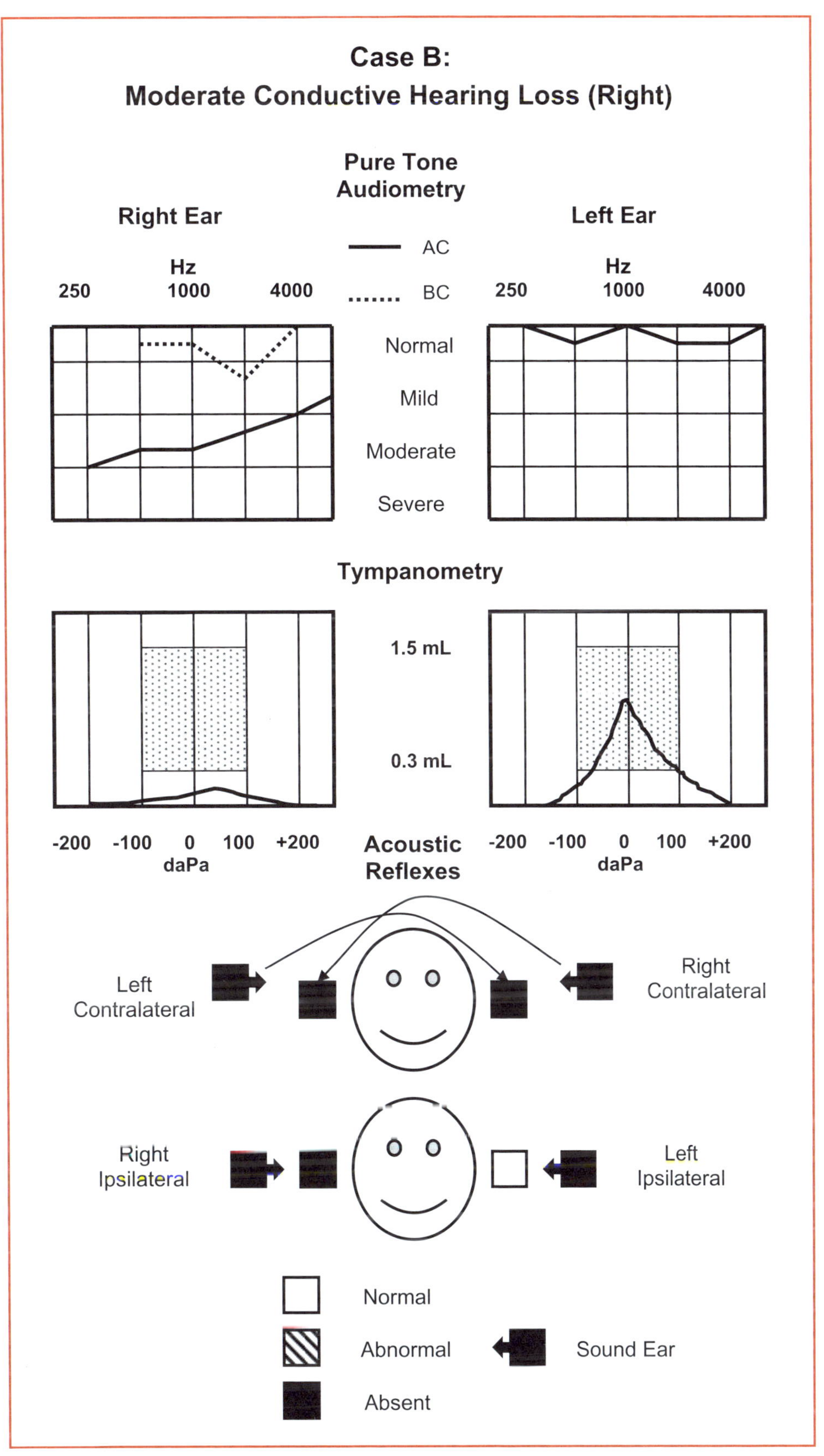

FIGURE 2–9. Relation among findings for the audiogram, tympanogram, and acoustic reflex findings for a patient with a moderate conductive hearing loss on the right ear.

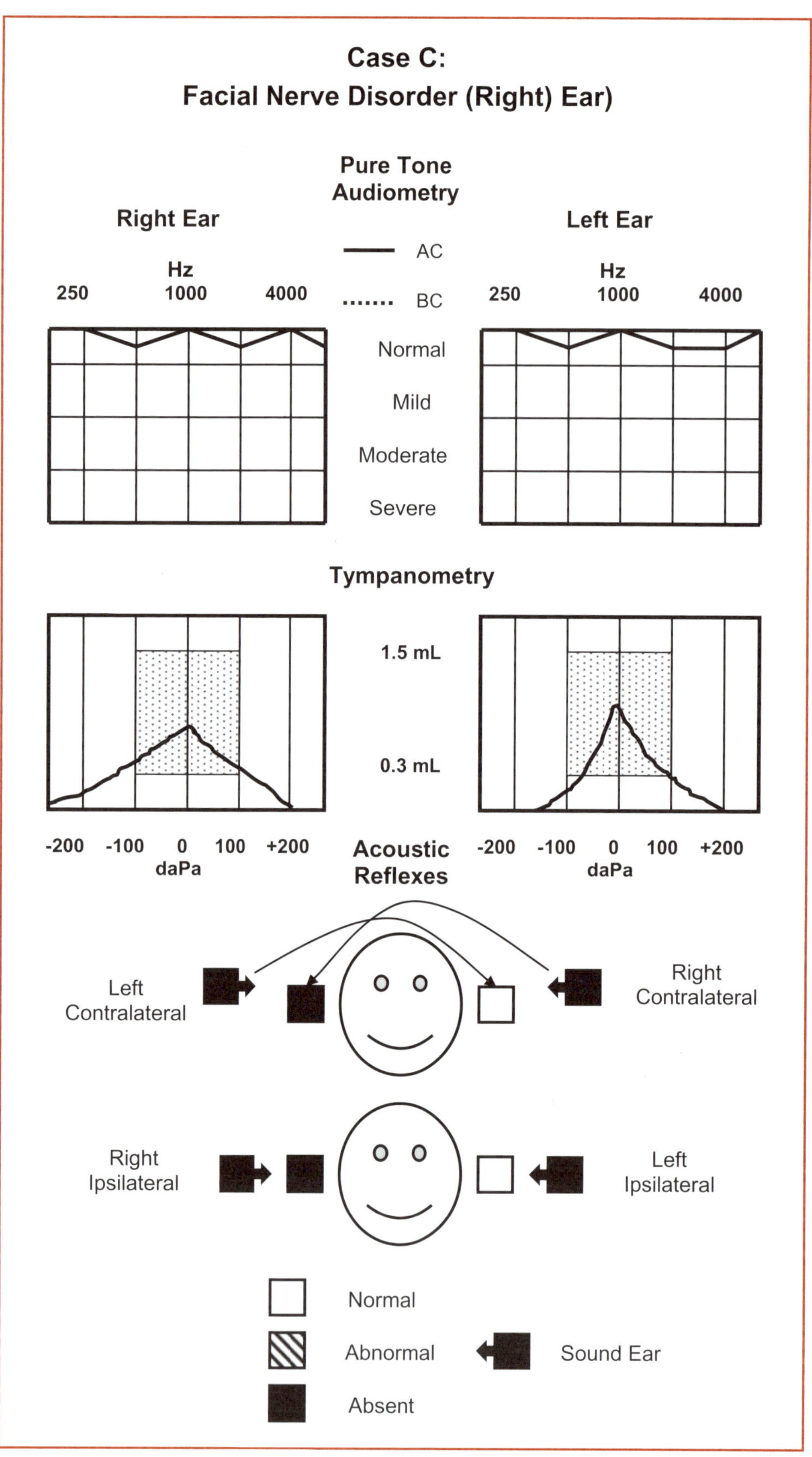

FIGURE 2–10. Relation among findings for the audiogram, tympanogram, and acoustic reflex findings for a patient with facial nerve dysfunction on the right side.

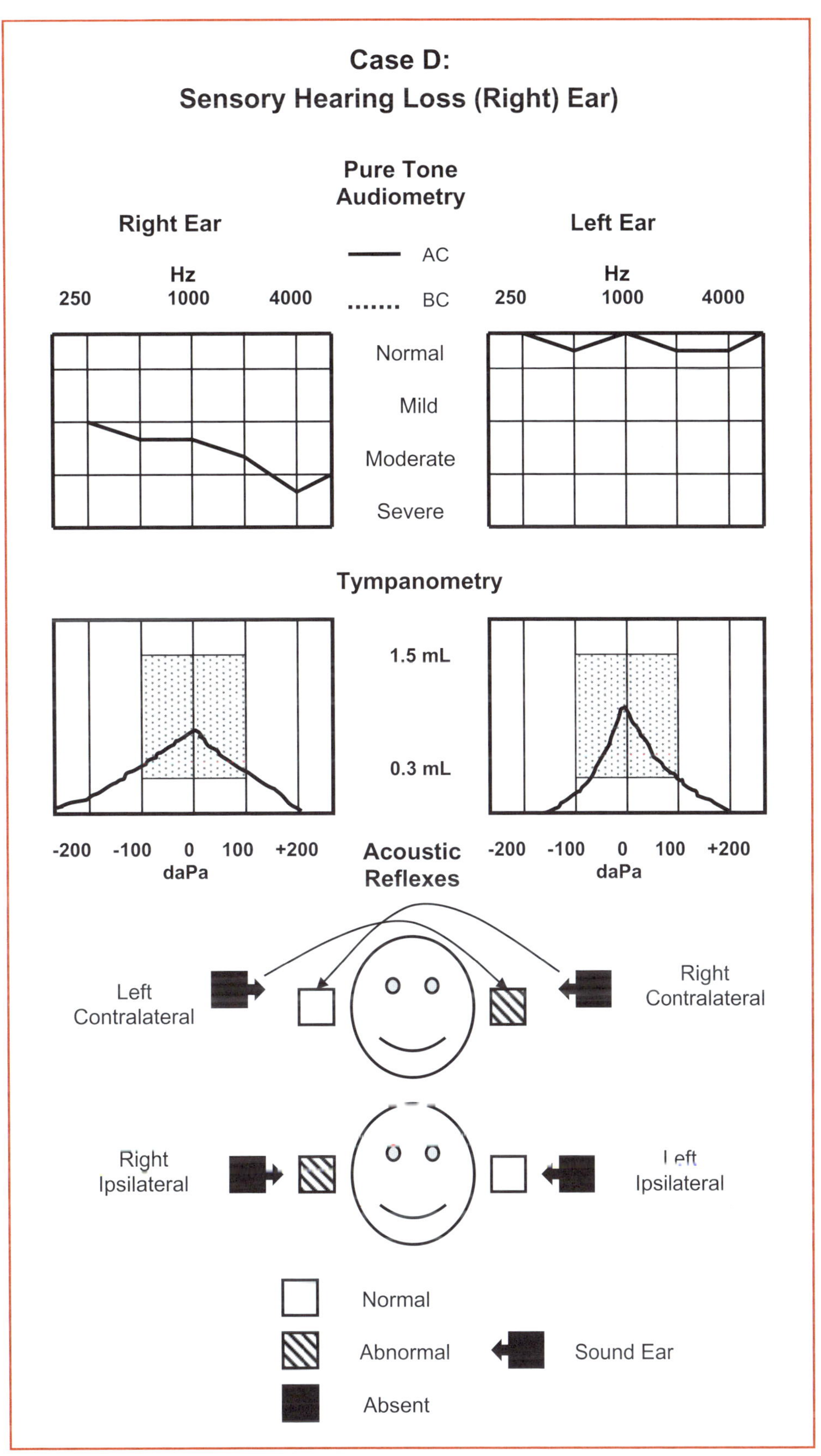

FIGURE 2–11. Relation among findings for the audiogram, tympanogram, and acoustic reflex findings for a patient with sensory hearing loss on the right side.

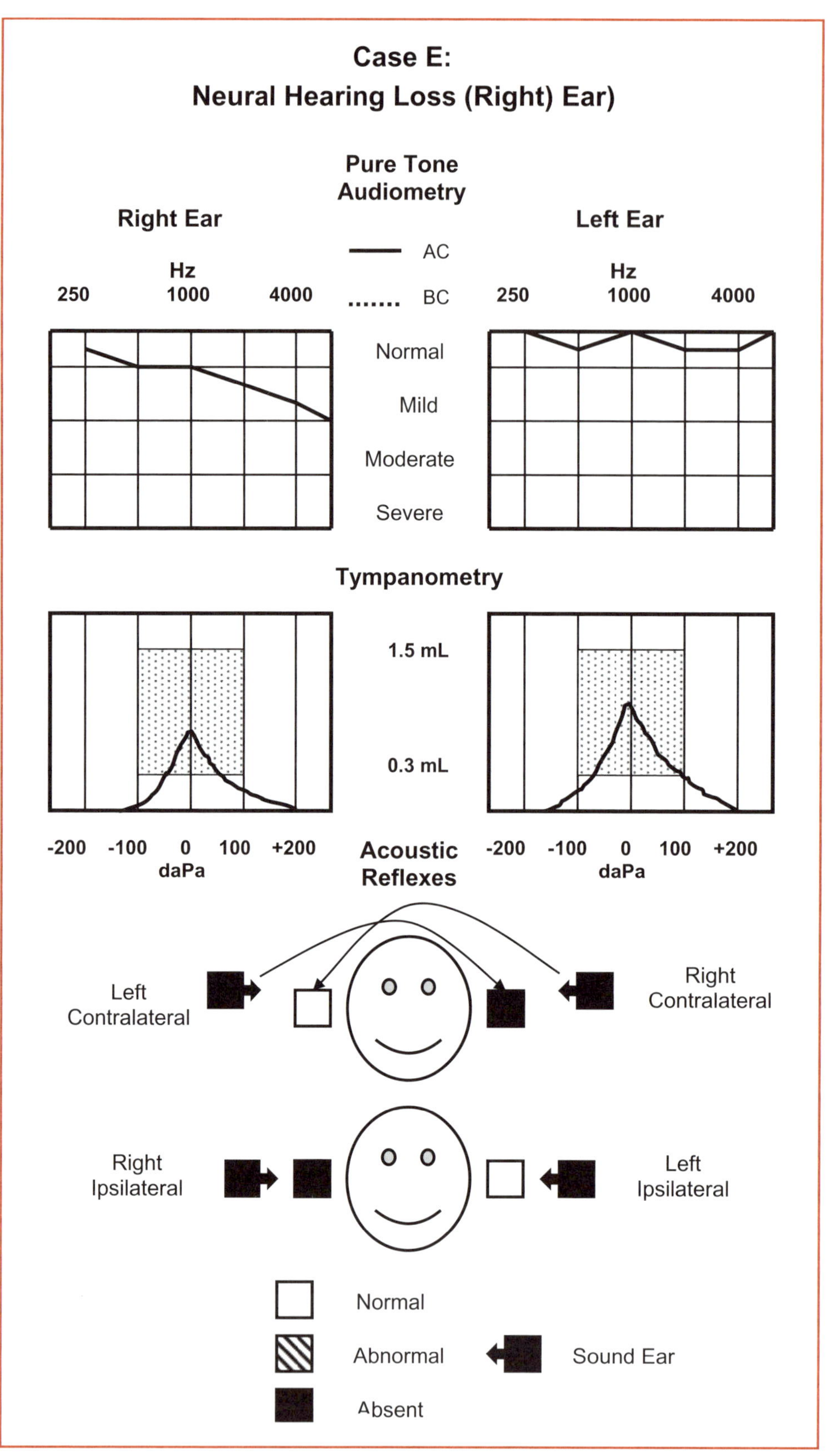

FIGURE 2–12. Relation among findings for the audiogram, tympanogram, and acoustic reflex findings for a patient with neural (eighth cranial nerve or retrocochlear) auditory dysfunction on the right side.

Case F: Inverted L Acoustic Reflex Pattern (Neural)

Just as severe conductive loss can extend the vertical acoustic reflex pattern to an inverted L pattern, a marked neural abnormality can extend a diagonal pattern to an inverted L pattern. The diagonal component of the pattern is produced directly by abnormality of the eighth cranial (acoustic) nerve affecting sound stimulation of the involved ear. With a large acoustic tumor compressing the brainstem as well as the eighth cranial nerve, an additional crossed (contralateral) acoustic pathway within the brainstem is involved. In other words, the inverted L neural pattern is consistent with a larger tumor involving the eighth cranial nerve and brainstem, whereas the diagonal neural pattern is found usually in smaller tumors affecting only the eighth cranial nerve.

Case G: Horizontal Acoustic Reflex Pattern (Brainstem)

The horizontal acoustic reflex pattern (Figure 2–13) is encountered in patients with brainstem auditory dysfunction but entirely normal peripheral auditory function. The presence of normal ipsilateral acoustic reflexes and normal tympanometry unequivocally rules out conductive hearing loss, sensory hearing loss, neural auditory dysfunction, and facial nerve disorder. The only appropriate anatomic explanation is brainstem auditory disorder. Whenever the horizontal acoustic pattern is found clinically, it is very important to rule out technical problems, and to verify that the appropriate stimulus intensity is being presented to each ear through the contralateral stimulus transducer. If supra-aural earphones are used for contralateral stimulation, collapsing ear canals must also be ruled out. The horizontal acoustic reflex pattern is a strong sign of brainstem auditory dysfunction in patients at risk for central auditory nervous system dysfunction, including those with suspected auditory processing disorder (APD). As noted at the beginning of this chapter, acoustic reflexes offer a completely objective auditory measure not influenced by the many listener variables (e.g., motivation, cognition, age, language, attention) that might compromise behavioral measures of auditory function. The horizontal acoustic reflex abnormality strongly suggests the need for a comprehensive assessment of central auditory function and, depending on the outcome of the assessment, referral to a neurologist or neuro-otologist for medical evaluation.

Case H: "Uni-Box" Acoustic Reflex Pattern (Brainstem)

A rare auditory finding first described by Jerger, Jerger, and Hall in 1979, the uni-box pattern is characterized by an abnormality in only one contralateral acoustic reflex condition (Figure 2–14). All pathologic explanations other than an isolated unilateral brainstem auditory abnormality can be convincingly ruled out by the presence of normal acoustic reflexes in the other three acoustic reflex conditions, plus normal tympanograms and usually normal hearing sensitivity bilaterally. As with the horizontal pattern, observation of the uni-box acoustic reflex abnormality should prompt a comprehensive assessment of central auditory function and, in many cases, referral for neurological or neuro-otological diagnostic evaluation.

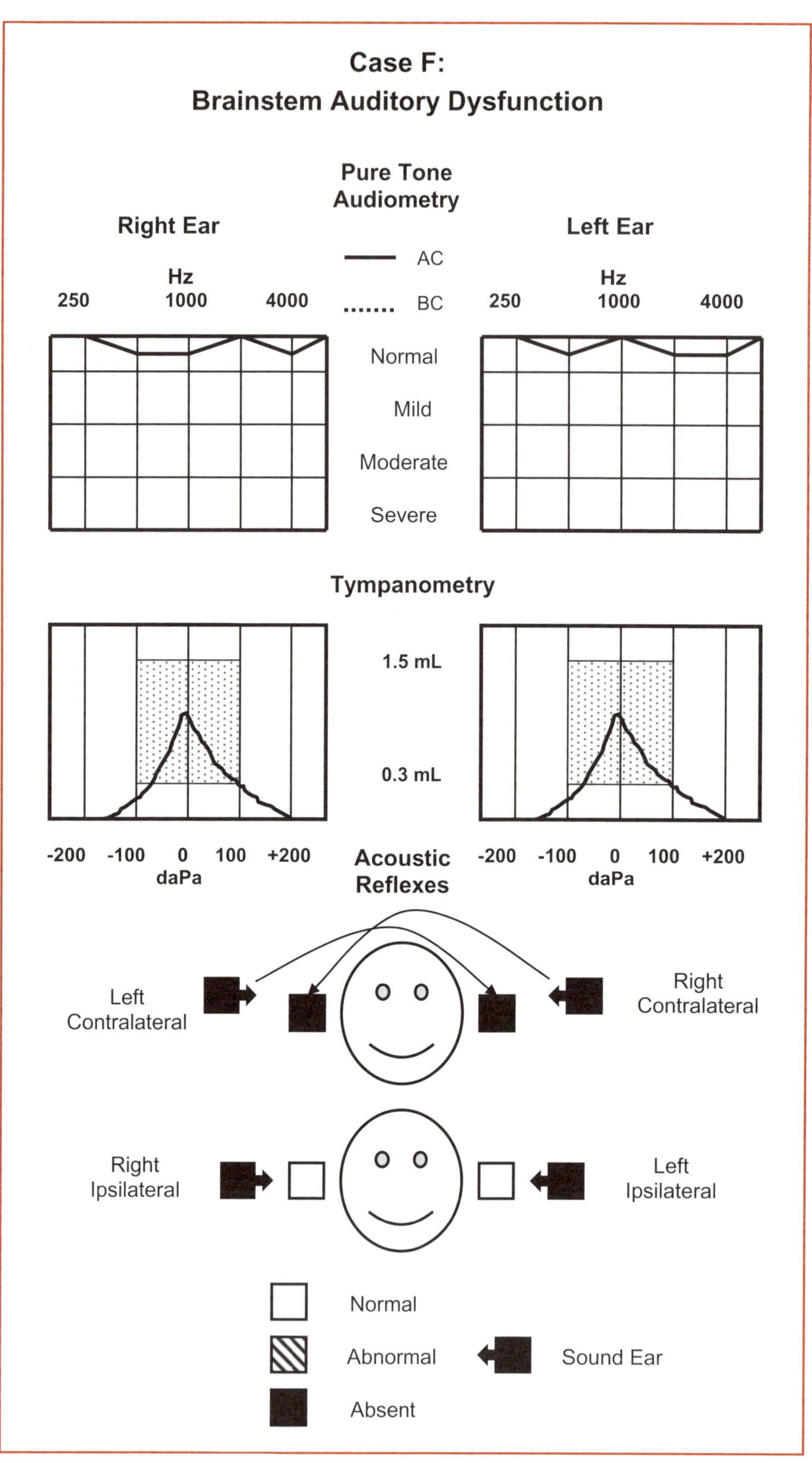

FIGURE 2–13. Relation among findings for the audiogram, tympanogram, and acoustic reflex findings for a patient with brainstem auditory dysfunction.

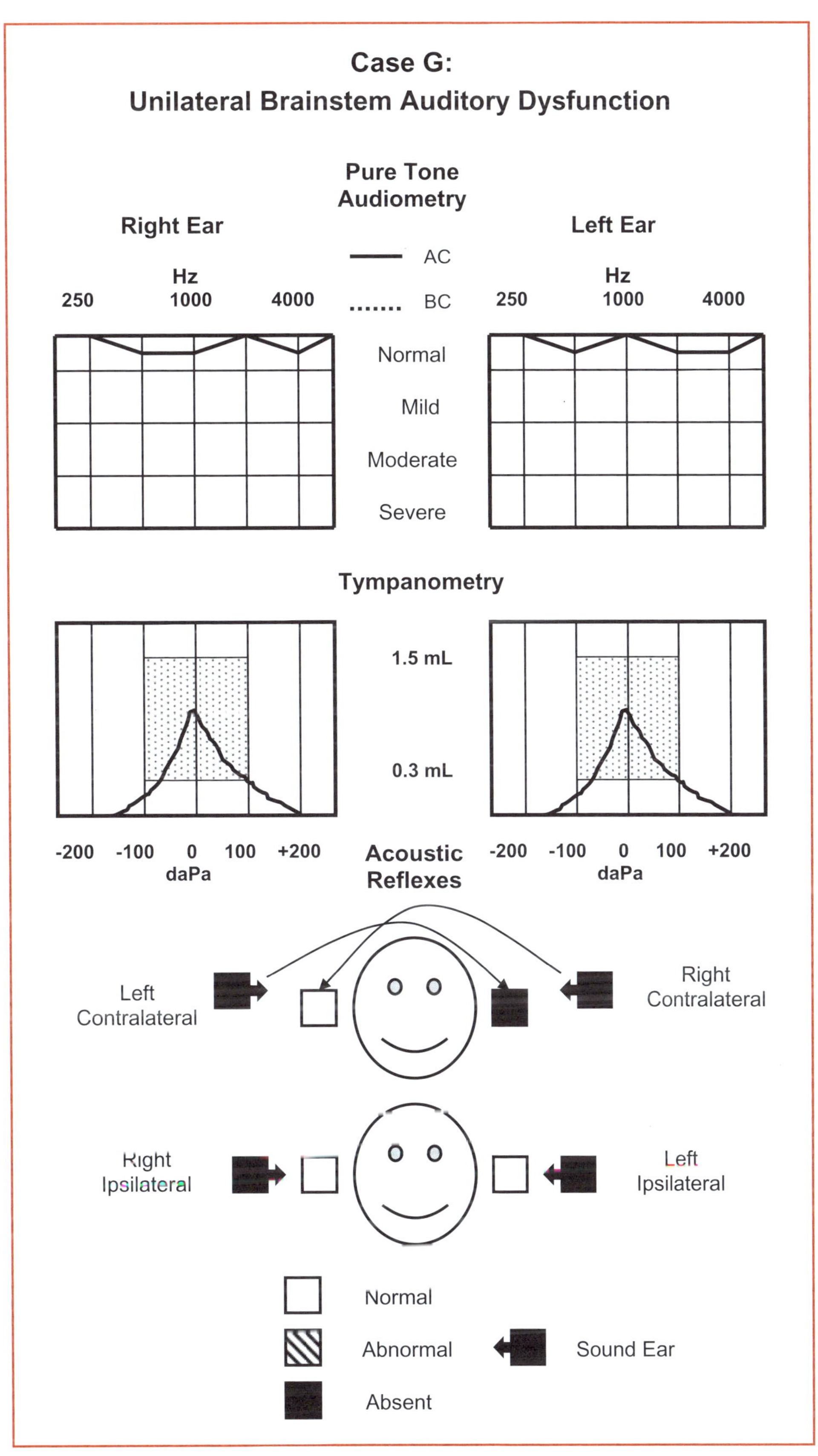

FIGURE 2–14. Relation among findings for the audiogram, tympanogram, and acoustic reflex findings for a patient with isolated unilateral brainstem auditory dysfunction.

3

Otoacoustic Emissions

INTRODUCTION

Ironically, otoacoustic emissions (OAEs) contribute importantly and in a truly unique way to the diagnosis of auditory dysfunction, yet they have essentially no value in defining the degree of hearing loss. This apparent paradox in no way minimizes or detracts from the role of OAEs in clinical audiology today. In terms of anatomic site sensitivity and specificity, that is, detection and verification of outer hair cell dysfunction, OAEs have no rival in the audiologic test battery. Because most hearing loss in children, including newborn infants, is secondary to cochlear abnormalities and, in particular, outer hair cell damage and/or dysfunction, OAEs are well suited for hearing screening of infants, preschool and school age children, and even adults. OAEs are also an attractive screening option because the technique is relatively inexpensive and simple, that is, OAE measurement just requires insertion of a disposable or reusable probe into the ear without the need for electrode application. Clinical technology for recording OAEs was introduced in the late 1980s, about 10 years after the discovery by Dr. David Kemp that the cochlea, and specifically the outer hair cells, is capable of motility and the generation of energy that can be detected as sound in the external ear canal. Now multiple manufacturers market small, handheld, battery powered devices designed for automated OAE measurement and analysis. In fact, the emergence of automated OAE technology in the late 1990s contributed importantly to the rapid growth and international expansion of universal newborn hearing screening (UNHS).

In this chapter, we review the application of transient evoked otoacoustic emissions (TEOAEs) and distortion product otoacoustic emissions (DPOAEs) in the detection of hearing loss and for the diagnostic auditory assessment of infants and young children. The chapter is focused only on this topic. No attempt is made to explain the mechanisms of OAEs, to describe in any detail OAE measurement, analysis, and interpretation, or to review the vast and rapidly growing basic and clinical literature on OAEs. And the application of OAEs in the identification and diagnosis of auditory dysfunction in adult patient populations is not included herein. Mechanisms and adult clinical applications of OAEs are thoroughly covered in another new book within the Plural Core Clinical Concepts Series, entitled *Otoacoustic Emissions: Principles, Procedures and Protocols* (2010) by Sumitjarit Dhar and James W. Hall III, , and other textbooks devoted to the topic of otoacoustic emissions (e.g., Hall, 2000; Robinette & Glattke, 2007).

SCREENING FOR HEARING LOSS

Introduction

Since the initial reports appeared in the early 1980s, many hundreds of published papers have described successful hearing screening of newborn infants with OAE technology. Over the past 25 years, untold millions of babies worldwide have now undergone OAE-based hearing screening. Even a cursory review of the literature reveals published articles reporting experiences from dozens of developed and developing countries in establishing newborn hearing screening programs with otoacoustic emissions. The advantages of OAE technology for newborn hearing screening were appreciated almost immediately following Kemp's discovery of sound-evoked sounds emitted by the inner ear. Advantages repeatedly confirmed by evidence generated in clinical trials include:

- Simplicity of technique
- Relatively brief test time
- Cost-efficiency
- Availability of handheld devices
- Automated OAE detection and analysis
- Sensitivity to peripheral auditory dysfunction
- Specificity to outer hair cell dysfunction

A full review of the vast literature on OAEs in newborn hearing screening is far beyond this chapter. Briefly, hundreds of early studies provided information on features of the test protocol for OAE measurement that can enhance efficiency and accuracy of hearing screening. During this era —approximately a 15-year period from the early 1980s to the late 1990s—hearing screening was conducted manually with OAEs. That is, the tester was responsible for verification of adequate test conditions, for example, assuring that stimulus quality (spectrum, intensity levels, stability) was adequate throughout the screening session, and for visual inspection and then analysis of OAE response parameters (e.g., amplitude, noise floor, signal-to-noise ratio). Nowadays, hearing screening with OAEs is almost always performed with automated instrumentation that essentially replaces the human factor in OAE analysis with statistical algorithms for ensuring reliable measurement and interpretation. Still, as summarized below, the operator (person conducting the screening) can exert an important influence on the outcome of hearing screening. What follows next is a brief summary of the transient evoked and distortion product OAEs, including an overview of measurement, analysis techniques, and the advantages of newborn hearing screening with OAEs. The emphasis of the discussion is not on details of test protocols or the intricacies of response analysis but, rather, on guidelines for deciding which screening technique is preferable (OAE versus automated auditory brainstem response [ABR]) and practical strategies for minimizing refer rates. Again, a companion Plural book (*Otoacoustic Emissions: Principles, Procedures and Protocols* (2010) is devoted entirely to the mechanisms of OAEs and to a detailed review of techniques for measurement, analysis, and interpretation in varied pediatric and adult clinical populations.

OAE Test Protocols for Newborn Hearing Screening

Dozens of parameters are incorporated into transient and distortion product OAE test protocols used in hearing screening. Most test parameters are unique to either TEOAEs; for example, the type of stimulus (click versus tone burst) and the single stimulus intensity level (e.g., 80 dB SPL) for TEOAEs and, for DPOAEs, the two frequencies (F_1 and F_2), the intensity level paradigm (L_1 versus L_2), the number of test frequencies per octave, and the F_2/F_1 ratio. Some analysis criteria are common to each OAE technique, such as the definition for the presence of an OAE as a difference of 6 dB between OAE amplitude and the noise floor at that frequency. Other analysis criteria are quite different for TEOAEs versus DPOAEs (e.g., reproducibility only for TEOAEs).

At least three general guidelines are helpful in selecting an OAE protocol for newborn hearing screening, or really hearing screening of any patient population. First, the protocol must be based on evidence generated by clinical research with the population to be screened. Before selecting a protocol for infant hearing screening, the clinician must verify that test performance of the protocol has been evaluated in clinical trials, and that the protocol is sufficiently sensitive to hearing loss and yields acceptably low refer rates. All manufacturers of OAE instrumentation include within the devices default or recommended protocols for infant hearing screening, with references to peer reviewed or manufacturer-sponsored studies of test performance with the protocol. The user has the responsibility of documenting the test performance (e.g., sensitivity, specificity, negative and positive predictive value) of the protocol he/she will use in a clinical newborn hearing-screening program. When automated OAE devices were first introduced for newborn hearing screening, there was a tendency for manufacturers, representatives, or distributors of specific brands of OAE equipment or even users to make rather arbitrary changes in parameters of protocols in an attempt usually to reduce test time and minimize failure rate. Some users actually boasted about modified test protocols that yielded refer rates as low as 0% for well baby hearing screening programs. Clearly, if no infants are failing a hearing screening procedure then the protocol lacks sensitivity to hearing loss and/or the pass criteria are excessively lax. Now, with many years of clinical experience with different OAE devices marketed by a variety of manufacturers, clinically proven test protocols are typically available and readily accessible to users of devices.

Another guideline for selection of a test protocol is the availability of pass/refer criteria that are derived from clinical studies conducted with adequate normative data—that is, a normative database developed for the test protocol in a test environment and general patient population comparable to the test setting where the device will be used, such as well baby nursery, intensive care nursery, hospital room, audiology clinic, or medical office. Importantly, the database should be developed with a large series of newborn babies whose normal hearing status is later confirmed independently with behavioral audiometry and, perhaps, other techniques (e.g., tympanometry, ABR).

Finally, it is advisable for a prospective user, or multiple likely users of OAE instrumentation, to perform trial hearing screenings with the specific type of device in the nursery setting where it would be used if purchased. Different brands of devices may have similar specifications, comparable track records in newborn hearing screening, and even similar appearances. Nonetheless, sometimes prospective users quickly develop a preference for one of the devices based on documented variables, such as lower refer rates, shorter test times, simple probe fit, and longer battery life, as well as rather intangible variables or impressions, like ease of operation and a brief learning curve for mastering the device and achieving successful results.

Pass versus Refer Criteria

One of the major factors influencing hearing screening with transient or distortion product OAEs, and a factor under the control of the tester, is the criterion employed for a pass versus refer outcome. Criteria include the minimum OAE amplitude required for definition of a response, the maximum noise floor permitted for definition of acceptable test conditions, the difference between OAE and noise floor (in dB) constituting a pass outcome, the test frequencies screened, and the proportion of test frequencies that must meet the criteria for a pass outcome out of the total number of test frequencies presented. Criteria also sometimes include parameters within the test protocol, such as the number of stimuli presented (sometimes defined as the minimum and/or maximum number) and allowable test time (sometimes defined as the minimum and/or maximum time in seconds). For TEOAEs, these criteria are typically applied to findings within predefined bands of frequencies, often half-octaves centered around an audiometric frequency, such as 750 to 1250 Hz. In the early years of newborn hearing screening with TEOAEs, a common criterion for a pass or a refer outcome was reproducibility of separate responses (A and B waves) to even and odd click presentations, typically for the overall TEOAE (whole) response. For example, criteria for a pass outcome might be a reproducibility of 50%, or 70%. Because reproducibility was calculated for the entire response, over a frequency region extending from below 500 Hz to higher than 4000 Hz, infants with hearing loss in a selected frequency region (e.g., just the high frequencies) could yield a pass outcome. Unfortunately, hearing screening with TEOAEs was often conducted with default test parameters and manufacturer recommended pass/refer criteria, with no reference to the source of the evidence in support of the criteria, that is, specific investigations or clinical trials.

Recent clinical practice in TEOAE screening commonly defines the presence of a response as a signal-to-noise ratio of at least 6 dB, or an overall minimum amplitude (wideband) response of 6 dB, with a reproducibility of 50% or greater. For DPOAE screening common criteria recommend that the signal-to-noise ratio should be at least 6 dB with a minimum response level of –5 dB SPL in the presence of an acceptable low noise floor of –4 dB SPL or less at three of the four test F_2 frequencies (2, 3, 4, and 5 kHz). Lower frequencies (e.g., 0.5 to 1k Hz) are commonly omitted because they are very prone to have excessive noise levels that compromise test efficiency and reliability.

Simple Steps for Minimizing Refer Rate

The foregoing discussion leads logically to a summary of modifications for newborn hearing screening strategies and techniques that typically minimize the refer rate, that is, steps that reduce the proportion of babies with normal auditory function who fail the hearing screening with otoacoustic emissions. Practical steps for reducing refer rates of infant hearing screening with OAEs are summarized in Table 3–1. Among these many programmatic and technical variables affecting OAE hearing screening of healthy newborn infants, two are perhaps most important for minimizing refer rates. One is the time after birth when OAE hearing screening is performed. Hearing screening with OAEs on day 2 after birth, rather than the first day, yields many benefits including more stable and symmetrical test results, fewer measurement artifacts, shorter test time, and lower refer rates and false alarm outcomes (e.g., Del Buono et al., 2005; Sadri, Thornton, & Kennedy, 2007). Over 30 years ago, Balkany et al. (1978) reported that almost all newborn infants have evidence of vernix caseosa (a lotionlike substance that covers the body at birth) within the ear canals, and for the majority of infants the vernix was sufficient to obscure a view of the tympanic membrane. The proportion of infants passing OAE hearing screening may increase dramatically (e.g., from less than 20% to over 90%) when vernix caseosa occluding the external ear canal is removed by cleaning, or the vernix naturally dissipates within 2 to 3 days after birth. Related to the problem of vernix within the external ear canal soon after birth, and its influence on the pass/fail rate for OAE screening, is the possibility of middle ear effusion, or middle ear cavities containing mesenchyme and not fully pneumatized at birth. The other major factor is the skill and experience of hearing screening personnel. Clinical information on newborn hearing screening with OAEs accumulated for over 25 years clearly indicates that refer rates are lowest when screening personnel are properly trained, understand the purpose and importance of hearing screening, and have acquired experience in recording OAEs in hearing screening of hundreds of babies.

Combined OAE and Admittance/ Reflectance Technologies

Within recent years, several groups have reported clinical investigations of instrumentation permitting hearing screening with a combination of OAEs and acoustic admittance and/or reflectance techniques. Clinical devices for simple and integrated measurement of OAEs and immittance/admittance/reflectance would contribute substantially to improved accuracy of newborn hearing screening. The middle ear, of course, plays a critical role in OAE measurement influencing both activation of the cochlea by the stimulus presented to the ear and also the outward propagation of OAE-related energy from the cochlea to the external ear canal. Put simply, OAEs are highly dependent on the status of the middle ear and markedly impacted by middle ear dysfunction. Preliminary evidence suggests that OAE amplitude is increased by several dB when measurements are made with compensation for middle ear pressure (Hof, Anteunis, Chenault, & van Dijk, 2005). The relationship between OAEs and

Table 3–1. Practical steps for reducing the refer rate for newborn hearing screening with otoacoustic emissions (OAEs)

Program Factors

- A small number of well-trained and dedicated persons who have extensive hearing screening experience with the technology (e.g., DPOAEs or TEOAEs) and the specific screening device(s) used in the program perform hearing screenings for all the infants.
- When a professional with interest in and knowledge of early detection of hearing loss in children (e.g., an audiologist or a pediatrician) oversees and monitors the hearing screening program and has the responsibility for assuring that screening personnel are adequately trained, the proportion of infants screened approaches 100%, and refer rates are consistently low.
- The hearing screening program and protocol are consistent with recommendations of the American Academy of Pediatrics and the Joint Committee on Infant Hearing Screening (JCIH).
- Infants undergo hearing screening:
  - In the quietest possible environment
  - While sleeping (usually after a regularly-scheduled feeding)
  - Toward the end of their hospital stay, relatively soon before discharge

Technical and Technique Factors

- Adequate test performance (e.g., pass/fail rates) and operation (e.g., test time) of the OAE device(s) used for hearing screening are supported with evidence from clinical trials.
- Steps are taken to keep the infant comfortable and to facilitate sleep to minimize physiological noise.
- Ambient noise in test is minimized (e.g., unnecessary equipment is shut down).
- The probe fits securely within the external ear canal with a probe design and size appropriate for newborn infants.
- Cords from the probe to the OAE device are routed away from the infant and from cables and wires that may be connected to the infant to reduce physiological and electrical sources of artifact.
- Manufacturer recommendations for stimulus verification are followed, such as:
  - Target stimulus intensity level(s) is (are) verified.
  - For TEOAEs, a flat spectrum of the stimulus is verified.
  - Stability of stimulus intensity throughout OAE measurement is verified.
- For infants who yield a refer outcome for one or both ears:
  - After trouble shooting to rule out technical problems (e.g., no stimulus, blockage of probe ports), hearing screening is attempted a second time.
  - The external ear canal is manipulated to minimize the negative effect of vernix caseosa.
  - The probe tip is examined for vernix and other debris that may occlude one of the ports (for stimulus presentation or response detection by the microphone).
  - Reinsert the probe tip with the pinna held in one hand.
- Infants yielding a refer outcome with OAE screening (first step above) undergo hearing screening with automated auditory brainstem response (AABR) before hospital discharge.

middle ear compensation is perhaps readily understood when we consider the rationale for the clinical approach for acoustic stapedial reflex measurement at the tympanogram pressure peak, rather than atmospheric middle ear pressure. Acoustic reflexes are more likely to be detected and, if present, amplitudes will be larger when measured at the ear canal pressure producing the highest compliance. In patients with negative middle ear pressure, acoustic reflexes are measured with adjustment for the negative pressure. Similarly, OAE measurement is associated with higher amplitudes and more confident detection when made with compensation of negative middle ear pressure. As an example, Keefe and colleagues at Boys Town National Research Hospital (2003) in an investigation of a series of 1045 ears found that OAE amplitudes decreased, and ABR latencies increased, with increasing high frequency admittance reflectance. Specifically, 28% of the variance in the amplitudes of OAEs and 12% of the variance in the latencies of ABR wave V was accounted for by reflectance data. Without doubt, the accuracy and test time of hearing screening with otoacoustic emissions will be enhanced by the development and utilization of devices permitting tympanometry and OAE measurement in combination. Other investigators (e.g., Prieve, Calandruccio, Fitzgerald, Mazevski, & Georgantas, 2008; Uchida et al., 2006) have also described a decrease in the DPOAE and TEOAE amplitude levels (approximately 4 dB) with abnormal middle ear measures, including static admittance, tympanogram peak pressure, and resonance frequency.

OAE Screening with Telehealth Technology

Telemedicine technology offers an exciting opportunity to conduct hearing screenings, and even diagnostic audiology procedures, from a remote clinical location. The advantages of this strategy are probably obvious. As an example, children in rural areas and those lacking audiology services can undergo hearing screening with the findings analyzed and interpreted by an audiologist located many miles away, perhaps even in another country in another continent of the world. In this way, children who have traditionally had no access to audiology services may benefit from hearing screening and diagnosis by highly qualified audiologists using the latest instrumentation. Krumm and colleagues (2008) extended their ongoing investigations of the application of telemedicine techniques to newborn hearing screening with DPOAEs and ABR. The subjects (18 males and 12 females) ranging in age from 11 to 45 days were screened remotely (160 miles away) with an integrated test system communicating with a computer network via a broadband network connection. No difference was found in findings for on-site, face-to-face hearing screening versus hearing screening remotely with telemedicine technology. In other words, hearing screening with DPOAEs and ABR conducted remotely was validated against the conventional approach for hearing screening with these technologies.

Newborn Hearing Screening with OAE and ABR Technology

Introduction. A more basic and essential clinical question is: "Should infant hearing screening be performed with OAEs or with automated ABR?" The answer to this question depends in turn on the answers to a series of other questions. One simple question that can almost always be answered confidently in advance of a decision regarding the approach to be taken for infant hearing screening is: "How long after birth do the children remain in the nursery or, put another way, how soon are the babies discharged?" If the answer is "less than 24 hours" then either an ABR screening approach or a two-step OAE plus ABR combination of technology is essential. Longstanding evidence confirms the unacceptably high failure rates for OAE screening within the first day after birth (e.g., Hergils, 2007; Kok, van Zanten, Brocaar, & Jongejan, 1994). The timing of screening after birth is reviewed further in a later section on nonpathologic factors influencing OAEs. On the other hand, if infants to be screened are exclusively healthy (not at risk for hearing loss) and screening will be conducted in a well baby nursery, or at least not in an ICN (NICU), then OAEs are certainly an appropriate and feasible screening technique.

Selected excerpts from the most recent report of the Joint Committee on Infant Hearing (JCIH,

2007) provide valuable, and widely accepted, guidance on newborn hearing screening with OAE and ABR:

- "Physiologic measures must be used to screen newborns and infants for hearing loss. Such measures include OAE and automated ABR testing" (p. 903).
- "Both OAE and automated ABR techniques provide noninvasive recordings of physiologic activity underlying normal auditory function" (p. 903).
- "Neural conduction disorders or auditory neuropathy/dys-synchrony without concomitant sensory dysfunction will not be detected by OAE testing" (p. 903).
- "The JCIH recommends ABR technology as the only appropriate screening technique for use in the NICU" (p. 904).
- "Some programs use a combination of screening techniques (OAE and ABR) to decrease the fail rate at discharge" (p. 904).

Clearly, OAEs are an accepted technology option for newborn hearing screening. However, OAEs are not an appropriate screening option in the newborn intensive care setting where children with auditory neuropathy or other neurological auditory dysfunction are most often found. For this reason, ABR is the screening technique of choice in the NICU (or ICN) environment and population or, as summarized in one of the excerpts above and reviewed below, a combination of ABR plus OAE technologies is optimal for hearing screening of children at risk for various types of auditory dysfunction, including neural disorders.

Two-Step Hearing Screening with OAE and ABR. Within the past decade, evidence from multiple clinical investigations conducted all around the world confirms the value of combining OAE and AABR technologies for newborn hearing screening (e.g., Babac, Djeriç, & Ivankoviç, 2007; Benito-Orejas, Ramírez, Morais, Almaraz, & Fernández-Calvo, 2008; Calevo et al., 2007; Chiong et al., 2007; Clarke, Iqbal, & Mitchell, 2003; Granell et al., 2008; Gravel et al., 2005; Hall, Smith, & Popelka, 2004; Helge et al., 2005; Iwasaki et al., 2003; Johnson, White, Widen, Gravel, & Meyer, 2005; Korres, Balatsouras, Lyra, Kandiloros, & Ferekidis, 2006; H. C. Lin, Shu, Lee, H. Y. Lin, & G. Lin, 2007; Luo, Wen, Huang, Zhou, & Chen, 2007; Pedersen, Møller, Wetke, & Ovesen, 2008; Schönweiler et al., 2002; Srisuparp, Gleebbur, Ngerncham, Chonpracha, & Singkampong, 2005; Suppiej et al., 2007; Tatli et al., 2007; White et al., 2005; Xu, Li, Hu, Sun, & Shen, 2003). The accumulated evidence from these and other studies lead to several general conclusions. Although there is typically a high correlation in the outcome for the two techniques, refer rates are typically lower for AABR than for OAE techniques, with the advantage for AABR increasing as the test time of the hearing screening after birth decreases. Overall refer rates and false positive error rates are invariably lowest, and sensitivity and specificity highest, with a combined OAE and AABR approach for newborn hearing screening.

There are two general strategies for utilizing OAE and ABR technologies in newborn hearing screening. The most common approach is to begin hearing screening with one technique and then, if the outcome is refer to perform a second screening with the other technique (Hall, 2000; Norton et al, 2000). The term *two-step hearing screening* is often used to describe this two-stage sequence of hearing screenings. For healthy babies in the normal nursery, OAEs are often the primary screening technique. Of course, a large majority of the babies will pass the screening and no further screening or immediate follow-up assessment is necessary. Even healthy babies who pass an OAE hearing screening should be followed, of course, if they are at risk for a progressive or delayed-onset hearing loss. Family history of congenital hearing loss is an example of such a risk indicator. Healthy children who yield a refer outcome for OAE screening undergo, before hospital discharge, a second screening with automated ABR. We hasten to state here that AABR can certainly be utilized as the primary hearing screening technique, even with healthy babies in the normal nursery setting. A 20-year experience with AABR hearing screening (e.g., Stewart et al., 2000) confirms that refer rates are acceptably low (<4%), and also false positive failures (<1%) are well within recommended guidelines (e.g., American Academy of Pediatrics, 1999; JCIH, 2007). According to conventional protocol, a pass screening outcome with an AABR technique implies that hearing is adequate for speech and language acquisition, and the infant requires no additional screening or follow-up unless there is a risk indicator(s) for progressive or delayed-onset hearing loss. Recent clinical research (Johnson et al., 2005), however, raises the possibility that a small proportion (2%) of babies who fail an OAE hearing screening but then pass a secondary AABR hearing screening have a mild high frequency sensory hearing loss. Among this group, over three fourths of the infants subsequently had a mild sensory hearing loss (<40 dB HL) and the majority had a unilateral hearing loss. Thus, the likelihood of significant permanent hearing loss among infants who pass a click-evoked (35 dB nHL) ABR hearing screening is quite small.

Infants who yield a refer outcome for each of the screening technologies (OAE and AABR) are, of course, scheduled for follow-up diagnostic assessment. Hearing impairment is more likely for infants who do not pass two different and rather independent hearing screening technologies than for infants who yield a refer outcome for only one technique (e.g., OAEs). Ideally, babies who refer both OAE and AABR screenings are scheduled immediately, and before hospital discharge, for a diagnostic assessment within the next 2 months. As discussed in Chapter 5, there are a number of practical advantages to scheduling the diagnostic audiologic evaluation within the first few months after birth. Guidelines for the diagnostic test battery are reviewed in Chapter 7. For infants admitted to the intensive care nursery (ICN) or newborn intensive care unit (NICU), as noted above, current standard of care as defined by the 2007 JCIH is a primary hearing screening with ABR. Infants in the ICN or NICU who yield a refer outcome for ABR screening are then screened again, but with OAEs. The absence of an ABR in an infant who passes OAE hearing screening is a "red flag" for possible neural auditory dysfunction, including auditory neuropathy. Diagnostic audiologic assessment with a completed test battery (see Chapter 7) is indicated.

Combined OAE and ABR Hearing Screening. Another approach involving both technologies is more appropriately called *combined OAE/ABR screening*, rather than two-step hearing screening. With the combined approach, both OAEs and ABR are recorded from each child. As summarized in Table 3–2, examination of the pattern of findings for both techniques permits differentiation even in the nursery setting of the three most commonly encountered general types of auditory dysfunction. According to Hall et al. (2004), the advantages of this screening strategy are as follows:

- In-ear calibration of signal intensity for OAE and ABR (selected devices)
- Lower refer (<2%) and false positive rates (<0.9%) than with either technique alone
- High sensitivity (up to 100%) and specificity (up to 99.7%)
- Fewer diagnostic follow-ups with substantially lower overall cost for early identification of infant hearing loss
- Differentiation at birth of auditory dysfunction as conductive, sensory, or neural (e.g., auditory neuropathy)
- Faster and more appropriate management based on information on types of auditory dysfunction
- Earlier intervention for hearing impairment
- Higher likelihood of optimal outcome from intervention for hearing loss

School-Age and Preschool Screening

Introduction

Hearing screening of school-age children is a longstanding convention for detection of hearing

Table 3–2. Distinct patterns of findings for hearing screening with combined OAE and AABR technologies associated with common categories of auditory disorders

Type of dysfunction	*OAE*	*ABR*
External/middle ear*	abnormal	normal
Sensory (OHC)	abnormal	abnormal
Neural	normal	abnormal

*Including transient nonpathologic dysfunction including vernix caseosa within the external ear canal.

loss that will interfere with academic performance. And, parallel to the emergence of newborn hearing screening worldwide, audiologists and other health care personnel (e.g., nurses, pediatricians) have assumed the responsibility for hearing screening of children in the preschool years, especially in programs designed to ready underprivileged children for school (e.g., Head Start programs in the United States). Without question, many health care personnel regularly utilize OAE techniques for hearing screening of preschool and school-age populations. As evidence of this statement, detailed guidelines for hearing screening with OAEs are available from the Web site of the National Center for Hearing Assessment and Management, or NCHAM (http://www.infanthearing.org). Nonetheless, in contrast to the many hundreds of publications describing newborn hearing screening experiences around the world, few papers report findings for preschool and school-age hearing screening with OAEs.

A pure tone hearing screening approach is required in formal recommendations for preschool and schoolage children (e.g., American Speech-Language-Hearing Association [ASHA], 1997). Pure tone hearing screening techniques are associated with multiple practical problems, particularly in preschool and young school-age (e.g., kindergarten) children. Unacceptably high refer rates for pure tone hearing screening, up to 70% in the preschool population (e.g., Berg, Papri, Ferdous, Khan, & Durkin, 2006), may result from a combination of factors, such as inexperienced or poorly trained screening personnel, excessive levels of ambient noise in the test environment, and listener variables common in young children (attention, cognition, motivation) that sometimes preclude a valid screening outcome. Within recent years, clinical studies have documented the value and many advantages of OAEs as a hearing screening technique in pediatric populations. It is certainly reasonable to consider OAEs for hearing screening of preschool and school-age children, given the proven effectiveness and feasibility of OAEs as a hearing screening technique in newborn infants. The following brief literature review, supplemented by original data, argues strongly for DPOAEs as a primary hearing screening technique, coupled perhaps with tympanometry (see Chapter 2).

School-Age Children

Based on a study of 1003 children entering school in Australia (children in the first grade with an average age of 6 years), Lyons, Kei, and Driscoll (2004) concluded that:

> When the results of a test protocol which incorporates both DPOAEs and tympanometry were used in comparison with the gold standard of pure tone screening plus tympanometry, test performance was enhanced. The use of a protocol that includes both DPOAEs and tympanometry holds promise as a useful tool in hearing screening of schoolchildren, including difficult-to-test children. (p. 702)

Hall and colleagues (2004) conducted a study in a series of 372 children enrolled in kindergarten (139 males and 152 females, 5 years of age) to validate DPOAEs and tympanometry against the conventional standard, pure tone audiometry. Criteria for a pass outcome for hearing screening for each technique included:

- Pure tone screening: Response at 20 dB HL for 500 Hz, 1000 Hz, 2000 Hz, and 4000 Hz with a portable audiometer (Inter-Acoustics) with insert earphones
- Tympanometry: Type A (peak pressure with range of +50 to −150 daPa) measured with a portable device (GSI 38)
- Distortion product otoacoustic emissions: DP–NF difference ≥6 dB at 2000 Hz, 4000 Hz, 5000 Hz, and 8000 Hz measured with a handheld device (Bio-Logic AuDx or GSI Audio-Screener)

Screening was performed in a quiet classroom setting by a graduate audiology student. Overall refer rates (either or both ears) for each technique were: pure tone audiometry = 17%; tympanometry = 11%; and DPOAEs = 12.5%. Comparisons of findings among techniques are summarized in Table 3–3. Screening outcome for pure tone audiometry agreed with tympanometry and with DPOAEs for about three fourths of the children. Interestingly, about one out of 10 children who passed pure tone screening failed tympanometry (9%) and DPOAEs (10%) when these techniques

Table 3–3. Comparison of hearing screening results for pure tone, otoacoustic emission, and tympanometry techniques in a series of 303 kindergarten children (age 5 years)

	*Pure Tone Findings**	
	Pass	***Fail***
Tympanometry Findings*		
Pass	70%	15%**
Fail	9%	6%
DPOAE Findings		
Pass	69%	16%**
Fail	10%	5%
Tympanometry/DPOAE Findings		
Pass	62%	11%**
Fail	16%	11%

*Pearson chi-square significant at $p < 0.01$.

**None of the subjects had a hearing loss on follow-up assessment. This proportion includes could-not-test outcomes and failures at 500 Hz only apparently due to ambient noise.

were used alone. Furthermore, 16% of the children who passed pure tone audiometry failed a combined tympanometry/DPOAE screening approach suggesting that the combined approach offers enhanced sensitivity to peripheral auditory dysfunction. Also, under each of the screening comparisons, from 11 to 16% of the children who failed pure tone screening actually passed tympanometry, DPOAEs, or the combined method. At first glance this pattern might suggest the possibility of false negative errors with the newer techniques. However, follow-up and close inspection of the children in this quadrant of the two-by-two table confirmed that the failures for pure tone audiometry were accounted for by two explanations. Either the 5-year-old children were unable to volunteer valid pure tone screening responses (e.g., they could not be tested) or ambient noise contributed to a fail response for the lowest pure tone test frequencies.

The data from this study, and other investigations with school-age children (e.g., Lyons et al., 2004), suggest that from the perspective of screening accuracy alone either DPOAEs or a combination of DPOAEs and tympanometry is preferable to pure tone screening. Two other important clinical advantages of DPOAEs are remarkably brief test time and simplicity of technique. Average test time for DPOAE screening with high frequency signals (2000 to 5000 Hz) was 20 seconds (Hall et al., 2004). Of course, the technique requires very little instruction of the child, the same probe tip size can be used with almost all children, and DPOAE analysis and interpretation are automated. Also, studies over the years initially suggested (e.g., Nozza, Sabo & Mandel 1997; Spektor, Leonard, Kim, Jung, & Smurzynski, 1991), and have more recently confirmed (e.g., Georgalas, Xenellis, Davilis, Tzangaroulakis, & Ferekidis, 2008), the role of TEOAE in school-age hearing screening. Refer rates for OAE screening of school-age children are closely connected to prevalence of middle ear disease. For example, studies of OAE hearing screening in children enrolled in the Special Olympics confirm higher prevalence of hearing impairment than the general population and, correspondingly, higher refer rates (24 to 38%) for OAE screening (e.g., Hild et el., 2008; Neumann et al., 2006). Notably, Hild and colleagues (2008) and Neumann and colleagues (2006) in Germany reported that excessive cerumen was removed for approximately one half (48 to 53%) of the children. Thus, OAE screening inevitably detects the presence of peripheral auditory dysfunction (high sensitivity approaching 100%), but doesn't differentiate permanent cochlear versus potentially treatable middle ear disorders.

Preschool Children

Hearing status is recognized as an important variable in speech and language acquisition, prereading skills, and general readiness for academic success. In the United States, hearing screening is required by Head Start programs financially supported by the Federal government, and serving underprivileged children up to age 5. As Dille, Glattke, and Earl (2007) point out:

> Behavioral testing is not cost effective for screening efforts that include very young preschool children (<3 years) because of the

> requirement for special equipment and trained personnel. An objective test such as OAE screening is an ideal tool to consider. It is quick, affordable, and well tolerated. (p. 1790).

The rather modest, but expanding, published research findings on the test performance and practical benefits of OAE technology in school-age hearing screening can guide the approach taken for hearing screening of preschool children. In our experience, consistent with findings reported in the literature, failure rates for hearing screening with OAEs in preschool populations aged 6 months to 4 years (e.g., usually within the range of 10 to 25%) are comparable to those reported for school-age children (e.g., Allen et al, 2004; Allen, Stuart, Everett & Elangovan, 2004; Psarommatis, Valsamakis, Raptaki, Kontrogiani, & Douniadakis, 2007; Psillas, Psifidis, Antoniadou-Hitoglou, & Kouloulas, 2006). Of course, OAE hearing screening failure rates are directly related to varied factors including the population, such as age distribution of the children (e.g., mostly 4 years versus mostly younger children), the likelihood of middle ear disease, socioeconomic status and access to medical care, and also technology or technique factors, such as specific OAE technique (transient versus DPOAEs), the OAE test protocol and pass/fail criteria, ambient and physiological noise levels, and even the specific brand of device used to record OAEs (Dille et al., 2007).

Hunter et al. (2007) provide evidence of the impact of middle ear disease on failure rate of OAE screening in a study of American Indian children. Almost 30% of the 366 children aged 2 to 5 months yielded a refer outcome for DPOAE screening even for stimuli within a high frequency region (2500 to 4875 Hz). However, refer rates then declined to more typical ranges for older children (17% for children aged 6 to 12 months and 14% for children aged 13 to 24 months). The authors cite the need for alternative techniques (such as pure tone audiometry) for children with persistent otitis media with effusion. Among OAE techniques, failure rates may be lower for DPOAEs in comparison to TEOAEs (e.g., Dille et al., 2007). Because OAEs are almost always abnormal in children with common etiologies of peripheral hearing loss, the technique applied in isolation (e.g., without tympanometry) has high sensitivity but low specificity as a screening technique (Taylor & Brooks, 2000). However, when OAE and tympanometry technologies are combined, sensitivity remains high but there is also a marked increase in specificity, that is, the ability to distinguish at the time of screening middle ear versus cochlear auditory dysfunction (Ho, Daly, Hunter, & Davey, 2002; Lyons et al., 2004). Failure rates for OAE technology in preschool populations are typically lower than failure rates for pure tone hearing screening because a high proportion of the children who fail pure tone screening are unable to cooperate with the behavioral requirements of the technique (Sideris & Glattke, 2006).

Without doubt, a group from a major Head Start Center at Utah State University in the United States (Eiserman et al., 2008) has recently reported the most extensive data on OAE screening for hearing loss in early childhood. Subjects were 4519 children ≤3 years who were screened by trained, nonprofessional personnel. Employing a multistep approach, only 6% of the children required follow-up medical and/or audiologic evaluation, which confirmed seven children with permanent hearing loss. The remaining children who failed OAE screening had external or middle ear disorders requiring management or further monitoring.

ESTIMATION OF HEARING LOSS

Introduction

We'll begin with a brief overview of OAE analysis. Clinical audiologists tend to wrongly apply the approach to inspection and analysis of OAE used in newborn hearing screening to the diagnostic setting. Important steps in the analyses of OAE findings are summarized in Table 3–4. Notice that the simple categorization of OAE findings as "present" versus "absent," commonly used in hearing screening, is inadequate for diagnostic applications of OAEs. Diagnostic measure-

Table 3–4. Major steps in the analysis of otoacoustic emissions (OAEs)

- Perform analysis of OAE amplitude and noise floor (NF) level at all test frequencies. Avoid generic statements, e.g., OAEs are present or absent. The goal of analysis is to categorize OAE findings as:
  - Normal
  - Abnormal but present
  - Absent
- Verify adequately low noise floor (< 90% normal limits)
- Verify the reliability of DPOAE amplitude (+/–2 dB) from at least two runs
- OAE analysis
  - Is the OAE–NF difference >6 dB≥
  - No, there is no evidence of OAEs *or*
  - Yes, OAEs are present
  - If present, are OAE amplitudes within normal limits?
    - Yes? OAEs are normal.
    - No? OAEs are abnormal (but present).

ment of OAEs yields a wealth of information on auditory function that will be untapped with a dichotomous present versus absent analysis of findings. Each of the steps in Table 3–4 is important to assure that OAEs are actually recorded and, then, to extract as much diagnostic value as possible from the rather straightforward calculation of OAE amplitude as a function stimulus frequency. Diagnostic application of OAEs deviates from their use in hearing screening in two main ways. First, when OAEs are applied diagnostically the goal is to obtain information on outer hair cell functioning for many more test frequencies. For example, it is clinically feasible, and valuable, with school-age children and adults to record a DPgram for five or even eight frequencies per octave over the range of 500 to 8000 Hz. Also, instead of differentiation of the OAE as simply present or absent (e.g., pass versus fail), in diagnostic analyses OAE findings, for each test frequency, are minimally defined as: (a) normal (amplitudes within a designated normal region), (b) present but abnormal, or (c) not present (absence of OAE activity ≥6 dB above the noise floor). This approach for DPOAE analysis is illustrated with the replicated DPgram displayed in Figure 3–1. We urge the reader to apply the step-by-step process for analyses of OAEs for diagnostic purposes (listed in Table 3–4) to the findings shown in Figure 3–1, and to examples of DPOAEs the reader may have recorded clinically from various types of patients.

There are multiple diagnostic applications of OAEs in pediatric and adult populations, as summarized in Table 3–5. Indeed, OAEs are now a mandatory component of the pediatric diagnostic test battery. That is, measurement of OAEs in the assessment of infants and young children is standard of care (e.g., JCIH, 2007). Evidence reported in the peer-reviewed literature clearly supports the applications of OAE shown in Table 3–5. A comprehensive review of the OAE literature is far beyond the scope of this chapter. As already noted, a recent textbook in the Plural Clinical Concepts (CCC) Series (*Otoacoustic Emissions: Principles, Procedures and Protocol, Dhar & Hall, 2010*), is largely devoted to the diagnostic application of OAEs, including a literature review, and detailed discussion of measurement and analysis strategies.

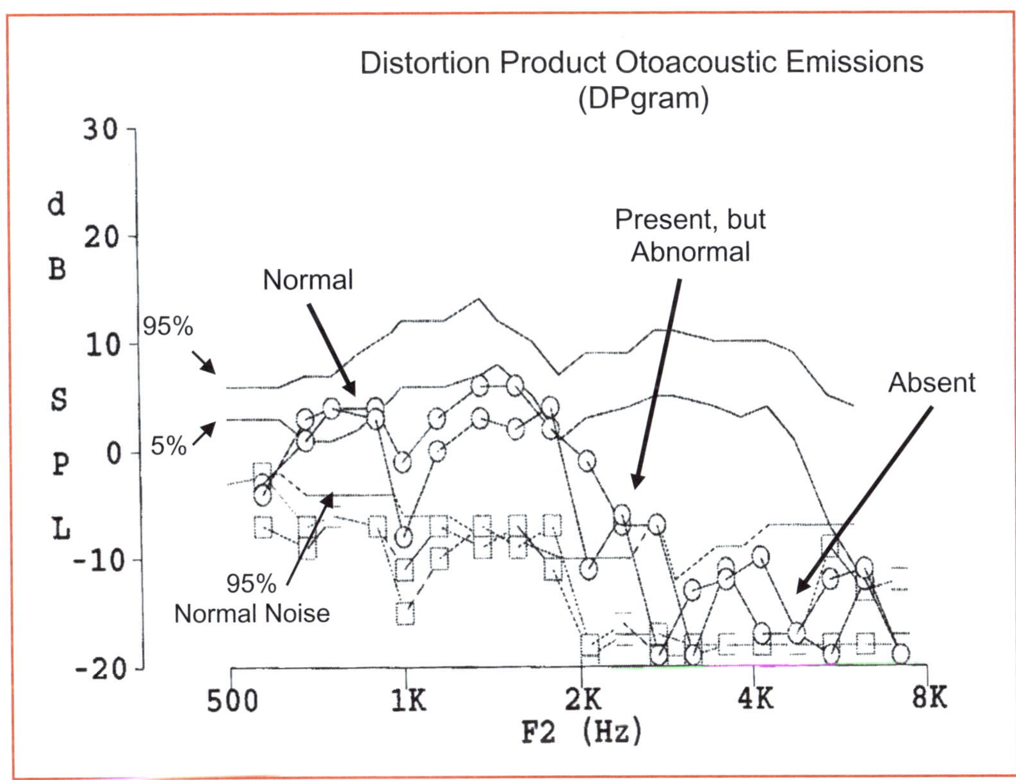

FIGURE 3–1. Amplitude of DPOAEs plotted according to stimulus frequency (F_2), a graph referred to as a *DPgram*. DPOAEs were recorded with a GSI 60 device.

Table 3–5. Applications of otoacoustic emissions (OAEs) in pediatric and adult patient populations supported by published evidence from clinical research. Applications are not listed in order of importance.

Pediatric Applications

- Newborn hearing screening
- Diagnosis of auditory dysfunction in infants and young children
  - Differentiation of site of auditory dysfunction
  - Identification of auditory neuropathy
- Monitoring ototoxicity*
- Preschool/school screenings*

Adult Applications

- Diagnosis of cochlear versus retrocochlear auditory dysfunction
- Identification of malingering
- Industrial and military hearing screening and conservation
- Identification and monitoring of auditory dysfunction in noise/music exposure*
- Diagnosis and management of tinnitus and hyperacusis*

*Evidence-based but underutilized clinical application.

Why have OAEs assumed such a valuable role in the diagnosis of auditory dysfunction? As listed in Table 3–6, the clinical advantages of OAEs are multiple, varied, and to a large extent not offered by other audiologic procedures available in clinical audiology today. Of course, no audiologic procedure, or really any diagnostic procedure in health care, is infallible or without limitations. Disadvantages of OAEs in the identification and diagnostic assessment of auditory dysfunction are also listed in Table 3–6.

Estimating Hearing Loss with OAEs

Hearing loss cannot be confidently or accurately predicted with OAE findings. Some of the most productive and highly regarded groups of hearing scientists, who have published widely on OAEs, have conducted well-designed clinical investigations of the relationship of OAE findings to hearing thresholds and, specifically, the precision with which OAEs predict the audiogram (e.g., Boege & Janssen, 2002; Dorn, Piskorski, Gorga, Neely, & Keefe, 1999; Gorga, Neely, Dorn, & Hoover, 2003; Martin, Ohms, Franklin, Harris, & Lonsbury-Martin, 1990). Dozens of investigations have been conducted with complex instrumentation in the laboratory setting, with precise manipulation of multiple stimulus parameters, repeated measurement of OAE input-output functions, examination of various OAE response parameters (amplitude, signal-to-noise ratio, threshold of detection), careful control of experimental and subject variables, with detailed analyses of data to determine test performance (such as hit and false alarm rates, cumulative distributions of OAE findings), and using statistical methods for data analyses, such

Table 3–6. General advantages and disadvantages of OAEs in identification and diagnosis of auditory dysfunction

Advantages
• Highly sensitive to cochlear (outer hair cell function)
• Site specific (to outer hair cells)
• Do not require behavioral cooperation or response
• Ear specific
• Highly frequency specific (multiple interoctave frequencies)
• Sound-treated environment not required for measurement
• Brief measurement time (less than 30 seconds for screening protocols)
• Portable (handheld devices)
• Relatively inexpensive
Disadvantages
• Susceptible to the effects of ambient and physiological noise
• Affected greatly by middle ear status; OAEs generally not present in patients with middle ear dysfunction, e.g., otitis media
• Evaluate cochlear integrity only for outer hair cells (not inner hair cells)
• May be abnormally reduced in amplitude or not detected with normal audiogram
• Not detected with hearing loss >40 dB HL
• Provide no information on the degree of hearing loss
• Not a measure of neural or CNS auditory function
• Not a test of hearing

as clinical decision theory, receiver operating characteristics (ROC) curves, and neural networks.

Two general approaches are taken in the reported investigations evaluating the estimation of hearing thresholds with OAEs. With one approach, some measure of the level of OAE activity, usually either the amplitude or the signal-to-noise ratio (SNR), produced by stimulation at a fixed stimulus intensity level (e.g., 80 dB SPL for TEOAEs or an L_1/L_2 stimulus paradigm of 66/55 dB SPL for DPOAEs) is plotted as a function of hearing loss. In studies utilizing DPOAEs, the OAE levels are plotted separately for a series of different stimulus frequencies (such as from 500 Hz up to 8000 Hz). The expected relation, of course, is decreased amplitude of the OAE (or the SNR ratio) as hearing loss increases. Unfortunately, for each stimulus frequency the correspondence between OAE level and hearing loss is associated with considerable variability, even under ideal measurement conditions. For example, inspection of published data, including graphs plotting OAE level in dB SPL as a function of audiometric threshold, indicates that at any given OAE amplitude (for example, a DPOAE amplitude of 0 dB SPL) for a stimulus frequency (e.g., 1000 or 4000 Hz), the predicted audiogram threshold data (plotted in 5 dB intensity increments) cover a range of 20 dB HL or more. Although data summarized statistically for relatively large groups of subjects appear to show promise for estimating the degree of hearing loss, for an individual subject (patient) the magnitude of error in estimating hearing loss from OAE level is clinically unacceptable.

Another approach for estimating hearing threshold is derived from analysis of the threshold for OAEs. First, input-output (I/O) functions are recorded for individual frequencies. OAE amplitude (the output) is recorded as stimulus intensity is either decreased or increased over a range of about 80 dB. For example, beginning with an intensity level of −10 dB stimulus intensity level is increased in 5 dB SPL steps and the TEOAE or DPOAE amplitude is recorded at each step up to a maximum stimulus intensity level of 70 or 75 dB SPL. OAE threshold is defined at the lowest stimulus intensity level that produces an OAE–NF difference of at least 6 dB. Figure 3–2 illustrates the relation of DPOAE threshold (in dB SPL) and behavioral hearing threshold (in dB HL), based on inspection of data reported by various investigators (e.g., Gorga et al., 2003). The diagonal line extending from −10 dB to 90 dB for pure tone and DPOAE threshold values indicates an ideal correlation between the two variables. The limitation inherent in estimations of hearing threshold from OAE data is readily apparent, and highlighted by two hypothetical data points. The circle represents a modest underestimation of hearing threshold. That is, the DPOAE threshold of −10 dB would imply better than average hearing level, but actual hearing threshold is about 10 dB HL. Although there is a discrepancy between the predicted and actual hearing level, it would probably not lead to misdiagnosis of sensory hearing loss or poor management decisions. Of course, the subjects in the above-noted investigations were carefully selected to assure a sensory hearing loss. As we have noted elsewhere in the chapter, patients with inner hair cell or neural auditory dysfunction may indeed have normal OAEs in the presence of significant hearing loss by pure tone audiometry. In other words, the trends illustrated in Figure 3–2 should not remove concerns about the possibility of serious and clinically significant underestimations of hearing loss by analysis of OAE findings. The more worrisome limitation associated with estimation of hearing loss by DPOAE (or TEOAE) thresholds, overestimation of hearing loss, is highlighted by the square symbol in Figure 3–2. Thresholds for OAEs may be markedly elevated or, in fact, OAEs may not be detected, in some persons with entirely normal hearing sensitivity. For the application of OAEs in hearing screening, the clinical consequence of this discrepancy is relatively minimal. An infant with an elevated OAE threshold would presumably undergo diagnostic audiologic assessment with a full test battery, including estimation of thresholds with frequency-specific ABR techniques (see Chapter 5). However, the not uncommon possibility of major overestimation of hearing loss by OAE thresholds argues strongly against abandoning pure tone audiometry in favor of OAE measurement for defining the degree of hearing loss.

Despite these obvious limitations inherent in precise prediction of hearing loss from OAE findings, it is clinically useful to appreciate the

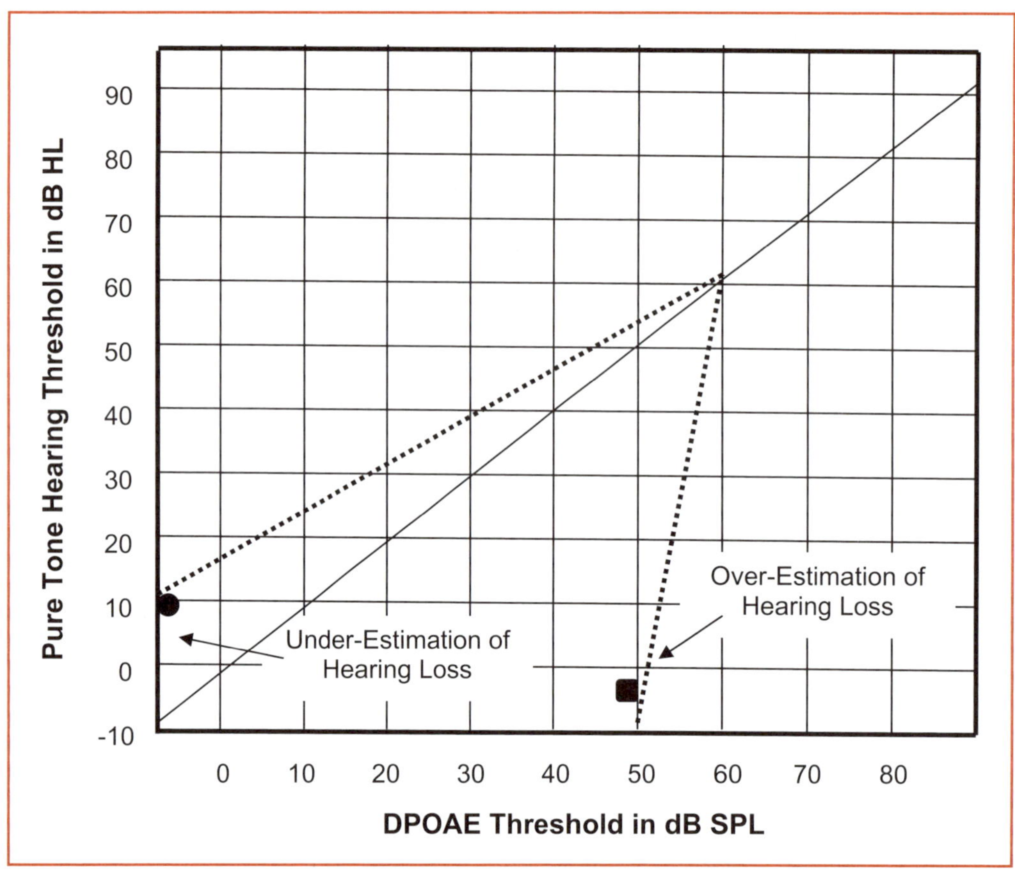

FIGURE 3–2. Relation between behavioral hearing threshold from the pure tone audiogram and the threshold for DPOAE derived from input-output functions (a graph of DP amplitude as a function of stimulus intensity level).

expected relation between hearing level and amplitude of OAE, or the presence versus absence of OAEs. OAEs can be exploited in the diagnosis of auditory dysfunction with adherence to a rather systematic approach for analysis and interpretation, as summarized in Table 3–7. The likelihood of recording normal OAE amplitude or detecting any OAE activity (exceeding the noise floor by at least 6 dB) at a particular frequency is shown schematically in Figure 3–3. In fact, the relation depicted in Figure 3–3 in some respects highlights the clinical value of OAEs in hearing assessment. A few points are quite apparent. Normal OAE findings, that is, OAE amplitudes that are within an appropriate normative region (e.g., between the 5th and 95th percentile for OAE data collected with the same equipment and test protocol from a carefully selected group of persons with normal auditory function) are expected only from persons with hearing sensitivity of 10 dB HL or better. With a hearing threshold decrease, even within a range usually defined clinically as "normal hearing sensitivity" (from 0 to 20 or 25 dB HL), the amplitude of OAEs steadily decreases. To be sure, OAEs may still be present, but are unequivocally abnormal based on analysis of amplitude relative to a normative region. The standard deviation for pure tone hearing threshold measurement is 5 dB. Hearing thresholds of 20 or 25 dB HL may be within the clinically normal region, implying for an adult patient at least that hearing sensitivity is still adequate for communication, and amplification or other management options are not indicated. However, from a statistical perspective a hearing threshold of 20 dB HL is four standard deviations below normal mean value and, by def-

Table 3–7. Guidelines for overcoming typical clinical limitations in the diagnostic application of otoacoustic emissions (OAEs)

Current Limitation	
Reliance on screening protocols	• Develop diagnostic test protocols.
Recording within limited frequency region	• Record OAEs for test frequencies over the widest possible range (e.g., 500 to 8000 Hz for DPOAEs) with multiple frequencies (5 or 8) per octave.
Simple pass versus fail outcome	• For each test frequency, categorize OAEs into one of three categories: (a) normal, (b) present but abnormal, and (c) absent.
Analysis limited to present or absent	• For each test frequency, perform close analysis of OAEs and noise floor rather than categorizing overall OAE as simply present or absent.
Inconsistent analysis techniques	• For each test frequency throughout OAE measurement, verify that noise level does not exceed the 95th percentile for normal noise levels (see suggestions for reducing measurement noise elsewhere in chapter). Calculate the difference (in dB) between OAE amplitude and noise floor (SNR) across the range of test frequencies. Presence of OAE is defined by SNR of ≥6 dB. • Assure that OAEs are reliable (perform a replicated measurement). OAE amplitudes recorded in separate runs should be within +/– 2 dB. Remember: "If your OAEs do not repeat, your test is not complete!"
Limited application of OAEs	• OAEs have clinical and diagnostic value in a variety of pediatric and adult patient populations (summarized elsewhere in the chapter). OAEs should not be applied only as a hearing screening technique with newborn infants.
Why record OAEs if an audiogram is available?	• The audiogram is not always in agreement with OAEs. OAEs provide diagnostic information not available from the audiogram. OAEs can be normal in patients with an abnormal audiogram and vice versa (as summarized in Table 3–8).

inition, abnormal. OAE amplitudes are abnormally decreased when hearing thresholds reach 20 to 25 dB, reflecting disruption in cochlear integrity, specifically outer hair cell dysfunction.

Let's consider this relation between OAEs and the audiogram from a clinical perspective. If, at the outset of an audiologic assessment, normal OAEs are recorded at all test frequencies (OAEs are not only present but amplitudes are within the normal region), then we would expect pure tone audiometry in the sound booth to result in hearing thresholds around 0 dB HL, and certainly no worse than 15 dB HL. The combination of normal OAE findings and even a mild sensory hearing loss is not expected, and must be investigated until an explanation is found. Possible reasons for discrepancies between OAE and pure tone findings are reviewed next. The reverse pattern of findings, that is, abnormal OAEs in a patient with entirely normal pure tone thresholds (hearing levels 15 dB or better) also requires an explanation. In short, the findings for OAEs and the pure tone audiogram must be scrutinized in combination. If findings for these two independent measures of auditory function are not in agreement, an explanation (technical problem, a possible cause based on patient history, or some type of auditory dysfunction) must be sought.

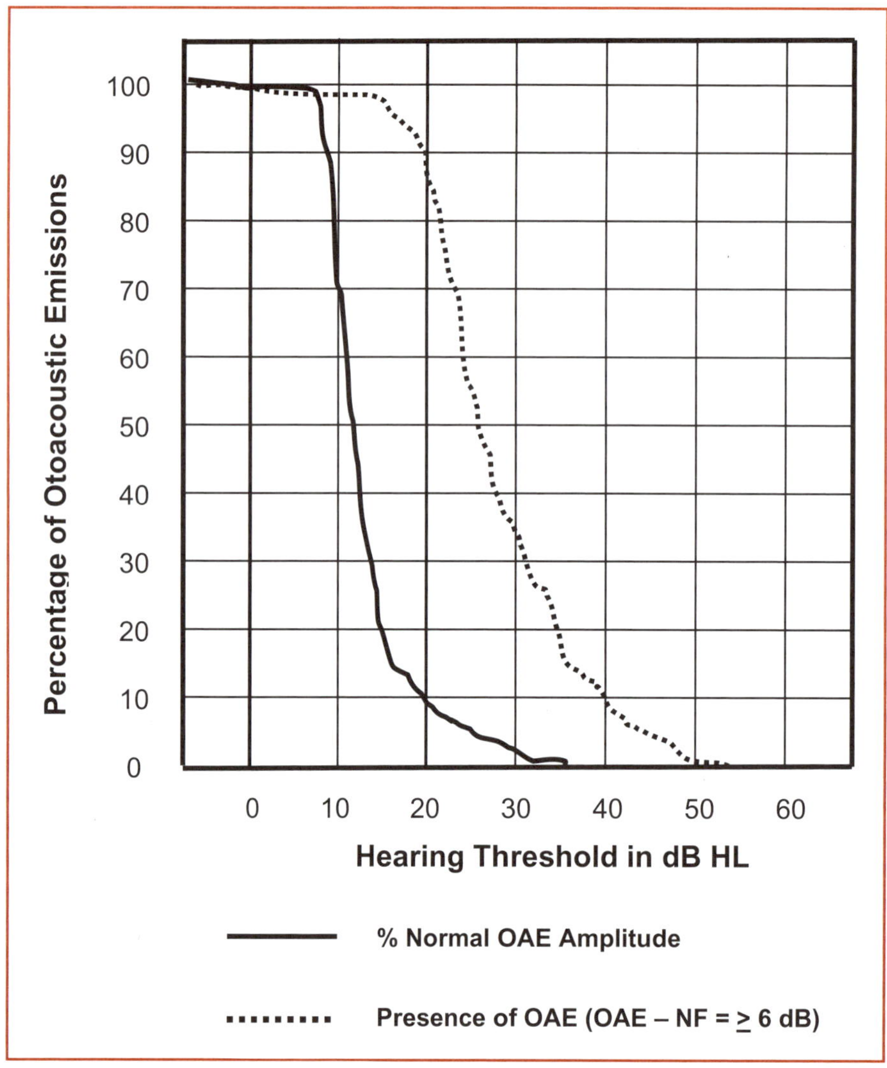

FIGURE 3–3. The likelihood of normal OAEs within the normal region (solid line) and the presence of OAEs (dotted line) as a function of hearing loss at a corresponding frequency.

Differences between OAE and Audiogram Findings

OAE findings are not always correlated with the audiogram. Rather, distinct discrepancies between the audiogram and OAEs are commonly encountered clinically. The discrepancy between OAE findings and the audiogram is not a reflection of a problem or weakness of either procedure. It's a good thing. Divergence among audiologic findings in general, and OAEs and the audiogram in particular, highlights the diagnostic value of individual audiologic procedures and the diagnostic value of the test battery approach in clinical audiology. If OAE findings simply mirrored the pure tone audiogram, OAE would have minimal clinical usefulness. Without doubt, some of the most interesting patients are those who demonstrate a difference, even a marked disagreement, between the audiogram and OAEs. Some of the common discrepancies between OAE and audiogram findings, and brief explanations, are summarized in Table 3–8.

Table 3–8. Two clinically common discrepancies between OAE and audiogram findings, with brief explanations

Discrepancy	
Abnormal OAEs with hearing sensitivity within normal limits	• Middle ear dysfunction: Propagation of OAEs from the cochlea to the external is dependent on integrity of the middle ear. Slight middle ear dysfunction that doesn't cause a deficit in hearing sensitivity may entirely preclude detection of OAEs. • Inner ear (outer hair cell) dysfunction: OAEs are more sensitive to outer hair cell dysfunction than the audiogram. OAE amplitude is typically reduced or OAEs are not detected with hearing sensitivity levels in the 15 to 25 dB region.
Abnormal audiogram with normal OAEs	• Inner ear (inner hair cell) dysfunction: OAEs are not affected by inner hair cell dysfunction, but hearing sensitivity is dependent on inner hair cell integrity. • Neural auditory dysfunction: OAEs are not affected by neural dysfunction. The OAEs are preneural in origin, whereas the audiogram is dependent on neural integrity, including synapse between inner hair cells and afferent eighth nerve fibers, eighth cranial nerve, auditory brainstem, and even auditory cortical regions. • Behavioral factors: Multiple listener variables, including attention, motivation, cognition, reliability, and psychoacoustical factors (e.g., decision criteria) can influence pure tone audiometry resulting in elevated thresholds. None of these factors affect OAE measurement.

CLINICAL CONSIDERATIONS AND CONCERNS

Subject (Nonpathological) Factors

Some of the major nonpathological factors influencing the outcome of hearing screening with OAEs are summarized in Table 3–9. Clearly, many of the factors can be controlled or manipulated, for example, scheduling the time after birth or after bath for infant hearing screening with OAEs.

As noted earlier in this chapter, ambient and physiological *noise* can have a deleterious influence on OAE detection and measurement. Noise levels in OAE recordings must be consistently monitored before and during OAE measurement and, as indicated, the following steps should be taken to minimize excessive noise.

- Eliminate extraneous noise sources in test room (such as other equipment)
- Close the door to the test room
- Insert the OAE probe deeply and snugly within the ear canal
- Secure the probe cord if necessary to prevent it from rubbing against the patient
- Instruct patient to remain quiet and still (as feasible) to reduce physiological noise associated with chewing, talking, etc.
- Position the test ear as far as possible from the OAE equipment
- Modify the protocol to limit test frequencies to those >2000 Hz (if necessary)

Potential factors that do not, in fact, exert an influence on OAEs include:

- Diurnal effects, that is, time of day of recording
- Body temperature
- Body position
- Anesthetic agents (with normal middle ear status)
- State of arousal (attention to stimulus)

Table 3–9. Factors influencing outcome of newborn hearing screening with otoacoustic emissions (OAEs)

Factor	*Influence*
Nonpathological	
Time after birth	Refer rates (percentage of infants failing hearing screening) are highest within the first 24 hours after the infant's birth, and then decrease steadily over the next 2 to 3 days. Refer rates are lower when hearing screening with OAEs is deferred until at least 48 hours after birth, and lowest when screening is performed on the 3rd or 4th day. The likely explanation is dissipation of vernix caseosa within the external ear canal and possibly fluid within the middle ear space. In developing countries, hearing screening performed weeks or even 1 to 3 months after birth at a regular follow-up visit to a public health facility minimizes refer rates, and maximizes the proportion of babies who undergo screening and who are identified with hearing loss.
Time of bath	Significantly lower refer rates are reported when the time period from bathing an infant and OAE measurement is at least 7 hours (e.g., Marques et al., 2008). Moisture in the infant ear can contribute to false-failure in OAE hearing screening.
Age	OAE amplitude is highest at term birth (40 weeks gestational age). Amplitude is relatively decreased in premature infants, and also decreases systematically with age from term birth through childhood. Age effects are presumably secondary to maturation of the middle ear and outer hair cells.
Gender	Transient OAEs are significantly larger in females than males at all ages, whereas there is no significant gender effect with distortion product OAEs.
Noise	OAEs consist of modest levels (usually <15 dB) of sound in the ear canal. Therefore, ambient noise in the test setting has a major impact on the detection of OAE activity, particularly for frequencies below 1500 Hz. All possible steps should be taken to minimize ambient noise within the external ear canal.
Ear probe placement	Depth and quality of ear probe coupling with the external ear canal affects the stability and intensity of the stimulus as well as the amount of ambient noise in the ear canal during OAE measurement. As a rule, a deeper and tight fit is desirable.
Ear canal status	Normal ear canal acoustics influence calibration and amplitude of DPOAEs for test frequencies in the region above 5000 Hz. TEOAEs are not affected by ear canal acoustics. Disorders and debris (e.g., cerumen, foreign objects) in the external ear canal can disrupt stimulus presentation and reception of OAE activity by the microphone within the probe.
Tester	
Background	The professional or educational background of the tester (e.g., audiologist, nurse, technician, volunteer) has no influence on screening outcome.
Experience	Infant hearing screening refer rates decrease directly with the experience of screening personnel. The efficiency of an infant hearing screening program is highest when many infants are screened by a few persons rather than many persons screening a few infants.
Instrumentation	Refer rates are influenced by different components of screening devices, such as the probe design (smaller and lighter is better), algorithms and configurations for detection of the OAE, and noise reduction. OAE refer rates are typically lower for DPOAE than for TEOAE technology.

Table 3–9. *continued*

Factor	Influence
Test protocol	Refer rates are lowest for test frequencies above 2000 Hz (reduced influence of noise), and lower for DPOAEs versus TEOAEs. Test settings, including stopping rules and signal-to-noise differences included in pass/fail criteria, influence refer rates and test times.
Pathological	
External ear canal	Stenosis and external otitis (infection) can affect ear probe placement and probe ports for stimulus presentation or OAE detection (microphone).
Middle ear disorder	Any middle ear dysfunction (e.g., negative middle ear pressure, otitis media) can minimize OAE amplitude or obliterate propagation of OAE activity from the cochlea to the ear canal. OAEs, particularly for high frequencies, can be recorded in patients with ventilation tubes if middle ear status is otherwise normal.
Cochlear dysfunction	
Outer hair cell	Abnormal or absent OAEs are characteristically found in outer hair cell dysfunction.
Inner hair cell	OAEs are typically not affected by isolated inner hair cell dysfunction.
Neural dysfunction	Since they are generated before the first synapse in the auditory system (preneural generators), OAEs are not influenced by neural auditory dysfunction.

Almost immediately following the clinical introduction of DPOAEs, there were concerns about the possibility of false negative hearing screening outcomes due to *artifact*. That is, under certain measurement conditions the presence of an artifact was misidentified as an apparent DPOAE, even in a person with no hearing (a "dead ear"), in a hard-walled calibration cavity or, in one study, even in the external ear canals of cadavers. Conditions or criteria contributing to the possibility of the confusion of an artifact for a response include: an inappropriately high stimulus intensity level, an inappropriate criterion for the presence of a response (e.g., difference between OAE amplitude and noise floor of ≤3 dB), reliance on specific frequency regions where standing wave interference is possible, deficiencies in equipment (close proximity of thin tubes used to deliver the stimulus and detect the OAE), and internal noise within the OAE system. The topic of OAE criteria and problems with artifact are reviewed in more detail in textbooks (Hall, 2000; Robinette & Glattke, 2007) and articles, among them some recent publications (Schmuziger, Lodwig, & Probst, 2006).

Pathologic Factors

Although we've made the point already, it bears repeating that normal OAEs can be recorded in persons with hearing loss, even persons with severe-to-profound hearing impairment. Some explanations for this apparent paradox were summarized in Table 3–9. The possibility, even probability, of normal OAEs or at least the presence of OAE activity (amplitudes reliably >6 dB the noise floor) is a diagnostic feature of auditory neuropathy. The topic of auditory neuropathy is discussed in some detail in the next chapter (Chapter 4) on electrocochleography. Well over 400 published papers report clinical experiences with, and research on, auditory neuropathy, including findings for otoacoustic emissions. Systematic auditory assessment with OAEs along with other procedures in populations of persons who are defined as deaf, for example students in schools for children with hearing impairment, has repeatedly revealed a rather sizeable proportion (10 to 15%) with evidence of OAEs and, therefore, the suspicion of auditory neuropathy. Based on these observations, routine screening for auditory neuropathy with OAEs is recommended.

Normal OAEs can also be recorded in persons with hearing loss secondary to inner hair cell dysfunction (e.g., Ohwatari et al, 2001). Routine hearing screening with OAEs of school-age children with documented hearing loss uncovers a small, but definite, proportion with a pattern of findings consistent with inner hair cell dysfunction. That is, in children with the presence of OAEs, pure tone audiometry documents a hearing loss. ABR confirms normal retrocochlear and brainstem auditory function, and also defines the degree of the hearing loss. Conversely, OAE abnormalities, including the absence of detectable OAEs, are the expected finding in children with cochlear dysfunction affecting the outer hair cells and secondary to a wide variety of etiologies.

4

Electrocochleography (ECochG)

INTRODUCTION

Each auditory measure has its strengths and weakness for identification and diagnosis of auditory dysfunction and hearing loss. And no auditory measure, whether behavioral, electroacoustic, or electrophysiologic, provides all the information needed for management of all patients of all ages. We must rely on a test battery and we must apply the cross-check principle for confident identification and comprehensive diagnostic assessment of patients, particularly children. The clinical value of an auditory measure is best judged by its contribution to the test battery and, especially, by the unique role it plays in defining the site of auditory dysfunction and in differentiating among specific auditory disorders. By this standard, electrocochleography (ECochG) has unquestionable diagnostic value.

ECochG is not useful in infant hearing screening. The literature contains no references to the application of ECochG in infant hearing screening, nor does the Joint Committee on Infant Hearing identify ECochG as a potential hearing screening technique. However, since its discovery over 80 years ago by Wever and Bray (1930), ECochG has acquired a reputation for contributing to the diagnosis of a diverse collection of auditory disorders, ranging from Ménière's disease to auditory neuropathy (AN). ECochG is valuable diagnostically to a large extent because its generators are relatively well defined and, therefore, ECochG findings are site specific. The three ECochG components and their origins in the auditory system are:

- Cochlear microphonic (CM): outer hair cells
- Summating potential (SP): inner hair cells, primarily
- Action potential (AP): distal auditory nerve fibers

In this chapter, we review three important clinical contributions of ECochG to the assessment of auditory function. Interestingly, the first contribution, the estimation of auditory sensitivity with ECochG, is mostly limited to selected countries outside of the United States of America. The second, application of ECochG measurement principles and techniques for enhancement of the ABR, is useful for patients of all ages, including infants and young children. The third contribution is the exploitation of ECochG site-specificity in the confirmation and diagnosis of AN.

TEST PROTOCOL

The overall goal in ECochG measurement is detection of one or more of the three components arising from the cochlea (cochlear microphonic and summating potential) and distal (cochlear end) of the eighth cranial nerve (action potential). With one exception, the test protocol for recording ECochG is quite similar to the probably familiar auditory brainstem response (ABR) test protocol (described with detail in the next chapter). The ECochG test protocol, including stimulus and acquisition parameters, is summarized in Table 4–1.

Table 4–1. Guidelines for electrocochleography (ECochG) test protocol

Parameter	*Suggestion*	*Rationale/Comment*
Stimulus		
Transducer	ER-3A	• Permits TIPtrode usage • Secures transtympanic electrode wire
Type	Click	• Produces robust response • Evaluates cochlear function in basal turn • Tone bursts can be used
Duration	0.1 ms	• Onset response • Longer tone burst duration to verify SP component, e.g., 2-10-2 cycle duration
Polarity	Alternating	• For recording SP component (cancels out CM)
	Single polarity	• When recording CM component (rarefaction and condensation separately)
Rate	7.1/sec	• Low rate enhances the N1 (AP) component • Very rapid rate is useful for SP delineation (e.g., >91/sec)
Intensity	70 to 90 dB nHL	• Produces robust response (no SP for intensities below about 50 dB)
Masking	None	• Never necessary • Detectable response always is generated by test ear
Presentation	Ear	• Monaural
	Mode	• Air conduction • Bone conduction may be useful in selected patients with conductive hearing loss
Acquisition		
Electrodes (options)*	TT-Ac	• Very large amplitude (4 to 20 μV) • Standard stainless steel subdermal needle for promontory site
	IEAC-Ac	• Noninvasive, but AP rarely exceeds 0.6 μV; TIProde for EAC
	TM-Ai	• Noninvasive and large amplitude ECochG (normally >1.0 μV)
	Fpz ground	• Convenient and used for ABR
Filter	10–1500 Hz	• Encompasses response • Lower high pass filter cutoff if possible for SP definition
Amplification	× 75,000	• Adequate for large response
Analysis time	5 or 15 ms	• Shorter time for ECochG • Longer time for ECochG/ABR and multichannel ECochG
Sweeps	<50 to >1500	• <50 for promontory electrode • >1500 for EAC electrode

*TT = transtympanic; EAC = external auditory canal; A = earlobe; i = ipsilateral to stimulus; c = contralateral to; TM = tympanic membrane.

The exception is the electrode type and location. The ECochG is a near-field response recorded by an electrode within the electrical field produced by activation of the auditory structures just mentioned. The electrode used to record the ECochG, therefore, must be located as closely as possible to the cochlea. Two electrode options permit near-field recording of the response. One is specially designed for noninvasive and safe placement by an audiologist of the tip of the electrode on the tympanic membrane. The other is a needle inserted by a physician through the tympanic membrane until the tip rests on the promontory (the bony medial wall of the middle ear space that is also the outer wall of the cochlea). In patients with normal hearing sensitivity, an ear canal electrode (e.g., the TIPtrode) can sometimes be effectively used to record ECochG components. However, the ear canal location is not within the electrical field associated with ECochG activity and the TIPtrode is technically not a suitable ECochG electrode. With an ear canal electrode, selected ECochG components (e.g., the cochlear microphonic or summating potential) are often not clearly detected even in persons with entirely normal auditory function and under otherwise optimal measurement conditions.

Rationale for each of the main stimulus and acquisition parameters is cited in Table 4–1. The reader is referred to the literature and the recent *New Handbook of Auditory Evoked Responses* (Hall, 2007) for more details about ECochG test parameters and measurement.

ESTIMATION OF HEARING THRESHOLDS

It is certainly reasonable to question: Why should ECochG be used for estimation of hearing thresholds when we have ABR and now also auditory steady-state response (ASSR)? Indeed, up until the mid-1970s, audiologists and otolaryngologists in major medical centers routinely applied ECochG for estimation of auditory thresholds in young and difficult-to-test children. With the advent and clinical introduction of the ABR, however, most clinicians quickly transitioned from ECochG to ABR as the technique of choice for electrophysiological threshold estimation. So, does ECochG offer a particular advantage for threshold estimation, perhaps in selected patients? The simple answer is "yes" . . . an enhancement of the signal-to-noise ratio (SNR). With an inverting electrode located close to the cochlea, that is, a "near-field" recording approach, ECochG can be recorded with amplitudes that greatly exceed the amplitude of the ABR wave V. For normal hearers, the amplitude for the action potential (AP) component of the ECochG is typically in the range of 1 to 2 μV with a tympanic membrane electrode option, and greater than 10 μV for transtympanic placement of a needle electrode on the promontory. A detailed discussion of ECochG measurement is beyond the scope of this chapter. The reader is referred to the *New Handbook of Auditory Evoked Responses* (Hall, 2007) for a recent comprehensive review of ECochG measurement.

For any patient, regardless of the type or degree of hearing loss, the ECochG AP component (ABR wave I) as recorded with a near-field technique (e.g., tympanic membrane or transtympanic membrane electrode placement) will be considerably larger than the ABR wave V. As stimulus intensity is decreased, the larger AP component will be more easily detected than wave V, as illustrated in Figure 4–1. At intensity levels close to auditory threshold, the ABR wave V disappears whereas the ECochG AP component remains clearly visible. As a result, ECochG estimates auditory threshold more accurately than ABR. ECochG is especially valuable in threshold estimation for patients with neurological dysfunction that affects the ABR. In some cases with neurological abnormalities, when ABR wave V or waves III and V are not detected, threshold estimation is entirely dependent on the identification of the AP component of ECochG at progressively lower stimulus intensity levels.

Outside of the United States, audiologists and physicians filling the role of audiologists record ECochG with a transtympanic (TT) needle technique for assessment of auditory sensitivity in children who are lightly anesthetized. In terms of surgical difficulty, the transtympanic technique is comparable to the insertion of ventilation tubes (grommets), with average differences between behavioral thresholds and ECochG estimations of

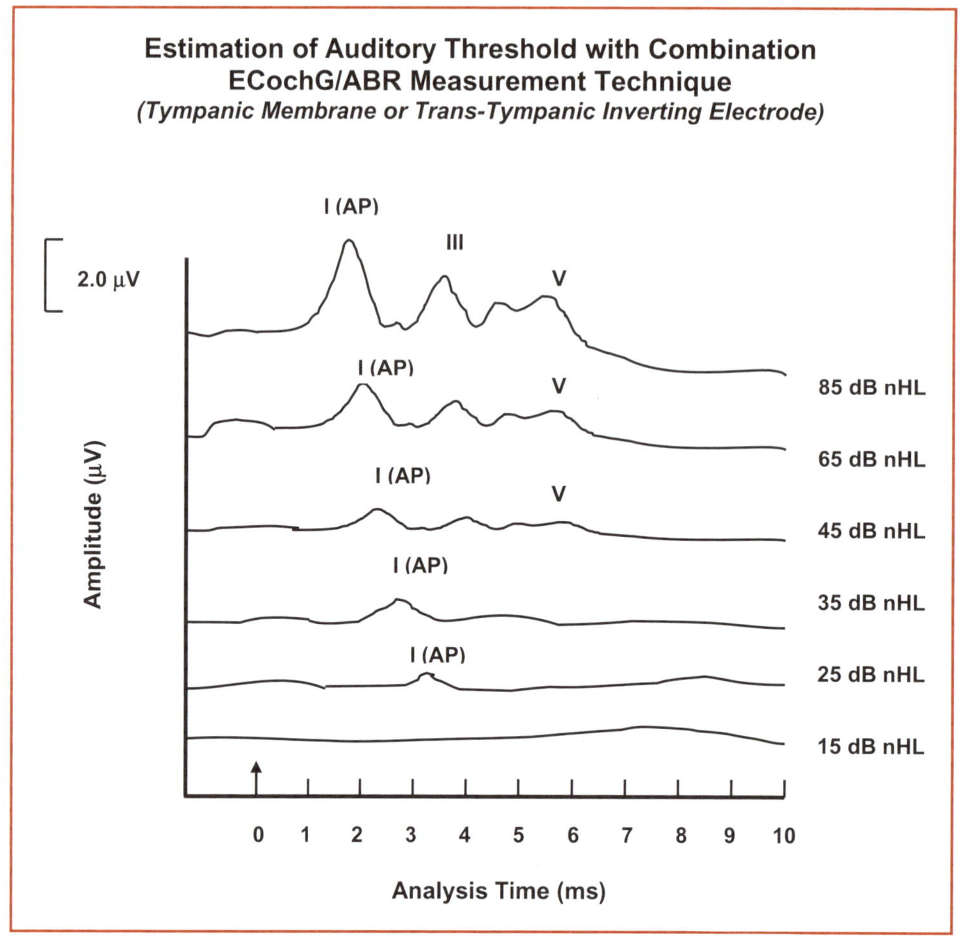

FIGURE 4–1. Combined ECochG and ABR technique producing prominent AP, i.e., ABR wave I, can be used to estimate auditory threshold.

threshold typically less than 6 dB at audiometric frequencies of 500 through 4000 Hz (Wong, Gibson, & Sanli, 1997). Because the AP component of ECochG recorded with the transtympanic electrode technique is 10 to 20 times larger in amplitude than ABR wave I recorded with a mastoid or earlobe electrode side, a response can be detected even in children with severe sensory hearing loss who yield no clear ABR (Schoonhoven, Lamore, de Laat, & Grote, 1999). Of course, frequency-specific ECochG responses can be elicited with tone burst stimuli as well as broadband click stimuli. An added advantage to ECochG as a measure of auditory sensitivity is the ability to detect and diagnose AN, as discussed next.

DIAGNOSTIC APPLICATIONS OF ECochG

Enhancement of ABR

With modification of a few ABR measurement parameters, ECochG principles can easily be applied to enhance the neurodiagnostic value of ABR. There are two major objectives to utilizing ECochG recording strategies in the measurement of ABR. One is to improve detection of the ABR wave I (ECochG AP component). This objective is accomplished by altering one or more of the following stimulus or acquisition parameters:

- Use a TIPtrode, a tympanic membrane electrode, or a transtympanic inverting electrode rather than a mastoid or earlobe inverting electrode
- Slow the stimulus rate to 11/second or less
- Record the ABR with a horizontal (versus ipsilateral) electrode array with the inverting electrode on the stimulus ear and the noninverting electrode on the opposite ear
- Increase stimulus intensity up to maximum level if necessary

A clear and reliable wave I (detected with an inverting electrode on the stimulus ear) verifies that the response is ear-specific (i.e., due to activation of the ear stimulated rather than the nontest ear) and also permits calculation of interwave latencies for neurodiagnostic analysis of the ABR. More precise and confident detection of retrocochlear and brainstem auditory dysfunction is possible with analysis of interwave latency values versus simply ABR wave V.

The second objective in applying ECochG recording strategies in the measurement of ABR is to detect or rule out AN in patients undergoing any ABR assessment. This is accomplished by routinely recording the ABR with both rarefaction and condensation polarity stimuli, rather than only one stimulus polarity or with alternating polarity stimulation. As illustrated in Figure 4–2, with single polarity stimulation (rarefaction and condensation) the cochlear microphonic is usually visible in the waveform immediately following the onset of stimulation. Polarity of the periodic waveform is entirely opposite in phase for cochlear microphonic activity evoked by rarefaction versus condensation polarity stimulation. Stated another way,

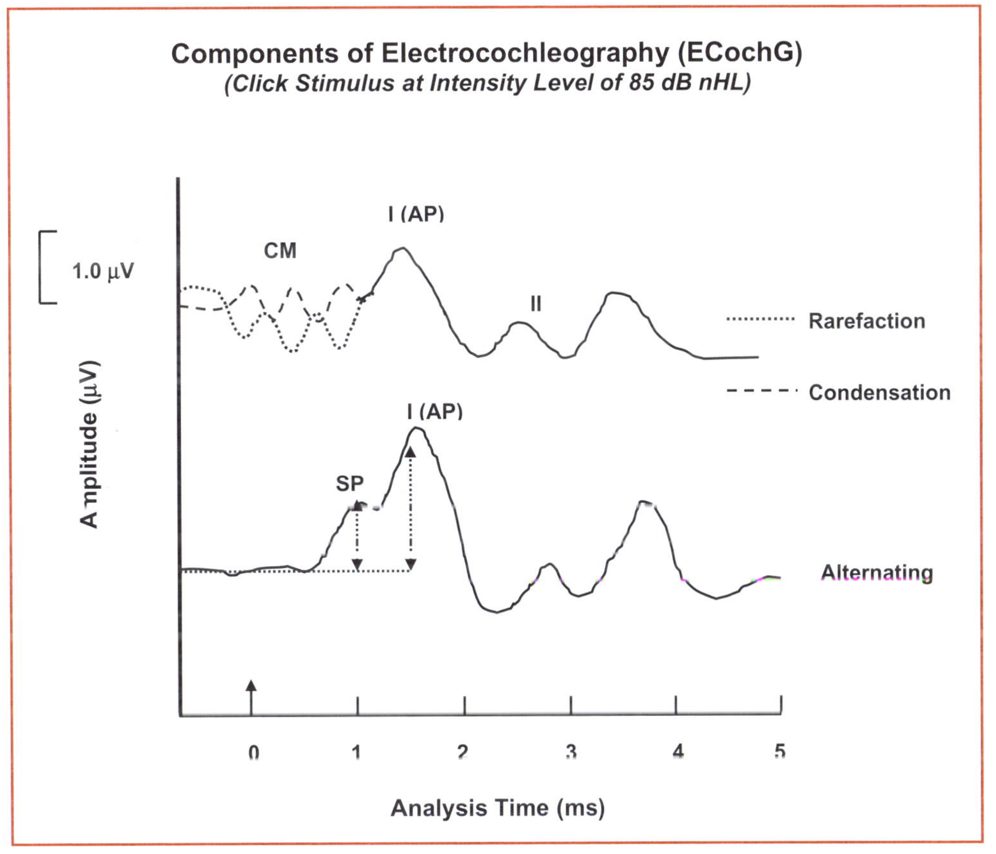

FIGURE 4–2. Different electrocochleography (ECochG) components (cochlear microphonic, summating potential, action potential) can be enhanced with different stimulus polarity conditions (e.g., rarefaction, condensation, or alternating).

when an ABR is recorded with a single stimulus polarity a cochlear microphonic may be apparent. Reversal of the waveform polarity (peaks become troughs and vice versa) when the response is evoked by the other stimulus polarity confirms the presence of cochlear microphonic. If, on the other hand, the waveform does not reverse polarity when stimulus polarity is reversed, then the activity is not cochlear microphonic. Importantly, ABR waves remain essentially unchanged when stimulus polarity is reversed. The clinical lesson here is to routinely and separately record ABRs with each stimulus polarity and then to analyze the resulting waveform to confirm the presence of cochlear microphonic. Of course, if reversing the stimulus polarity produces a total reversal of waveform polarity throughout the analysis time period, then the AN must be suspected. That is, the waveform consists of only cochlear microphonic and no evidence of an ABR. To double-check this outcome, the waveforms elicited separately by rarefaction and condensation stimuli can be digitally added together. All current auditory evoked response systems permit digital manipulation of waveforms, including addition and subtraction. If only cochlear microphonic activity is present in the waveform, then adding the tracings for each polarity will produce a flat line with no clear peaks or troughs. However, the presence of an ABR is confirmed if the addition of two waveforms has little effect on the appearance of the waveform. With some evoked response systems, it's possible to elicit an ABR with alternating polarity stimuli and then, after data collection is completed, to separate the waveforms resulting from each stimulus polarity. This feature permits quick confirmation of the presence of cochlear microphonic and an ABR, without carrying out signal averaging for two sets of stimuli.

Auditory Neuropathy

ECochG is often very helpful for the identification, and essential for the diagnosis, of auditory neuropathy, now referred to as *auditory neuropathy spectrum disorder* (ANSD). Advantages of ECochG techniques in the evaluation of AN are summarized in Table 4–2. To be sure, recognition of what has since 1996 been referred to as AN (Starr, Picton, Sininger, Hood, & Berlin, 1996) was directly related to the emergence of otoacoustic emissions (OAEs) as a clinical procedure. As OAEs began to be used regularly in the mid-1990s, especially in pediatric populations, audiologists around the world reported a seemingly incompatible combination of normal OAE findings in patients with no ABR or, in some cases, no behavioral or electrophysiological response to any type of sound. Although the site of lesion for this clinical entity was rarely verified in the early reports, the presence of OAEs argues for outer hair cell integrity and the absence of other responses was evidence of dysfunction within some other structure or region within the peripheral auditory system. There is growing appreciation that ECochG can contribute importantly to the diagnosis of AN, and to identification of the site of lesion.

Two recent investigations confirm the diagnostic value of ECochG in children and adults meeting current criteria for definition of AN. McMahon and Australian colleagues (2008) describe patterns for ECochG elicited with frequency-specific (tone burst) stimuli and recorded with a round window electrode technique. As the authors point out " . . . determining the site-of-lesion(s) in AN is important in understanding the physiological mechanisms that cause this disorder as it may ultimately be possible to develop a treatment or individual management plan for different manifestations of the disorder" (McMahon, Patuzzi, Gibson, & Sanli , 2008, p. 315). Each of the major ECochG components is attributed to a specific stage in the processing of information within the auditory periphery. Vibration of the basilar membrane produces activity within outer hair cells, reflected by the cochlear microphonic (and OAEs), and depolarization of inner hair cells (IHCs), reflected by the summating potential, or SP. Excitatory postsynaptic potentials (EPSPs) in afferent auditory nerve fibers, generated following the release of neurochemical transmitters within the synapse between the IHCs and the primary fibers, are in turn reflected by compound action potentials (CAP). By close analysis of the pattern of ECochG findings, McMahon et al. (2008) showed that 14 subjects with AN could be divided into those with pre- versus postsynaptic auditory dys-

Table 4–2. Advantages and disadvantages of ECochG in the diagnosis of auditory neuropathy (AN) in comparison to other electroacoustical and electrophysiological auditory measures

ECochG	• Cochlear potentials are generally present • Different patterns of summating and compound action potentials suggest different sites of lesion • CM present, sometimes enlarged, and may persist for several milliseconds	• Information on multiple anatomic sites (outer hair cells, inner hair cells, eighth CN) • Can differentiate pre- versus postsynaptic auditory neuropathy • Minimally affected by middle ear disease	• No information on central auditory nervous system • Invasive trans-tympanic ECochG is best for differentiating pre- and postsynaptic lesion
OAEs	• Present OAEs but may disappear over time	• Information on outer hair cell status • Measurement is quick and simple • Common technique in clinical audiology	• No information on structures other than outer hair cells • Not present in middle ear disease • May disappear over time in AN
Acoustic Reflexes	• Mostly absent but may be elevated in some cases	• Information on multiple anatomic sites (cochlea, eighth CN, auditory brainstem) • Independent of synchronous neural activity • Widely available in audiology clinics	• Not present in middle ear disease
ABR	• Absent at maximum intensities or grossly abnormal neural peaks at elevated intensities (peaks uncorrelated with hearing thresholds) • CM present and inverting with condensation and rarefaction polarity and may persist for several milliseconds	• Information on multiple anatomic sites (cochlea, eighth CN, auditory brainstem) • Important for diagnosis of AN (CM presence and absent or abnormal neural peaks) • Can be recorded in middle ear disease	• May be absent in other disorders
ASSR	• Absent or elevated responses uncorrelated with hearing thresholds	• Sensitive measure of neural activity	• May be absent in other disorders • No clinical role in diagnosing AN at this stage

Note. Clinical advantages shared by all electroacoustical and electrophysiological auditory measures are not cited. CM = Cochlear Microphonic; CN = Cranial Nerve.

function (seven subjects in each category). Santarelli, Starr, Michalewski, and Arlsan (2008) applied a transtympanic electrode approach in a study of eight patients with the diagnosis of AN. All showed either normal amplitude or unusually enlarged cochlear microphonic activity. Three patterns of

ECochG findings were described. One was the absence of a SP and and AP, which was considered representative of a presynaptic IHC abnormality. The second pattern, characterized by the presence of both SP and AP components of the ECochG, was attributed to a postsynaptic abnormality of a proximal (toward the brainstem) portion of the auditory nerve. With the third pattern, described as a postsynaptic abnormality of the nerve terminals near the synapse, the SP was present and followed by an absent AP, or an AP that was "broad" and poorly formed, small in amplitude, and delayed in latency. Differentiation of the SP and AP components was possible with the use of a rapid rate of stimulation (small interstimulus intervals) that led to reduction of the AP amplitude. These recent published studies, and accumulated clinical experience, document the diagnostic value of ECochG in the differentiation and precise description of varied patterns of AN.

CLINICAL CONSIDERATIONS AND CONSTRAINTS

Subject Factors

One major clinical advantage of ECochG is its relative independence from subject factors. ECochG components can be recorded in young children, even premature infants as young as 27 weeks gestational age. Body temperature is directly related to the amplitude of ECochG components, with decreased temperature resulting in reduced amplitude of the CM and AP. ECochG is not importantly influenced by subject attention, state of arousal, sedation, or anesthesia.

Pathologic Factors

Middle ear dysfunction resulting in conductive hearing loss will affect ECochG evoked with air-conduction stimuli. Typically, the CM and SP components are very small in amplitude, or not detectable, whereas the AP component is abnormally delayed in latency and reduced in amplitude in conductive hearing loss. As noted above, application of ECochG techniques during ABR recording (e.g., electrode selection) can enhance the detection of ABR wave I. The presence of wave I within the ipsilateral electrode array (with the inverting electrode on the ear ipsilateral to the stimulus) confirms that a bone-conducted ABR is ear-specific, even when masking is ineffective. ECochG is, of course, sensitive to cochlear auditory dysfunction. Absence of the CM is consistent with outer hair cell abnormality and absence of the SP suggests IHC abnormality. The value of ECochG in diagnosis of neural dysfunction was reviewed just above.

CONCLUDING COMMENT

ECochG plays an important role in the diagnosis of auditory dysfunction, particularly in infants and young children. With direct measurement of the ECochG, or relatively simple modifications of the ABR test protocol, the clinician can more precisely define the site of auditory dysfunction. Because ECochG measurement provides information on auditory function unavailable from other auditory procedures, it is an essential component of the pediatric audiologic test battery.

5

Auditory Brainstem Response (ABR)

SCREENING FOR IDENTIFICATION OF HEARING LOSS

Automated ABR

Background

Up until the mid-1980s, hearing screening was performed with a manual ABR technique and limited to infants at risk for hearing loss. Using essentially diagnostic equipment for recording ABRs, a skilled operator (typically an audiologist) placed electrodes and earphones on the infant, turned knobs and dials to create a test protocol that seemed to work in most cases, decided what stimuli and what stimulus intensity levels to use, and then analyzed the waveform by visually identifying major waves, calculating latencies and less often amplitude, and finally produced an interpretation (e.g., pass versus fail or normal versus abnormal). A serious, and obvious, practical limitation to this approach is the reliance on highly skilled operators (audiologists) for a relatively simple screening technique. Without automation of the technique, to at least identify the presence of a response, universal newborn hearing screening would not be feasible.

The first reports of infant hearing screening with automated ABR appeared in the mid-1980s (e.g., Hall, Kileny, & Ruth, 1987). Since then, automated ABR (AABR) devices have assumed an essential role in newborn hearing screening, and AABR is accepted as standard of care for early identification of hearing impairment (JCIH, 2007). The refer rates for AABR are well within the guidelines (≤4%) established by well-accepted organizations with an interest in pediatric hearing impairment, such as the American Academy of Pediatrics (1999) and the Joint Committee on Infant Hearing (JCIH, 2007). With the development of multiple instruments and algorithms for AABR have come new and improved and evidence-based test protocols—test protocols, that is, designed specifically for infants and young children and for optimal and confident detection of at least the ABR wave V component at either a screening intensity level (e.g., 35 dB nHL) or the lowest possible intensity level. AABR analysis is based on consistent statistical determination of response presence versus absence, rather than the judgment of the person conducting the test procedure. Different algorithms and strategies are used for automated detection of the ABR, including matching an infant's ABR to a normal template with statistical confirmation of the presence of a response or application of a statistical variance ratio approach (e.g., the F statistic) to differentiate response from non-response. Background information on AABR, especially details on a wide range of statistical methods for response detection, can be found within the literature and recent textbooks (e.g., Burkard, Don, & Eggermont, 2007; Hall, 2007). Those using AABR devices and/or coordinating infant hearing screening programs are advised to, minimally, review the device manual closely to understand the algorithms used for response detection and to review critically published clinical trials reporting evidence in support of the algorithms.

Clinical Findings

Well over a thousand published papers address the topic of pediatric application of ABR, including newborn hearing screening. During the past 20 years, many millions of babies around the world have undergone AABR screening in clinical programs for early identification of hearing loss, although the results are typically not reported in the literature. Findings for AABR hearing screening for selected recent published papers are summarized in Table 5–1. As reviewed in Chapter 3, the literature also includes hundreds of papers describing experience with otoacoustic emission (OAE) screening in dozens of countries around the world, most published during the past decade.

At least five important findings are consistently apparent from a review of recent literature on AABR (e.g., Hall, 2007; Stewart et al., 2000). First, the refer rate is acceptably low and almost always lower than the refer rate for OAEs, especially when screening is conducted within 24 hours after birth. Second, low refer rates for AABR are reported even when the hearing screening is completed within a few hours after birth (even before the baby's first bath). Refer rates for hearing screening with OAE technology decrease markedly as a function of time after birth. In contrast, age of the child within the first 2 to 3 days after birth is not a factor in ABR screening outcome. Third, hearing screening outcome is not dependent on the pro-

Table 5–1. Selected reports of automated auditory brainstem response (AABR) in newborn hearing screening reported since 2000 and arranged chronologically

Study (Year)	*N*	*Population*	*Device*	*Refer Rate*	*Comment*
Iley & Addis (2000)	44	WB	ALGO-2*	4.5%	Screening time of 5 minutes
Sininger et al. (2000)	4831 2348	HR WB	custom (Fsp) custom (Fsp)	<10% 14%	Excellent review of AABR screening technique
Stewart et al. (2000)	11,711	HR/WB	ALGO-2	<2%	Screening personnel and test time after birth are not factors in refer rate
Messner et al. (2001)	5771	WB	ALGO-2	5%	Only volunteers used for screening
van Strääten et al. (2001)	90	HR	ALGO-1 E	0%	Pass/refer rate decreased with gestational age
Vohr et al. (2001)	12,081	WB	ALGO-2	3.21%	TEOAE refer rate was 6.49%
Meier et al. (2004)	150	WB	ALGO-3	2%	TEOAE and DPOAE refer rate was 3%
Murray et al. (2004)	194	WB	ALGO-3	5.7%	Average screening time was 70.8 seconds
Suppiej et al. (2007)	206	HR	NR	NR	Sensitivity of 100% and specificity of 90.8%
Pedersen et al. (2008)	1627	WB	ABAER*	4%	Refer rate of 11% for TEOAE

*HR = high risk; WB = well babies with no risk factors; ALGO device by Natus, Inc. utilizing a template matching algorithm; ABAER = BioLogic automated ABR device; NR = not reported.

fessional credentials of the person who conducts the screening. That is, consistently low refer rates are reported for AABR performed by persons with a variety of job descriptions, such as technicians, nurses, volunteers, and audiologists. Fourth, as with any hearing screening technique, there is an indirect relation between screening experience and refer rate. That is, the lowest refer rates are invariably associated with the most experienced screening personnel. Fifth, AABR is the screening technique of choice for children in the neonatal intensive care unit, along with any infants at risk for neurological dysfunction, and is strongly recommended for these infants by the Joint Committee of Infant Hearing (JCIH, 2007).

ESTIMATION OF HEARING THRESHOLDS

Air Conduction Click-Elicited ABR Measurement

Rationale

Although various types of stimuli (e.g., versions of chirps, plops, logons, clicks, or tone bursts in noise, and even speech) can be used to elicit the ABR (Burkard et al., 2007; Hall, 2007), simple click and tone burst stimuli presented via air or bone conduction are by far the most commonly applied and clinically valuable. It is likely that current research on stimuli other than clicks and tone bursts will eventually lead to improvements in ABR measurement, that is, quickly recording highly frequency-specific ABRs. Pending the inclusion of alternative stimuli in the diagnostic evoked response test battery, however, there is ample evidence that clicks and tone bursts offer a clinically feasible approach for ABR measurement for neurodiagnosis of auditory dysfunction and for estimation of auditory thresholds. Since the discovery of the ABR over 35 years ago, click stimuli have consistently been viewed as necessary for neurodiagnostic ABR measurement. With the growth in clinical application of tone-burst ABR measurement for frequency-specific estimation of auditory thresholds, the relevance of including click stimuli in pediatric ABR measurement is questioned (e.g., Sauter, 2007).

Inclusion of click stimuli within the ABR test battery, along with but prior to tone bursts, yields multiple diagnostic dividends without appreciably increasing test time. Clinical experience shows that, for most patients, click-evoked ABRs can be recorded for a high intensity level and one or more lower intensity levels and for each ear in less than 4 to 5 minutes, and often in less time. Assuming the presence of a response, and adequate test conditions with minimal amounts of electrical noise and movement interference, an obvious ABR can be detected by averaging the response from as few as 200 or 300 stimulus repetitions (sweeps). With a typical stimulus presentation rate in the range of 21 to 37 clicks per second, only about 10 to 20 seconds is required to obtain the averaged waveform. This process is then immediately repeated to verify that the response is reliable, and then stimulus intensity is decreased and two more waveforms are quickly averaged. To be sure, the presentation of additional stimuli and extended signal averaging would result in a cleaner ABR waveform with less noise and better morphology. However, the overall objective with pediatric ABR measurement is not aesthetic waveforms but, rather, quick and accurate diagnosis of auditory dysfunction and frequency-specific estimation of auditory threshold. Gathering all of the information required to properly diagnose and manage a child's hearing impairment by limiting signal averaging to what is minimally required versus taking enough time to record a beautiful ABR is always a good clinical decision.

The investment of a few minutes of test time to record click-evoked ABRs yields remarkably high diagnostic dividends. In comparison to tone burst stimuli, particularly for lower frequencies, a click signal presented at a high stimulus intensity level is likely to produce a clearer and perhaps more reliable ABR. The findings of click-elicited ABR measurement guide the strategy that will be taken when recording tone burst ABRs. Analysis of the ABR evoked by click stimuli may facilitate decisions regarding the most appropriate initial tone burst frequency and the starting intensity level. The absence of a click-evoked ABR may prompt immediate recording of an auditory steady state response (ASSR). Or a normal click-evoked ABR may lead to the decision to record OAEs to verify cochlear integrity. Also, long-standing normative data exist for click-evoked ABR latency values, along with extensive age-corrected normative data for children. Finally, as reviewed below in the section on ABR analysis, calculation of click ABR latency values permits quick differentiation between normal auditory function somewhere in the high frequency region, a conductive hearing loss, a sensory hearing loss, neural dysfunction, and the ABR pattern suggesting auditory neuropathy.

A Practical Test Protocol

Detailed review of each of the stimulus and acquisition parameters employed in recording a click-evoked ABR is beyond the scope of this book and this chapter. The reader is referred to a recent textbook (Hall, 2007) for a thorough review of the topic. Essential test parameters for click-evoked ABR measurement are summarized in Table 5–2.

Table 5–2. Summary of a test protocol for ABR measurement via air-conduction click stimulation. Adapted from Hall (2007).

Parameter	*Recommendation*
Stimulus Parameters	
Transducer	Insert earphone (ER 3A). Supra-aural earphones should also be available for selected types of patients, e.g., children with aural atresia.
Type	Click
Duration	0.1 ms
Polarity	Rarefaction
Rate	>20 stimuli/sec (e.g., 21.1 or 27.3)
Intensity	Variable in dB nHL
Repetitions	Variable depending on signal-to-noise ratio (SNR)
Masking	Required only with no wave I in ipsilateral recording
Mode	Monaural
Acquisition Parameters	
Analysis time	15 ms
Prestimulus baseline	–1 ms
Electrodes	
Type	Disc type or disposable variety
Location	
Non-inverting	Fz (high forehead)
Inverting	Ai (ipsilateral earlobe)
Ground	Fpz (low forehead)
Filter settings	
High pass	30 or 75 Hz
Low pass	1500, 2000, or 3000 Hz
60 Hz notch	No
Amplification	× 100,000
Sweeps (# stimuli)	Variable depending on SNR

Source. Adapted from *New Handbook of Auditory Evoked Responses*, by J. W. Hall, III, 2007, Boston: Allyn & Bacon, Inc., p. 124. Adapted with permission.

The following discussion highlights the reasoning behind the recommended use of selected parameters for neurodiagnostic and threshold estimation applications of the ABR elicited with click stimuli. Insert earphones are the transducer of choice for ABR measurement in infants and young children. The numerous advantages associated with the use of *insert earphones* are summarized in Table 5–3. Clinical and research experience for over 35 years confirms unequivocally the effectiveness of click stimuli, produced by the activation of the transducer diaphragm by a *transient (0.1 ms) electrical signal*, for elicitation of the ABR. Although different polarity options (rarefaction, condensation, or alternating presentations of each polarity) are effective in eliciting the ABR, *rarefaction polarity stimuli* typically are best suited for activating the cochlea and auditory pathways. The ABR elicited with rarefaction polarity click stimuli has larger amplitudes and slightly shorter latencies, in comparison to the ABR elicited with condensation or alternating polarity stimuli (see Hall 2007 for explanation). However, if the ABR elicited with rarefaction polarity click stimuli is suboptimal, then it is advisable to utilize condensation polarity stimuli. Separate recordings evoked by rarefaction and by condensation stimuli will contribute to the differentiation of an ABR

Table 5–3. Clinical advantages associated with the use of insert earphones in clinical measurement of the auditory brainstem response in infants and young children

- Reduction of ambient noise during ABR measurement. Insert earphones are essentially sound attenuating earplugs. Reduced ambient noise in the ear canal will contribute to accuracy in threshold assessments. The advantage of reduced ambient noise applies also for bone conduction ABR measurement if insert earphones remain within the ear canal.
- Increased interaural attenuation of the stimulus (less concern about the stimulus crossing over from test ear to the nontest ear).
- Infection control and aural hygiene. Insert ear cushions are discarded after single use. Insert earplugs are disinfected before reuse. Acoustic tubes leading to ear cushions or plugs can be disinfected before each use.
- Minimization of ear canal collapse (a concern with compliant infant ear canals).
- Insert earphones remain in place, and insert cushions or earplugs within the ear canal, even for newborn infants with very small ear canals whereas supra-aural earphones usually need to be hand held.
- Accuracy and consistency in the delivery of sound to small infant ear canals, in comparison to large supra-aural earphones.
- Frequency response for insert earphones is relatively flat in comparison to that of supra-aural earphones.
- Diaphragm "ringing" is reduced for insert earphones in comparison to supra-aural earphones, creating less interference with identification of early latency evoked response components (e.g., cochlear microphonic or ABR wave I).
- Insert earphones are generally more comfortable than supra-aural earphones, an asset for relatively long threshold ABR measurement sessions.
- Concerns are eliminated about interference of stimulus artifact in ABR analysis when transducer box is placed 8 to 9 mm (the length of the acoustic tubing) away from all electrode wires.
- Insert earphones can be adapted for use with TIPtrode electrodes.

versus cochlear microphonic (CM) activity. Appearance of the ABR will remain similar when elicited with each of the two stimulus polarities, whereas the CM will appear completely inverted in polarity when elicited with each of the two stimulus polarities. With some evoked response systems, it's possible to record an ABR with alternating polarity stimulation, and then to view separately the waveforms elicited with rarefaction versus condensation polarity stimuli.

There is no magical *stimulus rate* for ABR measurement in infants and young children, but a few general guidelines should be considered. Children with normal auditory systems and hearing, even newborn and premature infants, will typically have a reliable and well-formed ABR that is evoked by stimulation at rates as high as 21 to 27 per second. Therefore, slower stimulus presentation rates offer no advantage and actually unnecessarily extend test time. Guidelines for minimizing test time when recording ABRs from children, including the recommendation for relatively fast stimulus presentation rates, will be reviewed next (Table 5–4). On the other hand, when stimulus presentation rate exceeds about 30 per second, there may be unwanted changes in the ABR waveform (e.g., poorer morphology) and with specific wave components (such as reduced amplitude for wave I). These changes are exacerbated for premature infants with immature auditory nervous systems. You'll notice that even integers (like 20 or 30) are not recommended for stimulus presentation rates. In order to minimize the likelihood of an interaction between the stimulus and 60 Hz electrical noise (or multiples of 60 Hz), it is customary to employ odd numbers for stimulus rate, like 21.1 or 27.3 per second, that are not evenly divided into 60 Hz or multiples of 60 Hz. Sometimes the quality of an ABR recording in a potentially electrically hostile setting (e.g., NICU or operating room [OR]) can be improved by a very slight modification in stimulus presentation rate (such as from 21.1 to 23.1/sec).

Without doubt, *stimulus intensity* is the most important measurement parameter manipulated by the audiologist who is performing an ABR assessment. Just as stimulus intensity is almost constantly changed during pure tone audiometry, the intensity of click and tone burst stimuli is increased and decreased often during an ABR assessment. And, as with pure tone audiometry, stimulus intensity calibration and verification are essential for the click and tone burst stimuli used with frequency-specific ABR measurement. Accuracy of electrophysiological estimations of auditory threshold is entirely dependent on careful calculation and documentation of click and tone burst stimulus intensity. However, calibration of transient click and tone burst stimuli with a typical sound level meter is not as straightforward as calibration of pure tone stimuli. Verification of click or tone burst stimulus intensity by the clinical audiologist and extrapolating pure tone audiometric thresholds from ABR thresholds can be accomplished with three rather simple steps. Because the same steps are taken in the verification of intensity level for air conduction clicks, bone conduction clicks, and air conduction pure tone stimuli, they will be described here, and then cited in the subsequent discussions of frequency-specific and bone conduction ABR measurement.

Step 1: *Before* Performing ABRs for Threshold Estimation. Obtain from a small group of normal hearing adults behavioral thresholds for all stimuli used in ABR measurement. Normative data for the stimuli used in ABR measurement should, ideally, be gathered soon after purchase of the evoked response system or, at least, before the system is used for frequency-specific ABR measurement with children. A group of five adults with normal auditory function must first be identified. Criteria for normal auditory function optimally include pure tone hearing thresholds of 5 dB or better for octave frequencies of 500 to 4000 Hz (measured in a sound-treated room using accepted clinical methods), normal tympanograms, and normal OAEs (probably distortion produced OAEs) throughout the frequency region. Then, thresholds are measured behaviorally from each of the normal subjects with each of the stimuli to be used in an ABR assessment, including air conduction clicks, bone conduction clicks, and air conduction tone bursts at 500, 1000, 2000, and 4000 Hz. The subjects don't need to be wired for ABR measurement. Stimulus intensity is varied with the evoked response system just as it would be for an audiometer, with the subjects indicating their

Table 5–4. Simple steps for minimizing test time in threshold estimation with the ABR, without sacrificing quality or quantity of data collected

• Be prepared to begin ABR as soon as the child is asleep. – Equipment is set up with patient information entered and initial protocol selected. – Electrodes are handy with electrode gel or paste. – Tape is cut and nearby. – Insert earphones are ready with proper size tips.
• Record ABR with measurement conditions that optimize the SNR, i.e, maximize the signal (ABR) and minimize the noise (all other electrical activity). – Sleeping, sedated, or anesthetized child – Low and balanced electrode impedance – Little or no electrical artifact – Deep fitting insert earphone to minimize ambient acoustic noise
• Use a stimulus presentation rate that speeds up data collection without deterioration of ABR morphology and prolongation of ABR latencies – For air conduction click stimulation, a rate of about 21.1/sec (wave I amplitude decreases at higher stimulus rates) – For bone conduction click stimulation, a rate of about 11.1/sec (to optimize chances of detecting a clear wave I) – For tone burst stimulation, a rate of about 37.7/sec
• Immediately troubleshoot if the ABR findings are different from what you expect.
• Think ahead to the next step in the assessment while signal averaging . . . *don't* do your thinking between periods of data collection.
• At high stimulus intensities: – Discontinue signal averaging as soon as a clear response is detected (usually <500 stimuli or sweeps). – Immediately replicate with even fewer averages.
• Calculate latencies and amplitudes while also collecting data at the next intensity level or the next test condition.
• Drop the stimulus intensity level down as quickly as possible to near threshold (e.g., from 80 dB nHL down to 40 dB nHL if the ABR has a wave I and wave V).
• After hearing thresholds are estimated with click stimuli, begin presenting subsequent tone burst stimuli at intensity levels 20 to 30 dB above anticipated ABR threshold.
• Don't replicate flat ABR tracings (when you have nothing you have nothing to repeat).

Note. By following these guidelines, it's possible with most patients to generate an electrophysiological "audiogram" in 30 to 45 minutes.

perception of the sounds by raising their hand. Importantly, behavioral thresholds for the ABR stimuli should be measured with the stimulus parameters to be used clinically in recording ABRs, (e.g., same rate, polarity, and duration) and in the environment or setting where the ABRs will be recorded clinically from children (e.g., in the audiology clinic, operating room, NICU, etc.).

The goal in collecting the normative thresholds for ABR stimuli is to replicate as closely as possible the conditions encountered when recording ABRs from children. Average thresholds for each of the stimuli, calculated from this small but carefully selected group of normal adult subjects, become 0 dB nHL. For example, if the average behavioral threshold for a 500 Hz tone burst in the OR setting is 30 dB (the intensity level on the screen of the evoked response system), then 0 dB nHL is viewed as the normal reference for the stimulus. The *nHL* refers to "normal hearing level," a biological dB unit for transient acoustic stimuli that are difficult to properly calibrate with a sound level meter. It is not equivalent to *dB HL*, the standard for intensity of signals in pure tone and speech audiometry.

If ABRs are recorded in diverse clinical settings, such as a quiet room in an audiology clinic versus an operating room or at bedside in a NICU, then a different set of normative data (different references for 0 dB nHL) is needed for each test setting. Variations in the "correction" for 0 dB nHL among settings are most obvious for lower frequency tone burst stimuli (e.g., 500 and 1000 Hz) because ambient noise is greater for the low frequency region. As a rule, separate normative data for the right and left insert earphones are not necessary, although verification of the consistency of findings for the right versus left insert earphones for one frequency is advisable. Special aspects of normative intensity data collection for bone conduction stimuli are reviewed below under the heading Bone Conduction ABR. The process of collecting normative threshold data for each of the stimuli used in pediatric ABR measurement requires at most a few hours, and usually only needs to be completed one time for an evoked response system, or one time for a set of transducers.

Step 2: *During* ABR Measurement. Analyze and describe the threshold for detection of the wave V component of the ABR in dB nHL. After first recording and analyzing the ABR elicited with high intensity click stimuli to differentiate among types of auditory disorders (see review above), the next goal in the estimation of auditory thresholds for air conduction tone burst stimuli necessary for an initial hearing aid fitting and, in some cases, recording a bone conduction ABR is to confirm or rule out the presence of a conductive hearing loss component. The top priority is to identify for each stimulus condition (e.g., 1000 Hz presented to the right ear) a reliable ABR wave V at the lowest possible intensity level. The minimal intensity level producing a reliable ABR wave V is typically estimated using 10 dB increments. Time permitting, more accurate estimations of thresholds will be made with 5 dB intensity increments. Sometimes the clinician is forced to make difficult decisions involving test time versus test precision, that is, whether to estimate more precisely auditory thresholds with 5 dB intensity increments at the cost of more test time or to use 10 dB intensity increments so that data are available for at least three, or even four, tone burst frequencies for each ear. This description of ABR threshold estimation is based on the assumption that wave V is the prominent component within the waveform. Usually, wave V amplitude is up to two times larger than the amplitude of wave I and wave III. However, in newborn infants (especially premature infants) and children with auditory brainstem dysfunction, the amplitude of ABR wave V may be reduced or wave V may not be clearly recorded. In such cases, ABR threshold estimation must be conducted cautiously by the identification of either wave I or wave III at progressively lower stimulus intensity levels.

Step 3: *After* Completing a Frequency-Specific ABR Assessment. Estimate pure tone behavioral thresholds from the minimal intensity level producing a reliable ABR wave V component. An ABR will not be elicited at stimulus intensity levels that are equivalent to behavioral threshold for the stimuli, that is, the intensity level at which the stimulus is just barely perceived. The stimulus intensity level must exceed behavioral hearing thresholds by at least 5 to 10 dB before the energy in the stimulus is sufficient to adequately activate the cochlea for the subsequent generation of action potentials synchronously in multiple afferent fibers within the distal (cochlear) end of the auditory (eighth cranial) nerve. If measurement noise (electrical and physiological) is low, if signal averaging is continued for thousands of stimulus presentations, and if stimulus intensity is increased in 1 or 2 dB increments, then it is possible to detect the emergence of an ABR wave V when the click or tone burst stimulus intensity is within 5 dB of behavioral hearing threshold. However, with clinical ABR measurement these ideal conditions are rarely encountered, and minimizing the time spent in estimating threshold for any one stimulus condition (ear and frequency) has a high priority in order to permit complete estimation of threshold for enough frequencies, at least three or four in each ear, for an accurate initial hearing aid fitting.

Clinical research and experience accumulated and reported for over 20 years (see Hall, 2007, and Stapells, 2000) confirms the reasonably close and predictable relationship between thresholds for the ABR elicited with tone burst stimuli and valid pure tone thresholds measured from cooperative children and adults with confirmed sensory hearing loss. Admittedly, the three-step process just described is somewhat cumbersome and opens the possibility of miscalculations in the estimation of auditory thresholds. Also, the process is based on the faulty assumption that for a given stimulus intensity level normal behavioral thresholds for adults are precisely equivalent to thresholds for infants. This assumption is clearly challenged by the well-known differences in ear canal acoustics, including resonance characteristics, associated with age-related differences in ear canal size and volume. Calibration of stimulus intensity in dB SPL within the ear canal of individual subjects, for example, infants undergoing ABR assessment, would appear to offer a distinct advantage for accurate estimation of auditory thresholds. Technology exists for in-ear documentation and adjustment of stimulus intensity to reach target values, utilizing miniature microphones within a probe assembly. The technique is, for example, already implemented regularly with clinical devices for measurement of OAEs. Nonetheless, pending the introduction of clinical evoked response devices permitting in-ear verification of stimulus intensity, abundant clinical evidence accumulated for over 30 years supports the reasonable (if not absolute) accuracy of biological verification of transient stimulus intensity in normal adult subjects with application of the data for estimation of auditory thresholds in children. Now that we've reviewed the steps required to verify stimulus intensity level in ABR measurement, we'll return to the discussion of the practical test protocol.

There are distinct differences in the need for, and techniques of, *masking* the nontest ear in ABR measurement versus conventional behavioral audiometry (e.g., pure tone and speech audiometry). Masking is not always necessary in ABR measurement. The consistent use of insert earphones for presentation of stimuli in ABR recording will minimize the need for masking. The following discussion focuses on the topic of masking during air conduction ABR measurement. The special features of masking during bone conduction ABR recording are reviewed in a subsequent section on Bone Conduction ABR. With air conduction ABR measurement, masking is not required when any of the following criteria are met:

- Air conduction stimulus intensity level does not exceed interaural attenuation (about 70 dB nHL).
- A clear and reliable wave I is identified in the ABR waveform.
- The latency of ABR wave V is within normal limits for the stimulus intensity level.

Crossover of the air conduction stimulation from the test ear to the nontest ear will not occur for lower intensity levels. When the ABR is elicited by stimulation crossing over to the nontest ear, there will be no wave I in the ipsilateral electrode array (Fz-Ai) and the time consumed by the crossover will produce an increase in ABR latencies. Conversely, masking is indicated in ABR measurement with air conduction stimulation when at a high (>70 dB nHL) intensity level the ABR is characterized only by a delayed latency wave V component.

Acquisition parameters for click-evoked ABR measurement in children (refer again to Table 5–2) are similar to those used for many years with adult neurodiagnostic applications of the ABR. Under all possible measurement conditions that tend to prolong wave latencies (e.g., immature nervous system, hearing loss, conductive components) an *analysis time* of 15 ms is adequate to encompass the entire click-evoked ABR waveform, including wave V and the broad negative trough following wave V, referred to sometimes as the SN_{10} wave (the slow negative wave around 10 ms). The inclusion of a prestimulus baseline period (e.g., –1 ms) provides a useful index of the quality of measurement conditions. Before stimuli are presented the averaged waveform should be essentially flat if measurement conditions are good. On the other hand, peaks and valleys in the prestimulus period indicate that considerable noise (nonresponse) activity is present within the waveform. The clinician should, in such cases, exercise caution in the analysis of the ABR waveform.

Nowadays, a variety of *electrode designs* are available for clinical ABR measurement of children, including newborn infants (see Hall, 2007, for details). Electrodes can be purchased from most manufacturers of evoked response instrumentation, with different styles and options highlighted in manufacturer catalogs of supplies (available in hard copy or electronic formats). A search of the Internet will also reveal independent manufacturers of electrodes and a wealth of different designs for various clinical applications. Disposable electrodes, available in many shapes and sizes, are often preferred for ABR assessment of infants and young children as the possibility of infection is minimized. With one disposable design, the entire electrode and lead is discarded after a single use. Alternatively, lead wires with snap-on devices can be reused with disposable electrode pads. Cost is a disadvantage of disposable electrodes. Reusable electrodes have been employed since the introduction of the ABR as a clinical technique in the early 1970s. Made of metal alloy, reusable electrodes are discs connected to a wire or lead that ends with a pin that plugs into an electrode strip or box. Most manufacturers include in their reusable electrode collection ear-clip electrodes that attach to the earlobe with a spring mechanism. Six clinical advantages of an earlobe versus mastoid electrode location are summarized in Table 5–5.

Electrode locations are simple and straightforward for conventional pediatric ABR assessments. An ABR can be recorded with as few as three scalp electrodes, as illustrated schematically in Figure 5–1). The *noninverting* (improperly referred to also as the "active" or "positive") *electrode* is

Table 5–5. Clinical advantages associated with the use of an earlobe (e.g., ear-clip) versus mastoid location for the inverting electrode in pediatric ABR measurement

- **Ease of application:** No tape is required as the electrodes are fitted within a spring clip that clings to the earlobe.
- **Consistency of placement:** Considerable force is required to dislodge the ear-clip electrodes, and they are easily replaced (again without the need for tape).
- **Lower impedance:** Interelectrode impedance is generally low because the ear-clip design makes contact with the skin on both sides of the earlobe (more surface area in comparison to other electrode designs).
- **Larger wave I amplitude:** ABR wave I is about 30% larger for earlobe versus mastoid electrodes.
- **Reduced postauricular muscle (PAM) artifact:** The mastoid electrode is located directly over the PAM, an ideal site for recording unwanted muscle artifact. The PAM response appears as a large wave in the 13 to 20 ms latency region. The earlobe electrode is located away from the PAM.
- **Reduced stimulus artifact in bone conduction ABR:** With a mastoid location for the inverting electrode, the bone oscillator placement on the temporal bone inevitably creates excessive electromagnetic stimulus artifact. Use of an earlobe-inverting electrode reduces problems with stimulus artifact in bone conduction stimulation of the ABR.

Note. Ear clip electrodes are available from manufacturers of evoked response systems and independent electrode manufacturers.

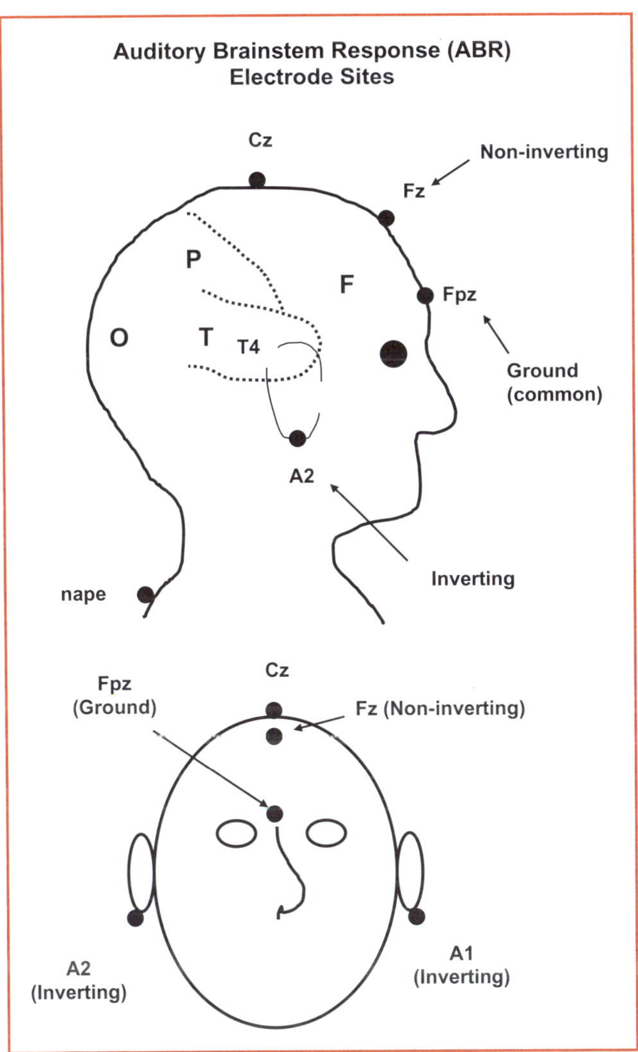

FIGURE 5–1. Locations of noninverting, inverting, and ground electrodes for pediatric ABR measurement.

placed on the high forehead in the midline (Fz). The *F* refers to *frontal* (it is located over the frontal lobe of the brain), and the symbol *z* is used to denote the midline (see Hall, 2007, for detailed discussion). For infants and young children, the Fz electrode location on the forehead offers a more convenient and secure placement site than the Cz (vertex or top middle of the head) location with no negative impact on ABR wave latency, amplitude, or morphology. The *inverting electrode* can be located in one of three locations: earlobe, mastoid, or nape of the neck. The earlobe site is adequate, and actually preferred, for most pediatric ABR recordings. Advantages of the earlobe versus mastoid location were noted above (see Table 5–5). However, with certain ABR applications in children (e.g., hearing screening and estimation of auditory thresholds with tone burst stimuli) the nape of the neck (a noncephalic site) also is an appealing option for the inverting electrode (see Figure 5–1). The amplitude of wave V is generally larger when an ABR is recorded with a noncephalic inverting electrode (in reality a true reference electrode inactive to brainstem auditory electrical responses), plus problems with postauricular muscle (PAM) artifact are eliminated. The ground (common) electrode can be located anywhere on the body, but a clinically common and convenient location is low and in the midline on the forehead (refer again to Figure 5–1). Deviations from the simple three electrode recording montage or array are noted in the following discussion about bone conduction ABR.

For pediatric ABR measurement, *filter settings* must encompass relatively low frequencies. The spectrum of the infant ABR is dominated by energy under the frequency of about 200 Hz. A recommended band pass filter for pediatric ABR recording is 30 to 3000 Hz. High pass filter settings (the low end of the frequency region) above 100 Hz are likely to remove spectral energy important for detection of the infant ABR, and for precise estimation of auditory threshold. Restricting the other end of the band pass filter is less concerning. The use of a low pass filter setting of 2000 Hz, or even 1500 Hz, may improve the quality of an ABR recording by removing unwanted high frequency electrical noise. A 60 Hz notch filter, introduced many years ago in an attempt to minimize electrical artifact associated with power lines and other electrical sources (such as fluorescent lights), rarely achieves this goal. Unfortunately, the 60 Hz notch filter removes spectral energy that contributes importantly to the infant ABR resulting in smaller ABR amplitude, and the notch filter may also distort latency measurements. Consequently, the notch filter should not be enabled during pediatric ABR recordings.

Finally, how many stimulus presentations (or sweeps through the analysis time) are required for pediatric ABR measurement? There is no absolute answer to this question. A common but ill-advised clinical practice is to consistently record (or average) ABRs with a fixed number of stimuli, for example, 2000. Asked why that number of stimulus repetitions was used, clinicians tend to justify the selection with remarks such as, "That's what is recommended in the equipment manual," or "That's what I was taught in graduate school." In fact, the answer to the question, "How many stimulus presentations are required in pediatric ABR measurement?" is best answered with the statement: Whatever number produces an adequate signal-to-noise ratio (SNR), assuming that the ABR is the signal and all other electrical and muscle activity is noise. As a rule, an adequate SNR is defined as ABR wave amplitudes that are two times larger than ongoing background noise within the recording (a SNR of 2:1). When the signal is large and/or noise is small, then less signal averaging and fewer stimulus presentations are required. The best example of that scenario is an ABR elicited with a high intensity stimulus and recorded from a normal hearing and very quiet child. Under these essentially ideal measurement conditions, the ABR is usually clearly observed after as few as 200 to 300 stimulus presentations. Ongoing signal averaging for many more stimulus presentations (like 2000) is simply a waste of valuable test time. At the other extreme, when an ABR is elicited with a stimulus intensity that is near threshold, and recorded from a person who is not quiet or in an electrically noisy area, then as many as 2000 stimuli or more may be needed to achieve an adequate SNR.

Bone Conduction Click-Elicited ABR Measurement

Rationale and Indications

In the late 1970s, within a few years after the ABR was introduced as a clinical procedure, papers appeared describing the clinical application of ABRs evoked with click stimuli delivered to the mastoid via bone conduction (see Hall, 2007, for review). Since then, over 30 years of clinical experience has confirmed the technical feasibility and clinical value of bone conduction ABRs, using commercially available auditory evoked response instrumentation. Bone conduction ABR measurements offer three main clinical advantages. First, the magnitude of an air-bone gap as determined by behavioral pure tone audiometry can be estimated with acceptable accuracy by bone conduction ABR findings. Second, bone conduction ABRs can be recorded from persons of all ages, including newborn infants and other young children who for a variety of reasons cannot be evaluated via behavioral audiometry. And, perhaps most important, as an electrophysiological measure that includes a component (wave I) that reflects activity of the eighth (auditory) cranial nerve on the side of the stimulus, bone conduction ABR permits confident ear-specific documentation of auditory function, usually without the clinical concerns or limitations associated with masking of the nontest ear. ABR measurement with bone conduction stimulation is an important procedure within the pediatric diagnostic test battery, and should be performed in any patient who is at risk for middle ear dysfunction by history and patients with medical or other audiologic evidence of middle ear dysfunction.

A Practical Bone Conduction ABR Protocol

The protocol described already for air conduction click-evoked ABR measurement can be modified for recording bone conduction ABRs. Selected parameters are critical for successful measurement of bone conduction ABRs, as summarized in Table 5–6. The initial, and obviously important, parameter in the test protocol is the use of a bone oscillator as the transducer for delivering stimuli to the skull. Existing bone oscillators (e.g., Radioear B-70) designed over 50 years ago for delivery of steady state (sinusoid) stimuli in bone conduction pure tone audiometry are not well suited for transduction of the transient stimuli (clicks) required for elicitation of ABRs. Because the bone oscillator is less effective for converting very short (0.1 ms) electrical signals to vibrations, the maximum stimulus intensity output for bone oscillators is limited to about 45 to 50 dB nHL. Also, the frequency response of the bone oscillator is dominated by energy in the lower audiometric frequencies and relatively reduced in the high frequencies (in comparison to air conduction trans-

Table 5–6. Protocol for bone conduction ABR measurement

Parameter	*Selection*	*Comment*
Stimulus Parameters		
Bone oscillator	B-70 or B-71	Dedicated for ABR measurement
Type	Click	Tone bursts can also be used
Duration	0.1 ms (100 μs)	
Polarity	Alternating	To minimize stimulus artifact
Rate	11.1/sec	Slower if wave I is not clear
Intensity	Variable	Maximum is about 50 dB nHL
Repetitions	Variable	Dependent on signal-to-noise ratio
Masking	Sometimes	Not needed if wave I is present
Mode	Monaural	Always delivered to mastoid
Acquisition Parameters		
Electrodes		
Non-inverting	Fz	High forehead preferred vs. vertex
Inverting	Ai	Ipsilateral earlobe or TIPtrode; two channel electrode array (Fz-Ai and Fz-A2) with contralateral inverting electrode helps to identify wave I (see Figure 5–1)
Ground	Fpz	Low forehead is convenient
Filters		
HP (high pass)	30 Hz	Bone conduction ABR contains substantial low frequency energy
LP (low pass)	1500 or 2000 Hz	
Notch	None	Notch filter reduces response energy
Amplification	× 100,000	
Analysis Time	15 ms	
Pre-stimulus baseline	–1 ms	Inspection of pre-stimulus time to estimate background noise
Sweeps (# stimuli)	Variable	Dependent on signal-to-noise ratio

ducers). The metal headband used to couple the typical bone oscillator to the head was not designed to fit the small heads of infants and young children, nor for a comfortable placement suitable for extended test times in sleeping infants. Unfortunately, a bone oscillator designed specifically for ABR measurement is not on the market. Clinical investigation confirms that the bone oscillator produces adequate energy within the 2000 to 3000 Hz region for activation of the ABR. However, the frequency response is not flat but, rather, characterized by peaks and valleys within that frequency range.

A logical and practical two-part question at this juncture is: "How can the B-70 bone oscillator be coupled to the small head of an infant, and where should the oscillator be located?" To answer the first part of the question, one option is to hold the bone oscillator against the skull with firm pressure. First of all, the bone oscillator should be placed in a posterior location on the temporal bone at a distance from the earlobe electrode (Figure 5–2A), or a TIPtrode electrode, rather than on the mastoid immediately behind the pinna. For infants with small heads, it is helpful to place a folded towel or a sponge between the headband and the infant's skull, essentially increasing the size of the head to match the size of the headband (Figure 5–2B). Or the bone oscillator can be coupled to the infant head by means of a soft headband with pressure adjusted with a Velcro strap. Clinical research confirms that click stimulation with a handheld bone oscillator is associated with a frequency response equivalent to that of a bone oscillator held with the conventional metal band. Importantly, the tester should avoid grasping the bone oscillator directly, as damping of the vibrations will result in a significant loss of energy and corresponding stimulus intensity. Instead, as illustrated in Figure 5–2C, the tester should hold the headband with the concave surface of the bone oscillator placed against the skull.

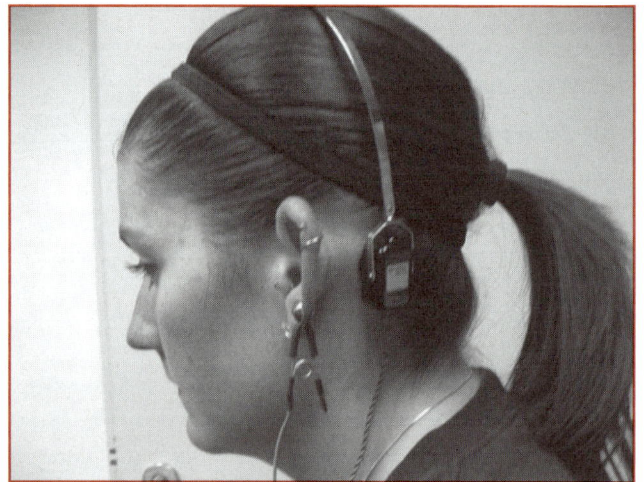

A

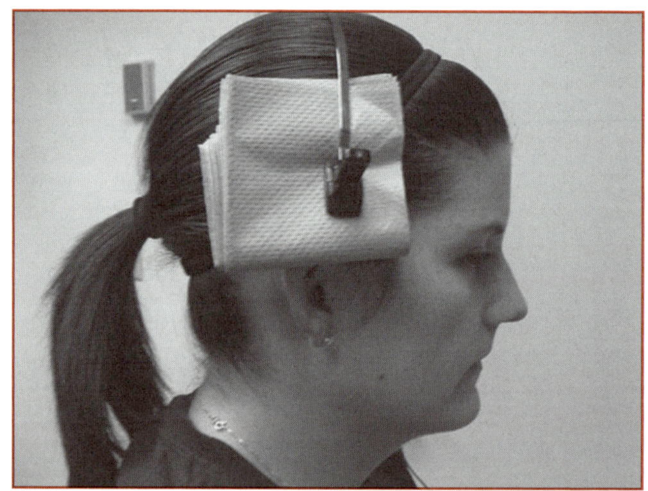

B

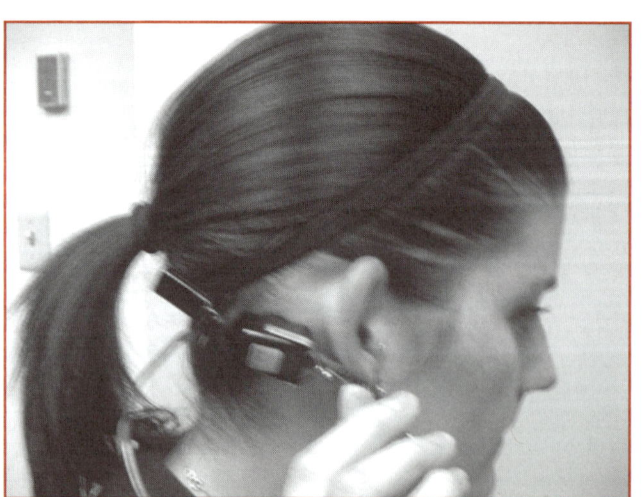

C

FIGURE 5–2. Photograph of techniques for coupling a B-70 bone oscillator to the head of an infant in pediatric ABR measurement, including placing the bone oscillator posterior on the temporal bone at a distance from the earlobe electrode (**A**), inserting padding (e.g., folded towel or a sponge) between the bone oscillator headband and the skull to achieve appropriate pressure (**B**), and handholding the oscillator against the head (**C**).

The simple answer to the question about where the bone oscillator should be located is "the temporal bone." In terms of effectiveness of stimulation, the optimal location for the bone oscillator is probably the mastoid region of the temporal bone. However, a mastoid placement of the bone oscillator often creates unacceptable amounts of stimulus (electromagnetic) artifact when the inverting electrode is located nearby and, especially, on the mastoid bone. The logical solution to the problem of excessive stimulus artifact in bone conduction ABR measurement is to separate the bone oscillator and inverting electrode as much as possible. A simple strategy for increasing the distance between the source of electromagnetic energy and the recording electrode is to rely on an earlobe or even an ear canal (e.g., TIPtrode electrode location) with the bone oscillator pressed to the head in a more posterior and superior location on the temporal bone (refer again to Figure 5–2A) than is customary for bone conduction audiometry, avoiding hair as much as possible. An added advantage of an earlobe or ear canal inverting electrode versus a mastoid site is the enhancement (by about 30%) of the wave I component of the ABR.

We have some good news about masking in bone conduction ABR measurement. It's rarely needed. The sutures of the skull are not entirely fused for children under the age of about 1 year. That is, the temporal bone is not fused to adjacent parietal, frontal, and occipital bones, and the skull base. Consequently, for infants there is minimal concern that bone conduction stimulation to one mastoid will cross over via the skull to the opposite site of the head and then activate the cochlea of the nontest ear. Also, as noted elsewhere in this chapter, wave I of the ABR reflects compound action potentials from fibers within the distal end of the eighth (auditory) cranial nerve. When detected with an inverting electrode near or on the ear (technically the mastoid) that is being stimulated, the presence of a reliable wave I confirms ear-specific ABR measurement. Of course, if the clinician has unequivocal evidence that the ABR is arising from stimulation of the test ear, then there's no need for masking of the nontest ear.

Alternating stimulus polarity is optimal for bone conduction ABR measurement. This is in contrast to the recommendation of rarefaction stimulus polarity in the test protocol for air conduction ABR measurement. Although rarefaction polarity stimuli are typically most effective for elicitation of the ABR, an alternative polarity approach is necessary to minimize the stimulus artifact associated with the close proximity of the bone oscillator and the inverting electrode. With alternating polarity stimulation, the signal averaging of the ongoing EEG activity during ABR measurement largely "cancels out" the alternating positive voltage and negative voltage electrical artifact that is detected by the inverting electrode, amplified, and processed by the evoked response system. Theoretically, amplitude of the ABR wave I component would be larger with rarefaction polarity stimulation. Clearly, for bone conduction ABR enhancement of wave I amplitude is a high priority. This advantage is usually offset by problems with stimulus artifact that interfere with confident identification of the ABR wave I. Another potential disadvantage of reliance on alternating polarity stimulation is the resulting absence of a cochlear microphonic (CM) response, and the possible failure to identify auditory neuropathy. However, because bone conduction ABR measurement is inevitably preceded by recordings of the ABR elicited with air conduction click stimuli, auditory neuropathy will already be either identified or ruled out before bone conduction ABR measurement begins. The amplitude of the ABR wave I component is affected by stimulus rate. As a rule, amplitude of wave I gradually decreases as stimulus rate is increased and, conversely, wave I amplitude will be enhanced by slower stimulus presentation rates. Generally, a reliable ABR wave I is clearly present with bone conduction stimulation at a rate of 11.1/second or 21.1/second. However, if the ABR wave I component is indistinct or not apparent at that rate, repeat measurement at a slower rate is indicated.

Before ABRs are recorded clinically with bone conduction stimulation, stimulus intensity in dB nHL must first be defined by the collection of behavioral thresholds from a small sample of normal hearers, as described above. Using a bone oscillator supplied by the manufacturer of the evoked response system (with proper impedance and other characteristics) and dedicated only to

ABR measurement, behavioral thresholds are obtained for click stimuli. In acquiring normative data for bone conduction thresholds, it's very important to simulate as closely as possible actual ABR measurement conditions. For example, the stimulus rate to be used in ABR measurement should be used also in collecting normative data for intensity level (i.e., defining 0 dB nHL). Normal thresholds should be measured with bone conduction stimulation in the same test environment(s) where pediatric ABR measurements will be made clinically (e.g., the NICU, the OR, and the audiology clinic). And, importantly, behavioral thresholds for bone conduction stimulation should be measured from normal hearing adults with insert earphones within each ear canal because bone conduction ABRs are likely to be recorded from children with insert earphones in place. What about the occlusion effect? you might ask. As you define normal thresholds for bone conduction stimuli, you will be assuring that normal subjects and patients alike benefit from the occlusion effect. Another important benefit of bone conduction ABR measurement in the occluded condition is the minimization of the influence of ambient noise on findings. That is, the insert earphones reduce the masking via air conducted ambient noise of bone conduction stimulation.

Acquisition parameters are essentially unchanged for bone conduction versus air conduction ABR measurement. As already noted, to minimize stimulus artifact during bone conduction ABR measurement the inverting electrode is best placed either on the earlobe or within the ear canal, and not on the mastoid bone. Bone conduction stimulation, particularly in children, elicits an ABR that is dominated by low frequency energy. Therefore, the high pass filter setting should be relatively low, such as 30 Hz or at most 75 or 100 Hz. Finally, because the maximum intensity level for bone conduction stimulation is only 45 to 50 dB nHL, response amplitude is typically modest and waves I and V are found within the latency region expected for air conduction stimulation at a low to moderate intensity level. Increasing the number of stimulus presentations (sweeps), and the associated signal averaging, may be necessary for confident detection of the bone conduction ABR in the presence of ongoing electrical and myogenic noise.

Frequency-Specific (Tone Burst) ABR Measurement

Rationale

Frequency-specific estimation of auditory thresholds, that is, an "electrophysiological audiogram," is essential for the initial hearing aid fitting of infants and young children who cannot be completely evaluated with pure tone audiometry. Minimally, reliable information on auditory thresholds is required for low (around 500 Hz) and high (around 4000 Hz) frequencies, and for each ear. Every attempt should also be made to estimate auditory threshold of a signal near the center of the speech frequency region, such as 1000 Hz, to permit definition of the configuration of the hearing loss. Frequency-specific estimation of auditory thresholds with ABR is strongly endorsed and recommended by peer-reviewed guidelines developed by state and national groups (e.g., JCIH). There is ample clinical evidence that the threshold estimation for ABRs elicited with click stimulation is woefully inadequate for accurate hearing aid fittings in infants and young children.

Limitations of click-evoked ABR findings for defining an audiogram are highlighted graphically in Figure 5–3. Superimposed on the audiogram of familiar sounds are three hearing loss configurations. The thick vertical line at 3000 Hz represents the region of the audiogram that contributes most to the generation of a click-evoked ABR. A child with the audiogram configuration indicated by the dashed line and labeled A, a significant hearing loss in the speech frequency region with a rising configuration, would be expected to yield a normal click-evoked ABR due to the relatively good hearing within the high frequency region. In other words, the hearing loss would go undetected if only a click-evoked ABR were recorded. However, the hearing loss would most certainly be identified and threshold determined by an ABR evoked with a low frequency tone burst (e.g., 500 Hz). The configuration would be adequately defined by threshold estimations also for ABRs elicited by 1000, 2000, and 4000 Hz tone burst stimuli. A child with the audiogram configuration indicated by the dotted line and labeled B would also be expected to yield a normal click-evoked ABR due the relatively good hearing in the 3000 Hz region, even though

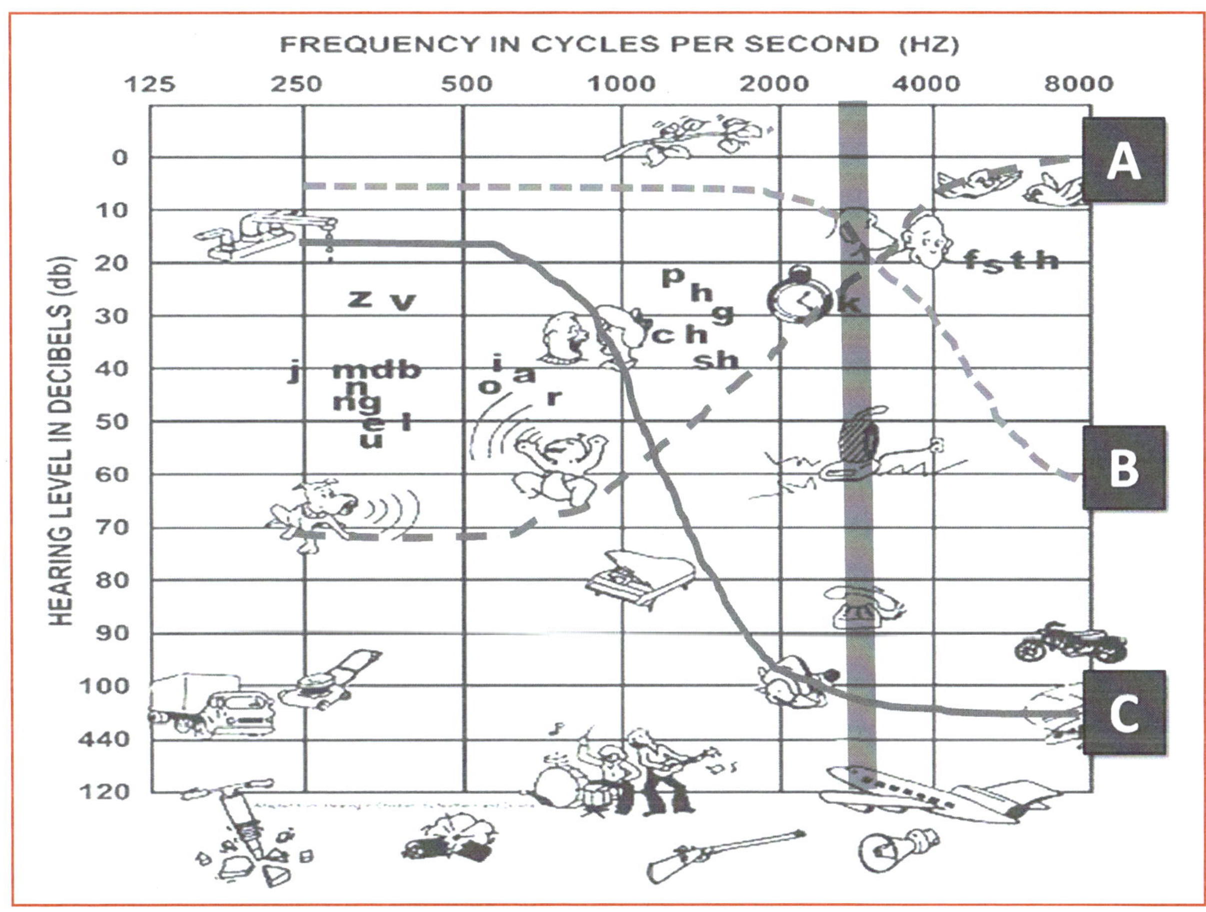

FIGURE 5–3. Audiogram of familiar sounds, with illustration of audiogram configurations associated with normal and abnormal click-evoked ABR recordings. Vertical line at 3000 Hz indicates the area primarily represented by a click-evoked ABR threshold.

there is a hearing loss for higher frequencies. Decreased hearing sensitivity for frequencies in the 4000 Hz region can, of course, affect speech perception (especially for consonant sounds), and consequently speech and language acquisition. In this case, threshold estimations based on ABRs elicited with 500 and/or 1000 Hz tone burst stimulation would confirm normal low frequency hearing sensitivity, whereas a 4000 Hz tone burst ABR would document the high frequency hearing loss. Finally, a child with the precipitous high frequency hearing loss indicated by the solid line (audiogram C) would probably not have a click-evoked ABR, even at maximum stimulus intensity limits. Hearing loss in the 2000 to 3000 Hz region, important for activation of the click-evoked ABR, exceeds maximum click stimulus intensity levels (90 to 95 dB HL). It would, however, be misleading and really inaccurate to describe the hearing loss as simply "profound," as hearing sensitivity is within normal limits for much of the speech frequency region. A hearing aid fitting that assumes this patient has a profound hearing loss at all speech frequencies would be inappropriate at best, most likely rejected by the child, and would create a risk of sound-induced cochlear damage. In summary, frequency-specific hearing threshold information is essential in pediatric diagnostic audiologic assessment, and only available from ABRs recorded with tone burst stimulation and not click stimuli.

A Practical Tone Burst ABR Protocol

An evidence-based and clinically proven test protocol for frequency-specific ABR measurement is summarized in Table 5–7. Estimation of auditory thresholds with ABRs elicited by multiple tone burst stimulation might seem daunting initially,

Table 5–7. A protocol used for measurement of frequency-specific ABRs

Parameters	*Suggestions*	*Comments*
Stimulus Parameters		
Transducer	Insert	Insert earphones offer many advantages in clinical ABR measurement, especially with infants and young children, as delineated in Table 5–3.
Polarity	Alternating	Instead of the usual rarefaction polarity, alternating polarity stimuli can be used to minimize the possibility of a frequency-following type response.
Ramping	Blackman	Ramping refers to how the rise/fall portions of the tone burst are shaped. Some nonlinear ramping or windowing techniques reduce spectral splatter and increase frequency specificity of tone burst stimulation. Blackman windowing is the best, and most current AER systems include it in their stimulus package.
Duration	Variable	The rise/fall and plateau times for the tone burst stimuli vary depending on the frequency. As a rule, it's desirable to use longer times for lower frequencies so as to include more cycles to increase the chance that the stimulus sounds like the desired frequency, and not a click. However, as discussed in this section of the chapter, the use of a very brief (0.5 cycles or 2 ms) 250 Hz tone burst will generate a more well-formed and distinct ABR, albeit not quite as frequency specific (an energy band within the frequency range of 100 to 600 Hz). The most common approach for signal duration is to use 2 cycles rise time, 0 cycle plateau, and 2 cycles fall time or, in milliseconds (ms): • 500 Hz: 4 ms rise/fall and 0 ms plateau • 1000 Hz: 2 ms rise/fall and 0 ms plateau • 2000 Hz: 1 ms rise/fall and 0 ms plateau • 4000 Hz: 0.5 ms rise/fall and 0 ms plateau
Intensity	Variable	Keep in mind that the intensity levels on the screen for your ABR system will usually not be defined in dB nHL, as they are for a click. More often, the values are in dB SPL. That is, 95 dB may be selected, but the intensity range for the tone burst frequency may go as high as 115 dB. Always obtain behavioral threshold data for each tone burst stimulus to be used for ABR recording (with the earphones specific to the evoked response system and in the room where ABRs will be recorded), and then develop biologic normative data for tone burst intensity. For example, if the maximum dial setting for a 500 Hz tone burst is 115 dB, but normal subjects have an average threshold of 30 dB for this stimulus, then at 115 dB on the dial the intensity level is really 85 dB nHL (referenced to the normal behavioral threshold for the stimulus). With most evoked response systems, these "correction factors" can be incorporated into the intensities displayed on the screen so that all intensity values are in dB nHL according to clinic normative data. It is then advisable to actually record ABRs for this 500 Hz stimulus from a few of these normal hearing subjects to estimate the lowest intensity level that produces an observable and reliable ABR wave V.

Table 5–7. *continued*

Parameters	*Suggestions*	*Comments*
Acquisition Parameters		
Electrode sites	Fz-Ai	Noninverting (positive) electrode is located in the midline on the high forehead (Fz) and the inverting electrode is located on the earlobe ipsilateral to the stimulus ear (Ai). With an ear-clip electrode design, the earlobe electrode is easily applied, impedance is low, and the electrode is removed from the mastoid region. The earlobe electrode records a larger wave I than the mastoid electrode, and is associated with less stimulus artifact in bone conduction ABR recordings. The ground electrode can be located on the low forehead (Fpz) or the contralateral earlobe (limits recordings to a single channel).
Filter settings	30 to 3000 Hz	A low frequency cutoff for the high pass filter (e.g., 30 Hz) is very important because the tone burst ABR is dominated by low frequency energy, especially in infants.
Analysis time	15 to 20 ms	For click signals and higher frequency tone burst signals, an analysis time of 15 ms is adequate to encompass the wave V component even under conditions associated with delayed wave V latency, e.g., low signal intensity level, hearing loss, very young age (immaturity of the auditory pathways). For tone burst signals of 1000 Hz and below, a 20 ms analysis time is recommended.
Sweeps	Variable	The number of sweeps (stimulus repetitions or number of signal averages for an ABR recording) is dependent on the signal-to-noise ratio. When the signal (ABR amplitude) is larger (e.g., at a high intensity level with a normal hearing patient) and/or when background noise is low (e.g., the patient is sedated or anesthetized), then relatively fewer stimulus repetitions are needed. On the other hand, when ABR amplitude is smaller (e.g., at lower signal intensity levels and/or in a patient with hearing loss) and noise is greater (a restless, unsedated child), more signal averaging (more stimulus repetitions) will be needed. As a rule, less stimulus repetitions are required for the second (replication) ABR run when the goal is to simply verify that the response is reliable (and not just artifact).

Note. The conventional ABR protocol for air conduction click signals must be modified to successfully record ABRs for tone burst signals. The main differences between protocols for click versus tone burst ABRs are noted under comments.

but reliance on an appropriate test protocol is a big step toward successfully performing this valuable clinical procedure. Some of the parameters in the test protocol for recording frequency-specific ABRs are found also in the test protocol for click-evoked ABR measurement, reviewed above. For example, the strong argument for delivering click stimuli to the ears with insert earphones, especially in pediatric ABR measurement, applies also to tone burst stimulation. And the careful verification with adult normative data of stimulus intensity for different tone burst stimuli at octave frequencies (e.g., 500 to 4000 Hz) follows the process as described above for click stimulation. Tone burst ABRs can certainly be elicited with single polarity stimuli (rarefaction or condensation), but for lower frequency stimulation (500 Hz) artifact or non-ABR activity in the waveform is minimized by the use of alternating stimulus polarity.

The rationale for using tone burst stimulus duration components of 2 cycles of rise time, 2 cycles of fall time, and no (0 cycles) plateau dates back to recommendations of Dr. Hallowell Davis (the "Father of Auditory Evoked Responses") in the 1970s. By establishing duration in terms of the same number of cycles, rather than equal milliseconds (for rise, fall, and plateau), the amount of energy is essentially equivalent for each tone burst frequency. The number of cycles per millisecond increases predictably from low to high frequency tone burst stimuli. For example, in a time period of 2 ms there is a single (1) cycle for a 500 Hz stimulus yet in the same 2 ms time period there are 4 cycles for a 4000 Hz tone burst.

The band pass filter settings for tone burst ABR measurement of infants and young children should extend down to a high pass cutoff of 30 Hz, or at most 75 Hz. As noted earlier, the spectrum of the infant ABR is dominated by low frequency energy whether the ABR is elicited with click or tone burst stimuli. The relative contribution of low frequency energy to the infant ABR is increased when the ABR is evoked with tone burst stimuli. The major feature of an ABR evoked by low frequency tone burst, particularly at low intensity levels (near threshold), that permits detection of the response is a long negative wave that follows the ABR wave V component. Low frequency energy in the ABR contributes to this broad negative wave. The recommendation to avoid the inclusion of a 60 Hz notch filter in infant ABR measurement is also made because of the predominance of low frequency energy, and the likelihood that energy in the ABR contributing to detection of the response will be removed by the filter. An extended analysis time is a critical parameter for successful tone burst ABR measurement. Latency of wave V and the following trough is encompassed within a 15 ms analysis time for click-evoked ABRs, even under conditions that tend to prolong ABR latency values (e.g., low intensity level, neurological immaturity, conductive hearing loss). However, a longer analysis time is necessary for detection in infants and young children of the important components of the ABR elicited by mid- and low frequency tone burst stimuli. ABR latency increases as tone burst frequency decreases because time is consumed while the stimulus travels from the regions of the cochlea near the base toward lower frequency regions nearer the apex. The time required for a traveling wave to go from the base to the apex of the cochlea is estimated at approximately 5 ms. Correspondingly, for a high intensity stimulus (e.g., 85 to 90 dB nHL) the normal latency of ABR wave V is about 5.5 ms for click stimulation and 8 to 10 ms for a 500 Hz tone burst. An analysis time of 15 ms is adequate for click stimuli and tone burst stimuli of 4000 and 2000 Hz. However, analysis time should be extended to 20 ms for lower tone burst frequencies (e.g., 1000 and 500 Hz). As just noted, confident detection of the wave V component of the ABR elicited by low frequency tone bursts is based on not only the appearance of the wave V peak but also the extended trough or negative-going wave after wave V. Indeed, as reviewed below the analysis of ABR waveforms for low frequency tone burst stimulation is often entirely dependent on the detection of the extended negative-going wave, rather than a peak in the waveform.

Analysis and Interpretation

Introduction

In comparison to the technique required to record a neurodiagnostic ABR from an adult patient (e.g., placement of electrodes and transducers, selection of the appropriate protocol and measurement parameters), there are certainly many similarities in recording pediatric ABRs for diagnostic purposes, including estimation of auditory thresholds. However, there are at least three distinct challenges associated only with ABR measurement in children. First, test time is inevitably a major factor affecting the success of ABR measurement and the likelihood of obtaining the results needed for timely and appropriate management. The clinician must take any and all possible steps to make the best use of test time, always guided by the question: "If the child wakes within the next few minutes, what information is essential for management decisions?" In addition, frequency-specific estimation of auditory thresholds may entail many ABR recordings. For example, assuming threshold information is needed for four different frequencies in each ear, and repeated waveforms will be recorded at multiple intensity levels, more than 50 separate "runs" will be performed in the process of the ABR session. Even if one minute of test time were consumed for each run, the total test session could exceed one hour. Clearly, steps must be taken to reduce test time without sacrificing the quality of findings.

Second, even though optimal measurement conditions are not certain for pediatric ABRs, they are actually more important than for adult ABRs. Most adult patients will, upon request, remain quiet for the time required for completion of a neurodiagnostic ABR performed at a high intensity level with less concerns about detecting a small signal amid background noise. Obviously, infants and young children, particularly those who are difficult to test, will not remain adequately quiet and physically immobile throughout a 30 to 45 minute period simply because we want them to. Special steps must be taken to ensure that test conditions are adequate, and the child is sleeping.

Finally, the results of the ABR will contribute to early intervention for a hearing loss that, without management, will lead to communicative disorders that might remain with the child for a lifetime. There are diagnostic alternatives to a neurodiagnostic ABR in an adult, such as a CT or MRI scan, whereas initial management of the child with hearing impairment is dependent entirely on the results of the electrophysiological diagnosis of hearing loss and estimation of auditory thresholds.

Analysis and interpretation of pediatric ABR waveforms and findings are quite straightforward and simple if three important assumptions are met. First, ABRs are recorded with an evidence-based and *clinically proven test protocol*. The stimulus and acquisition parameters described above (for air conduction and bone conduction click-evoked ABRs and tone burst evoked ABRs) are the product of over 30 years of clinical research and experience. Perhaps the best example of the development of an effective ABR test protocol during this time period is the rather dramatic decrease in failure (refer) rates for infant hearing screening with ABR technology. In the early years of screening with ABR of infants at risk for hearing loss—up to the mid-1980s—reported failure rates of 10 to 25% were not uncommon, and the failure rates described in selected papers were as high as 50% (see Hall, 1992, for review). That is, half of the babies screened (usually at 35 dB nHL) yielded no reliable ABR wave V. As each of the ABR test parameters was systematically and critically evaluated in formal studies or altered in a trial-and-error fashion by clinicians in an attempt to improve ABR detection, the infant hearing refer rate consistently decreased. With the ABR test protocols described herein, infant hearing screening refer rates are as low as 5 to 6% for at-risk children, and below 2% for well babies with no risk factor for hearing loss. Consistent success in pediatric ABR measurement will be greatly enhanced by strict adherence to these or other evidence-based protocols, and by the immediately adaptive modification of parameters during ABR recording as indicated by patient status (e.g., quiet versus active, normal hearing versus hearing impaired) and measurement conditions (like electrical noise, ambient acoustic noise).

Second, in pediatric ABR measurement it is assumed that the child is in a quiet *physical state* and *state of arousal*. A child in deep sleep, either natural or induced by sedation or anesthesia, is optimal. ABR amplitude, even for the normally robust wave V, is only one half of a millionth of a volt (0.5 μV) under the best of test circumstances, that is, when the ABR is evoked with a high intensity click stimulus from a neurologically mature patient (>18 months old) with normal hearing sensitivity and normal brainstem function. Under other test conditions, ABR wave V may be considerably smaller in amplitude and difficult to detect with confidence. Complicating matters further, muscle and electrical artifact during ABR recording may be more than 100 to 1000 times larger in amplitude than the largest component within the waveform. Movement interference will always complicate ABR measurement, analysis, and interpretation. Excessive ongoing muscle artifact may make it impossible to detect any ABR activity, rendering the findings invalid and not useful clinically. If the two assumptions are met, an optimal protocol and optimal test conditions, then even a neophyte to pediatric ABR measurement (or a graduate audiology student enrolled in an auditory evoked response course) will have little difficulty recording quality ABR waveforms and confidently analyzing them. On the other hand, if the protocol is flawed (e.g., one of the parameters is inappropriate) and/or the child is producing unacceptable amounts of muscle article, then even an experienced clinical audiologist will encounter serious obstacles in analyzing the ABR waveform and accurately estimating auditory thresholds.

Finally, ABR waveforms must be *reliable*. That is, the major ABR waves, or at least wave V, in two separately averaged waveforms (two runs) recorded with the same test parameters must be very similar. With some auditory evoked response systems, it's possible to derive a measure of correlation or consistency of ABR recordings by comparing waveforms evoked during the same averaging run for rarefaction versus condensation stimuli presented as alternating polarity stimuli. Waveform repeatability or reliability is one major factor contributing to the clinical feasibility, and the early clinical appeal, of the ABR. Under optimal test conditions, two superimposed ABR waveforms appear almost as a single line. Several mottos are helpful to guide the clinician who is performing ABR assessments clinically, particularly in infants and young children: "If the waveform does not repeat, your ABR assessment is not complete." In other words, a true ABR waveform will be highly repeatable from one run to the next. If the response morphology appears different for the two runs, that is, a wave is present in one run but not another or there is a significant difference in latency of a wave from one run to the next, then the clinician must assume that no response is present. The clinician should then take steps to improve ABR reliability and morphology. The test protocol or conditions must be modified in an attempt to obtain a repeatable ABR. Another simple phrase raises another practical issue in pediatric ABR assessment, particularly for frequency-specific threshold estimation: "If the ABR waveform is not reliable, you could be liable." The implications of this statement are probably clear. Important, really life changing decisions regarding management of hearing loss, including amplification and cochlear implantation, are made on the basis of ABR findings. If these decisions are incorrectly made on the basis of ABR waveforms that are not reliable and, perhaps, an apparent ABR that is not really a response, then the clinician could be exposed to serious legal liability, failure to diagnose a hearing loss.

Steps in ABR Analysis

Once these three assumptions are met, that is, (a) appropriate protocol, (b) quiet patient, and (c) reliable response, waveform analysis continues as follows:

- Major ABR waves (V, III, and/or I) are identified.
- The need for masking the nontest ear is ruled out (see guidelines above and in the discussion of bone conduction ABR measurement).
- Using a cursor, absolute latencies are calculated for major waves. Latency calculations may be more accurate if two reliable waveforms are first digitally added together. The resulting waveform is essentially a product of signal averaging for the combined number of stimuli used to evoke each waveform. Waveform manipulation, such as addition of waveforms, should not be carried out until the data for all the recorded waveforms are first saved. Generally, wave V latency is calculated from the last data point before the most precipitous drop in the waveform, rather than from the peak of the wave (see Hall, 2007, for details).
- Using absolute latencies for major waves, relative ABR latencies (i.e., interwave latencies) are calculated. Minimally, the latency interval between wave I and V is calculated, but additional diagnostic value can be derived from analysis also of the wave I–III and wave III–V latency intervals.
- If amplitude data for ABR waves are also of interest, one cursor is placed on the peak of the wave and a second cursor is placed in the lowest point in the preceding (for wave I and III) or following (for wave V) trough or negative-going portion of the waveform.
- Absolute and relative ABR latencies for a patient are compared to age-appropriate nor-

mative data. Interaural symmetry for latencies is also determined.

These analysis steps should be carried out while ABR measurement is ongoing, rather than after the assessment is completed and the patient is no longer available. For example, calculation and analysis of absolute and interwave latency values for the ABR waveforms elicited initially with high intensity click stimulation can be done while ABRs are recorded for lower intensity levels. There are two main advantages of immediate "on-line" versus delayed "off-line" ABR data analysis. As noted in the introduction to this section, the findings of the click-elicited ABR recordings will often contribute to decisions regarding subsequent ABR recordings. That is, the outcome of click ABR recordings will determine what comes next in the ABR assessment (e.g., bone conduction measurement) or, perhaps, what other audiologic procedures should be performed (e.g., OAEs or tympanometry). Also, with on-line ABR analysis serious measurement problems can be detected early and corrected while the patient remains "hooked up." Identification of problems affecting ABR analysis and interpretation after the ABR assessment is finished and the patient has left the clinic is unacceptable clinical practice. Failure to recognize and adequately address measurement problems when the ABR is recorded, under sedation or anesthesia, and detection of the problems later are likely to create a serious dilemma for the clinician, that is, inadequate information to make appropriate and timely management decision versus the risk and financial cost associated with another ABR assessment under sedation or anesthesia.

Analyses of ABR Waveforms for Air Conduction Click Stimulation

Analyses of ABRs elicited with air conduction click stimulation depend largely on calculation and interpretation of latency data. Representative ABR waveforms elicited with click stimuli, and the corresponding test protocol, are illustrated in Figures 5–4A and B. Test time documented by the evoked response instrumentation is shown in Figure 5–4B, along with ABR test parameters. Notice that the time required to record two clear and reliable ABR waveforms for the high intensity level (85 dB nHL) was less than a minute.

As illustrated in Figure 5–5, analysis of click ABR latency values for several intensity levels quickly allows for the differentiation between normal auditory function somewhere in the high frequency region, a conductive hearing loss, a sensory hearing loss, neural dysfunction, and the ABR pattern suggesting auditory neuropathy.

Decisions based on cursory inspection and the analysis of ABR waveforms initially evoked with click stimuli are summarized in Table 5–8. Information from the click-evoked ABR can contribute to more efficient use of precious test time, and can increase the likelihood of an accurate and prompt diagnosis of auditory dysfunction. Estimation of mild or moderate hearing loss can be accomplished with either frequency-specific ABR techniques or with auditory steady-state response (ASSR). However, if there is no click-evoked ABR at maximum signal intensity levels (usually 95 to 100 dB nHL) and/or an ABR is identified only at maximum click intensity levels but not consistently for tone burst stimulation at maximum intensity levels, then ASSR measurement is advised in an attempt to estimate actual auditory thresholds for persons with severe to profound hearing loss. In a small but important proportion of children, the ABR will not be recorded due to severe hearing loss (>80 dB HL), yet auditory thresholds in the region of 80 to 120 dB HL can be estimated with the ASSR. The ASSR is discussed in detail in the next chapter (Chapter 6). Of course, some children with profound hearing loss will have no evidence of an ABR or an ASSR, even for stimulation at intensity levels as high as 120 dB HL. This latter finding in infants can contribute to prompt and conclusive decisions regarding candidacy for cochlear implantation. When auditory evoked response findings point toward cochlear implantation, important clinical and nonclinical (e.g., health insurance) steps can be initiated to expedite the process while the child is undergoing a critical (and in the United States mandatory) period of amplification. This clinical approach, that is, beginning with ABR and then turning to ASSR as needed, is consistent with the view of the 2007 Joint Committee on Infant Hearing (JCIH, 2007) that the ASSR is a supplementary procedure for pediatric diagnosis of hearing loss.

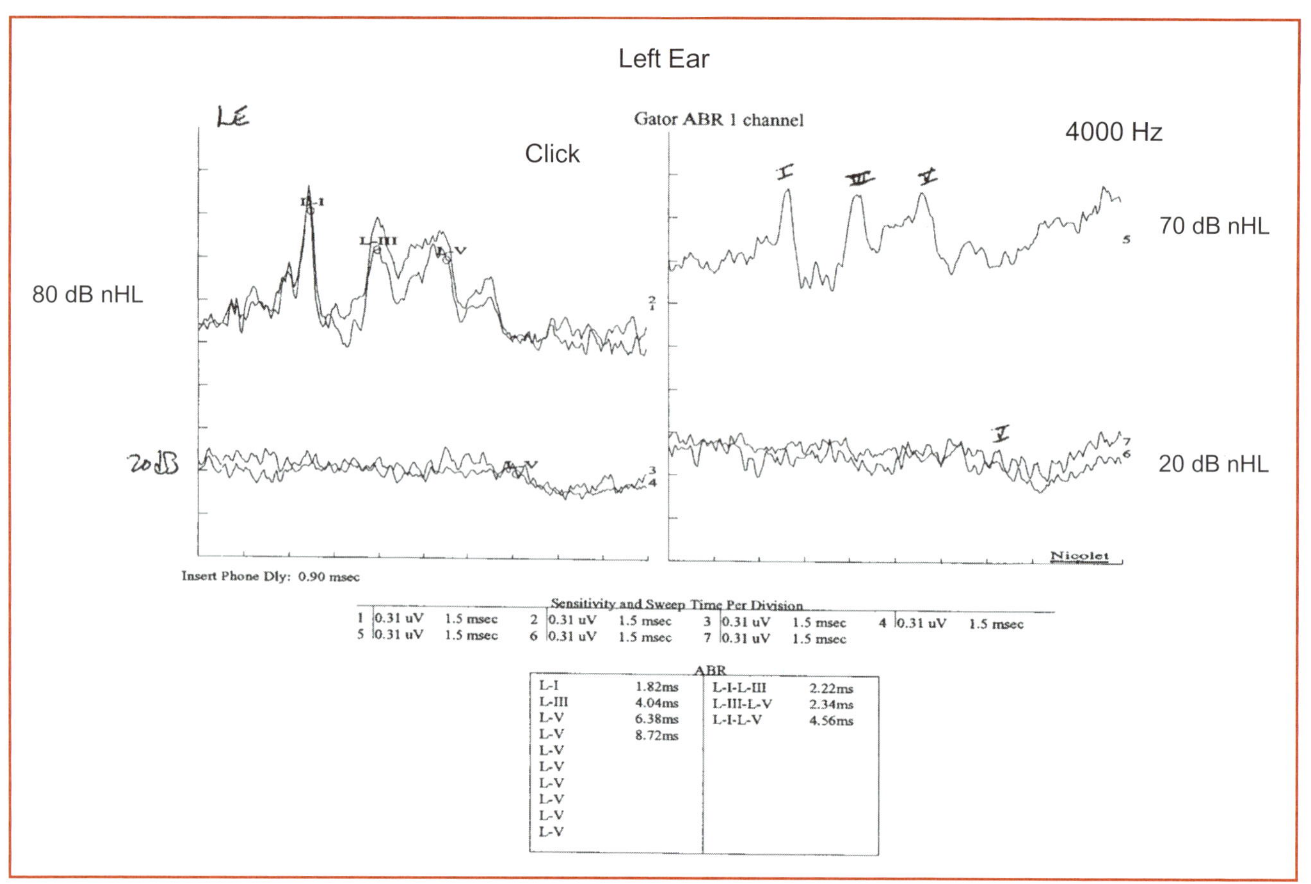

A

UF DEPT. COMMUNICATIVE DISORDERS
SPEECH AND HEARING CLINIC
PO BOX 100174
GAINESVILLE,FL 32610-0174

Gator ABR 1 channel

AMP	Elect	Mode	Sns	Lff	Hff	Notch	Artifact	REM	Remarks
1	Fz-A1	Run	50uV	30	3K	Off	90	1	
2	Fz-A1	Run	50uV	30	3K	Off	90	2	
3	Fz-A1	Run	50uV	30	3K	Off	90	3	
4	Fz-A1	Run	50uV	30	3K	Off	90	4	
5	Fz-A1	Run	50uV	30	3K	Off	90	5	
6	Fz-A1	Run	50uV	30	3K	Off	90	6	
7	Fz-A1	Run	50uV	30	3K	Off	90	7	

ACQ	Comm	Sweep	Time	Delay	Rate	Trigger	Stim
1	A	2000	15ms	-1ms	21.1	Inter	Gated
2	A	2000	15ms	-1ms	21.1	Inter	Gated
3	A	2000	15ms	-1ms	21.1	Inter	Gated
4	A	2000	15ms	-1ms	21.1	Inter	Gated
5	A	2000	15ms	-1ms	21.1	Inter	Gated
6	A	2000	15ms	-1ms	21.1	Inter	Gated
7	A	2000	15ms	-1ms	21.1	Inter	Gated

MISC	Type	Ch#	Accept	Reject	Filter	Fsp/SNR	Date	Time	Add	Sub	Inv	Filter	Smooth
1	Sum	1	386	0	Butter	7.30	06/10/2004	10:22	no	no	no	no	no
2	Sum	1	209	0	Butter	1.88	06/10/2004	10:22	no	no	no	no	no
3	Sum	1	349	0	Butter	0.43	06/10/2004	10:23	no	no	no	no	no
4	Sum	1	676	0	Butter	0.97	06/10/2004	10:23	no	no	no	no	no
5	Sum	1	328	0	Butter	3.96	06/10/2004	10:24	no	no	no	no	no
6	Sum	1	301	0	Butter	0.60	06/10/2004	10:24	no	no	no	no	no
7	Sum	1	453	0	Butter	1.19	06/10/2004	10:25	no	no	no	no	no

STIM	Trans	Type	Pol	Dur	Level	Freq	Pla	Ramp	Env	Noi	NLev	dB	Trans	Type	Pol	Dur	Level	Freq	Pla	Ramp	Env	Noi	NLev	dB
1	Insert	Click	Rar	100us	80					Off		nHL	Insert	Off								Off		nHL
2	Insert	Click	Rar	100us	80					Off		nHL	Insert	Off								Off		nHL
3	Insert	Click	Rar	100us	20					Off		nHL	Insert	Off								Off		nHL
4	Insert	Click	Rar	100us	20					Off		nHL	Insert	Off								Off		nHL
5	Insert	Tone	Alt		100	4KHz	0cy	2	Blk	Off		nHL	Insert	Off								Off		nHL
6	Insert	Tone	Alt		50	4KHz	0cy	2	Blk	Off		nHL	Insert	Off								Off		nHL
7	Insert	Tone	Alt		50	4KHz	0cy	2	Blk	Off		nHL	Insert	Off								Off		nHL

B

FIGURE 5–4. Representative ABR waveforms elicited with click and 4000 Hz stimuli (**A**) and the corresponding test protocol (**B**) used to make the recordings. The arrow in Figure 5-4B indicates the time that elapsed while recording each of the waveforms in Figure 5-4A.

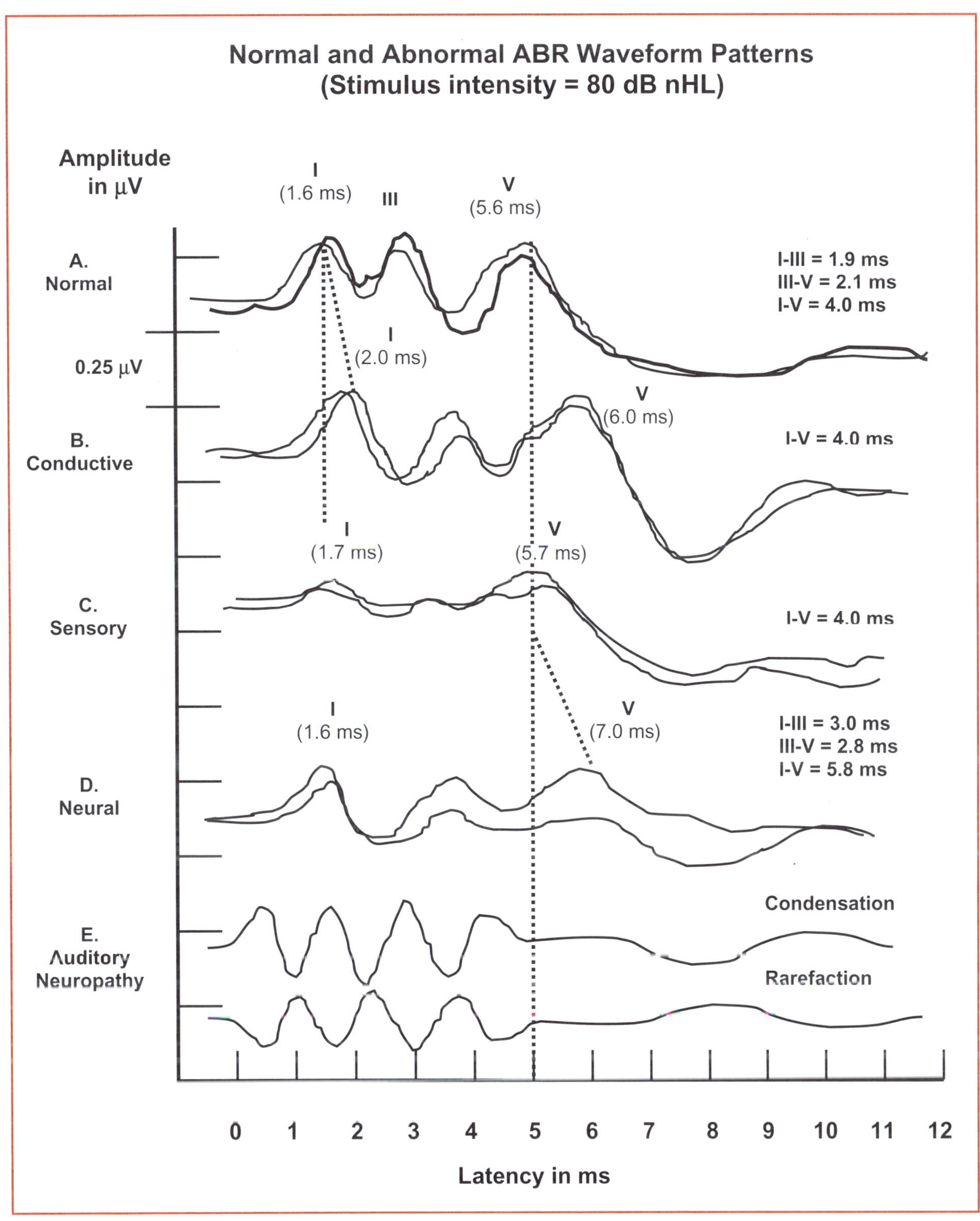

FIGURE 5–5. Illustration of representative ABR waveforms recorded with click stimulation for different types of auditory dysfunction. Basic ABR analyses calculations are shown for the normal (*top*) waveform.

Table 5–8. Clinical decisions made from the initial analysis of an ABR elicited with high- and low-intensity click stimuli

ABR Pattern	
Normal latencies and amplitudes	• Record tone burst ABR and or otoacoustic emissions (OAEs) to confirm normal auditory sensitivity • Begin a frequency-specific ABR recording with a 500 Hz tone burst
Delayed wave I latency at high intensity	• Suspect conductive auditory dysfunction • Prepare to record a bone conduction ABR • Consider tympanometry if it hasn't already been performed • Consider a referral to otolaryngology
Normal for high intensity but abnormal or absent ABR for low intensity	• Suspect a mild or moderate sensory hearing loss • Estimate auditory thresholds with tone burst signals • Verify sensory auditory dysfunction with OAEs
Abnormal or no ABR for high intensity level	• Suspect severe sensory hearing loss • Record an ABR for the maximum click stimulus intensity level • Consider recording an auditory steady-state response (ASSR)
No clear ABR	• Suspect auditory neuropathy (auditory neuropathy spectrum disorder) • Record an ABR with rarefaction and condensation stimulus polarity • Inspect waveforms for evidence of cochlear microphonic (CM) activity • Record OAEs to verify integrity of outer hair cells

Note. The clinical decisions assume that technical explanations for abnormal ABR findings have been ruled out with diligent trouble shooting.

Analyses of ABRs for Bone Conduction Stimulation

The foregoing step-by-step description of the analyses of ABRs elicited with air conduction stimulation applies, of course, also for bone conduction ABRs. There are, however, several additional and critical steps in the analysis of ABRs elicited with bone conduction stimulation. First and foremost is the identification of a wave I component in the ipsilateral electrode array, that is, the ABR recorded with a noninverting electrode in the Fz location and an inverting electrode close to the ear (e.g., on the earlobe). A clear and reliable ABR wave I in the ipsilateral electrode array serves as a biological marker confirming that the bone conduction ABR is ear specific, that is, generated by activation of the test ear. The ABR wave I reflects compound action potentials in the distal (cochlear) end of the eighth cranial (auditory) nerve, in the region of the spiral ganglion. The presence of an ABR wave I with the inverting electrode on the test ear verifies that the test ear was activated by the click stimulus, and solves the so-called masking dilemma (Figure 5–6). The presence of a wave I in the ipsilateral channel also, therefore, eliminates the need for masking of the nontest ear. This statement is true even for patients with serious bilateral conductive hearing loss, the classic example of the masking dilemma.

How can the presence of wave I in a bone conduction ABR recording be confidently identified and confirmed? Two easily implemented strategies are helpful in confirming an ABR wave I following bone conduction stimulation. Once the wave I to V latency interval has been calculated for an ABR elicited with high intensity air conduction click stimulation, this value can be used to estimate the general latency region for the wave I in a bone conduction response (refer again to Figure 5–6). Let's say the wave I–V interval for a high intensity click stimulus is 4.0 ms. As soon as an ABR has been recorded for relatively high intensity (e.g., 40 to 45 dB nHL) bone conduction

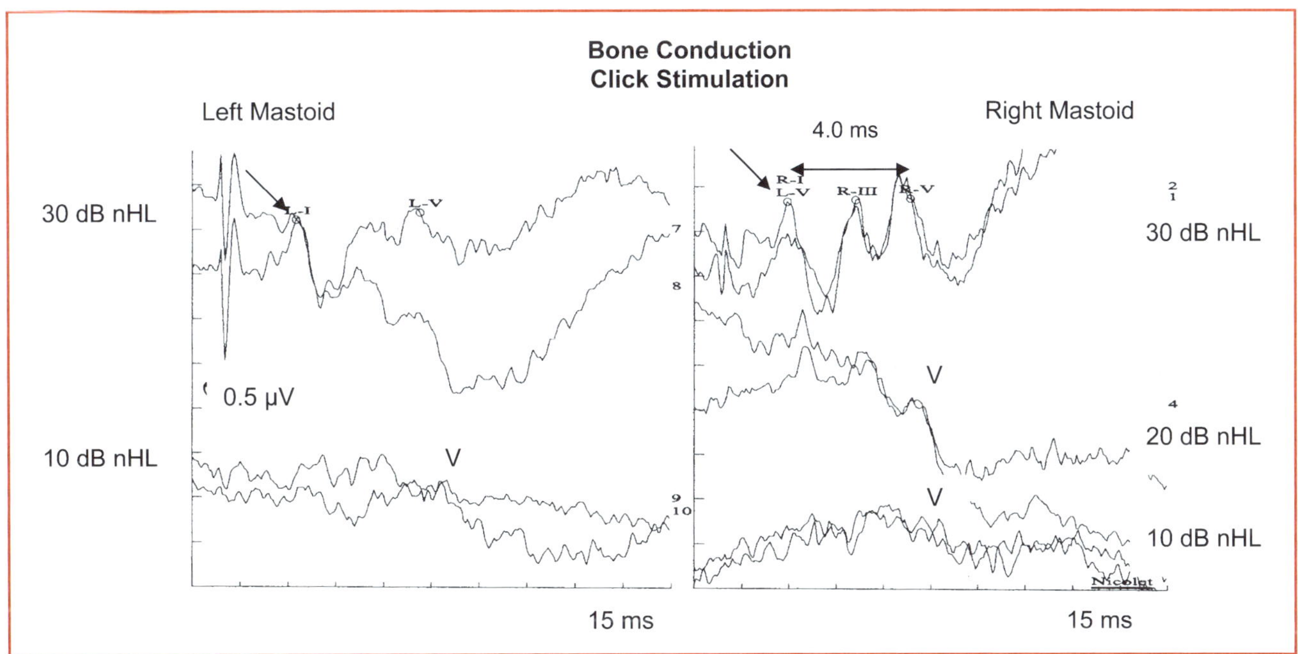

FIGURE 5–6. ABR waveforms evoked with bone conduction stimuli presented to the left and then right mastoid region and recorded with an ipsilateral electrode array. Electrode locations were illustrated in Figure 5–1. The detection of an ABR wave I (*see arrow*) with an electrode on the ear ipsilateral to the bone conduction stimulus confirms activation of the test ear (cochlea) and minimizes the need for masking of the nontest ear. The general latency region for wave I can be estimated by subtracting the wave I–V interval from an ABR elicited with high intensity air conduction click stimulation from the wave V in the ABR elicited by bone conduction stimulation.

stimulation, or even during the ABR recording, place one cursor on the wave V component, and then move a second cursor toward the earlier portion of the waveform until the displayed interval between cursors is 4.0 ms. The wave I component in the bone conduction ABR should be in the same general region. An apparent wave I that is more than 0.5 ms earlier or later than this region is highly suspect until it can be demonstrated in two or three replicated waveforms. Another commonly employed strategy for confirming the presence of wave I in an ABR elicited with bone conduction is to simultaneously record the response with a second (contralateral) electrode array, with the same noninverting electrode (Fz) for each channel and also an inverting electrode on the contralateral ear (such as on the earlobe). When the ipsilateral and contralateral waveforms are displayed on the same screen, a wave component should be detected in waveform recorded with the ipsilateral electrode array, but not in the waveform recorded with the contralateral electrode array. A wave I should be present only in the ipsilateral array. The appearance of a possible wave I in both ipsilateral and contralateral waveforms, or only in the contralateral waveform, argues against the presence of a true ear-specific wave I for the bone conduction ABR. As noted in the discussion of protocols above, the protocol used for recording bone conduction ABR is largely focused on enhancing the likelihood of generating a clear wave I component.

Analyses of Frequency-Specific ABRs (Tone Burst Stimulation)

Confident identification and analysis of an ABR waveform for tone burst stimulation is really dependent on developing the ability to recognize variations in ABR patterns. As illustrated earlier in Figure 5–4A, normal ABRs elicited with high frequency tone burst stimuli (e.g., 4000 Hz) at high intensity levels are very similar in appearance to click-evoked ABRs. The waveform includes the major components (wave I, wave III, and wave V). Each highly repeatable wave has a rather distinct peak and a latency within the region expected for click-evoked ABRs. For lower frequency tone burst stimuli, and at lower intensity levels, there are predictable alterations in waveform morphology. Wave I is less likely to be present. For tone burst stimulation, and at lower intensity levels, threshold estimation is dependent entirely on identification of a reliable wave V. Wave V latency increases systematically as tone burst frequency decreases from 4000 Hz to 500 Hz. Also, for lower frequencies and lower intensity levels wave V appears not as a sharp peak but, rather, as a broad and rounded wave. Near auditory threshold, identification of the response is based mostly on the detection of a shallow negative wave in a latency region slightly beyond the wave V observed for higher intensity levels.

Often it's not possible to identify a clear peak for precise calculation of latency. Confident analysis of ABRs for tone burst stimulation is aided by arranging waveforms for progressively lower intensity levels so a clear wave V for a higher intensity level can serve as a clue to the likely latency for a less distinct wave V at a lower intensity level, as illustrated in Figure 5–7. Although precise calculation of wave latency values isn't essential for accurate analysis and meaningful interpretation of tone burst ABRs, for confident identification of wave V it is very helpful to have in mind general expectations of normal latency values. Normative data for the latency of wave V for ABRs elicited with tone burst stimulation (500, 1000, and 4000 Hz), and also click stimuli, are displayed in Table 5–9. Data were compiled from a group of children age 18 months and older who had entirely normal ABR findings and later confirmation of normal hearing sensitivity. None of the children had clinical evidence or a history of neurological dysfunc-

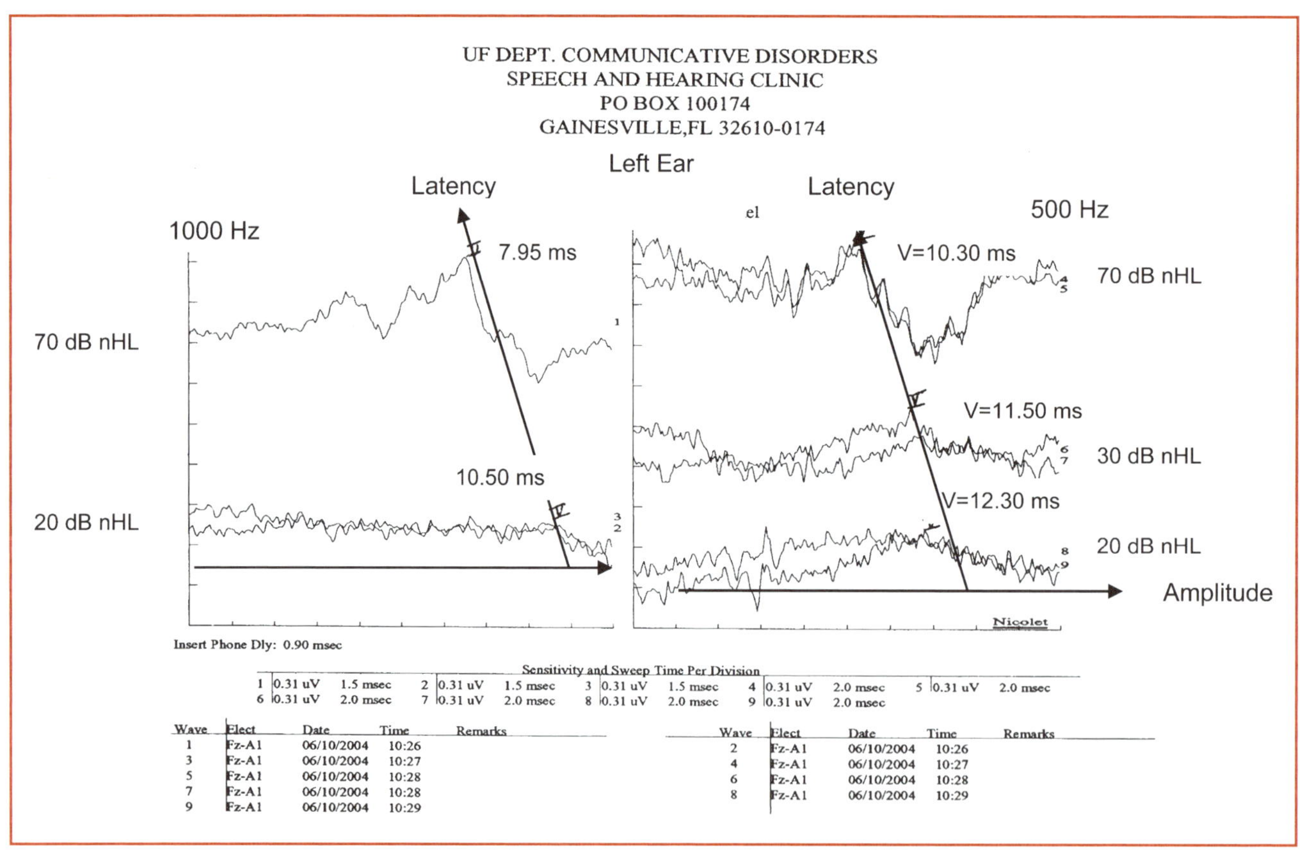

FIGURE 5–7. ABR waveforms elicited with 1000 Hz (*left portion*) and 500 Hz (*right portion*) tone burst stimulation at a high and lower stimulus intensity level.

Table 5–9. Summary of latency values for ABRs elicited with click and tone burst stimuli at selected intensity levels

		LATENCIES (ms)							
		80 dB nHL						*20 dB nHL*	
		I		*III*		*V*		*V*	
		L	*R*	*L*	*R*	*L*	*R*	*L*	*R*
Click Stimulus	*n*	26	26	25	26	26	26	25	24
	mean	1.64	1.70	4.06	4.09	6.18	6.16	8.72	8.72
	min	1.40	1.5	3.4	3.65	5.54	5.54	7.85	7.58
	max	1.91	2.0	4.37	4.46	6.71	6.62	9.92	9.92
	95% CI	1.59–1.69	1.65–1.75	3.97–4.15	4.01–4.17	6.06–6.30	6.07–6.26	8.52–8.92	8.45–8.99
		70 dB nHL						*20 dB nHL*	
4 kHz Tone Burst	*n*	16	15	16	15	22	18	17	16
	mean	1.92	1.97	4.31	4.24	6.50	6.47	8.19	8.04
	min	1.46	1.55	3.92	3.98	5.90	6.02	7.4	7.3
	max	2.36	2.24	4.79	4.58	7.37	7.73	8.99	8.78
	95% CI	1.80–2.40	1.89–2.06	4.21–4.41	4.16–4.32	6.35–6.66	6.26–6.67	7.99–8.40	7.86–8.22
1 kHz Tone Burst	*n*	4	4	3	2	10	8	10	6
	mean	3.46	3.63	6.01	6.24	7.98	7.66	10.15	9.70
	min	3.14	2.96	5.81	6.18	7.4	7.22	8.84	8.57
	max	3.94	4.56	6.30	6.30	9.74	7.66	11.48	11.22
	95% CI	3.11–3.81	2.95–4.31	5.72–6.30	6.12–6.36	7.57–8.39	7.42–7.90	9.62–10.69	8.89–10.50
		70 dB nHL V		*40 dB nHL V*		*30 dB nHL V*		*20 dB nHL V*	
		L	*R*	*L*	*R*	*L*	*R*	*L*	*R*
500 Hz Tone Burst	*n*	10	12	12	14	15	12	12	11
	mean	9.67	9.53	10.22	10.03	11.51	11.45	12.10	11.65
	min	8	6.68	7.46	7.82	10.1	8.09	9.74	8.09
	max	11.50	11.62	12.82	11.58	13.54	13.22	15	13.78
	95% CI	8.89–10.45	8.64–10.41	9.48–10.96	9.50–10.56	10.93–12.08	10.62–12.27	11.18–13.02	10.55–12.75

Source. Data from R. Kelley and J. W. Hall III, 2007.

tion. ABR measurement was carried out while the children were lightly anesthetized with one of two common agents (propofol or sevoflurane).

In reviewing the waveforms for lower frequencies and intensity levels in Figure 5–4A and Figure 5–8, and in clinical practice, one may at times have doubts about the actual presence of an ABR versus nonresponse activity. How can an ABR be confirmed under less than optimal conditions, or when very close to auditory threshold response amplitude is modest and morphology is poor? A handful of strategies are helpful in proving that a response is present and, therefore, that estimations of auditory threshold are accurate:

- When in doubt about the presence of a response at a specific intensity level, increase the intensity by 5 or 10 dB. The presence of a response is confirmed by a larger and clearer wave V with a slightly earlier latency. The value of this technique for response confirmation is illustrated by the waveforms for the 500 Hz tone burst stimuli in the right panel of Figure 5–7.
- The ABR recorded at the lowest intensity level before the response disappears should always be duplicated, or even "triplicated," to verify that it really is a response. To further verify the presence of a response, after the data are saved, the two or three waveforms can be digitally added. This simple process will enhance the detection of the response while simultaneously minimizing random (not stimulus related) background activity.
- Detection of a response at intensity levels near threshold is sometimes challenging because the amplitude is very low relative to the amplitude of the response for higher stimulus intensity levels. To verify that a response is present, the size of the waveform displayed on the computer screen can be increased without actually changing the amplification of the evoked response system, or the absolute amplitude of the response. As a rule of thumb, three or four sets of ABR waveforms (e.g., two waveforms per intensity level) should be displayed on a screen at one time. If it's desirable to display more waveforms, or two separately display waveforms for different sets of stimuli (e.g., left versus right ear click stimuli, or two different tone burst stimuli), a "split screen" option is available with most evoked responses systems. When viewed using the split screen option, the vertical dimension of each wave appears to increase and peaks are easier to detect visually.
- An appropriate sensitivity setting for the display of waveforms on an evoked response system is 0.25 to 0.30 μV. If all of the ABR waveforms appear flattened, and wave V is very difficult to detect at lower intensity levels, consider modifying the default sensitivity or display gain for the system.
- With the low frequency cutoff for the high pass filter (e.g., 30 Hz) required for infant and tone burst ABRs, changes in state of arousal during sleep, sedation, or anesthesia may introduce broad nonstimulus EEG activity (apparent waves) in the recording. Taking a minute to complete a recording with 1000 to 2000 averages in a no stimulus condition will verify whether the slow wave activity is really a response. The no stimulus condition can be produced by decreasing the intensity level to the lowest possible value, by removing the insert earphone from the child's ear at the end of the ABR session, or even by unplugging the earphone cable from the evoked response system. Of course, if a wave is apparent in a no stimulus condition, then the presence of a similar wave at low stimulus intensity levels must be viewed with suspicion.

CLINICAL CONSIDERATIONS AND CONSTRAINTS

Nonpathologic Factors

The possible influences of subject factors and other nonpathologic factors on the ABR are summarized in Table 5–10. Among these factors, age and body temperature have the most pronounced influence on the ABR. For children under the age of 1.5 years (18 months), ABR findings must always be analyzed and interpreted in the context of age-related normative data. Absolute and interwave latency values, in particular, decrease substantially as a function of neurological and audiological development and maturation. Before consulting normative data for the chronological age of an infant, it's important to first verify whether the child was born full term (at about 40 weeks gestational age) or born prematurely.

Table 5–10. Summary of nonpathologic and auditory ("pathologic") factors that may influence the outcome of ABR measurement in children

Factor	*Influence*
Nonpathologic	
Age	Latency, particularly for wave V and interwave latencies, decreases and morphology changes from premature infancy through 18 months post-term birth. Analysis of ABR findings for children under the chronological age of 18 months (corrected for premature birth) must be done with age-corrected normative data.
Gender	Differences in ABR findings for males versus females are insignificant in children before puberty.
Body Temperature	Hyper- and hypothermia exert important and indirect influences on ABR latencies. Wave V latency and the wave I–V latency interval increase by approximately 0.2 ms for every degree of temperature decrease from normal body temperature (37.0°C or 98.60°F). A corresponding decrease in ABR latency is associated with increased body temperature (hyperthermia).
State of Arousal	State of arousal, including attention, sleep, and sedation, has no significant effect on the ABR
Movement	Bodily movement, including myogenic artifact, has a significant negative influence on the quality of ABR recordings.
Drugs	Most drugs have no effect on the ABR, including sedatives commonly used in children (e.g., chloral hydrate and Versed). Selected anesthetic agents (e.g., propofol and sevofluorane) produce a modest increase in ABR interwave latency values. Nitrous oxide, a gas that is sometimes used to induce anesthesia can inflate the middle ear space and produce a transient (intraoperative) conductive hearing loss producing a prolongation of absolute ABR latencies.
Auditory	
Middle Ear Dysfunction	Even a modest degree of conductive hearing loss may produce a delay in absolute ABR latencies, beginning with wave I. Conductive hearing loss has no important effect on ABR interwave latencies. Middle ear dysfunction has no influence on ABRs evoked with bone conduction stimulation.
Sensory (Cochlear) Dysfunction	High frequency cochlear auditory dysfunction and resulting hearing loss typically is associated with poorer waveform morphology and reduction of wave I amplitude. With moderate to severe sensory hearing loss, wave I may be absent. An ABR is rarely recorded with sensory hearing loss exceeding 80 dB HL within the 1000 to 4000 Hz frequency region. Isolated low frequency sensory hearing loss with preservation of hearing above 2000 Hz has little or no effect on the ABR. A click evoked ABR can be recorded if hearing sensitivity is within normal limits at some frequencies (including interoctave frequencies) within the region of 1000 to 4000 Hz.
Neural	An abnormal ABR will typically be recorded in retrocochlear and neural auditory dysfunction. The pattern of ABR abnormality will depend on the location and extent of the lesion or dysfunction. A tumor in the cerebello-pontine angle (CPA) characteristically results in an ABR characterized by normal wave I latency and amplitude, and either a delay of interwave latencies or absence of ABR wave III and/or wave V.
Auditory Neuropathy	The neurophysiologic signature of auditory neuropathy (also now known as auditory neuropathy spectrum disorder [ANSD]) is the absence of all ABR components with evidence of cochlear microphonic (CM) activity for single polarity (rarefaction and condensation) click stimuli.

Note. The influence of stimulus and acquisition parameters on the ABR is not listed in the table.

The ABR is generally mature by 18 months after term birth. Therefore, if a child is born prematurely by, for example, 2 months (born at a gestational age of 32 weeks rather than 40 weeks), then we would not expect the child's ABR to be mature or adultlike until age 20 months after birth.

Most audiologists do not collect extensive normative data for ABR analysis of infants and young children. The practical problem associated with the development of an "in-house" normative database is verifying that infants and young children really have normal hearing sensitivity (and normal neurological status). The verification of normal auditory function for a newborn infant must be deferred until valid findings are available for an independent (non-ABR) measure of hearing sensitivity, that is, behavioral audiometry. In most clinical settings, audiologists will refer to a normative database collected by a research center and either published in the literature or distributed in some other way (e.g., by the manufacturer of an evoked response system). Soon after the introduction of the ABR as a clinical procedure for estimation of auditory function in young children, audiology centers at major pediatric hospitals reported normative ABR latency data covering the age range of about 30 weeks gestational age through preschool years. Modern auditory evoked response systems often include normative databases that, after the entry of the child's age and calculation of latencies of the waves, automatically creates graphic displays of a child's latencies relative to normal expectations. A collection of published normative databases, in the form of tables showing mean normal latencies and some measure of variability (e.g., standard deviation) for a range of ages in months, can be found in the appendices of auditory evoked response textbooks (e.g., Hall, 2007), and via the Internet. An example of ABR normative data for children older than 18 months was shown earlier in Table 5–9. These data were collected at the University of Florida Audiology Clinic with the test protocols already reviewed, and are summarized in Table 5–2 (click stimulus) and Table 5–7 (tone burst stimuli). Importantly, before analyzing ABR findings for a child with reference to a specific normative database, it is important to verify that the test parameters you used in recording the ABR are in general agreement with those used in developing the normative database. Consistency or general agreement is most important for selected test parameters, including stimulus presentation rate, stimulus intensity, earphone design, and filter settings.

To illustrate the process of analyzing ABR latency data from a child with respect to a normative database, inspect again the findings displayed in Figure 5–4A and Figure 5–7 for click, 4000 Hz, 1000 Hz, and 500 Hz stimuli. The first question to be asked before ABR data are analyzed is: "How old is the patient?" The child whose findings are displayed was a 2-year-old boy undergoing ABR assessment of hearing because of a marked delay in speech and language development. In the top portion of Figure 5–4A, wave I, wave III, and wave V are marked for the ABR evoked by click (left panel) at an intensity level of 80 dB nHL and a 4000 Hz tone burst (right panel) stimulation at an intensity level of 70 dB nHL. Latency values in milliseconds are shown in the boxed table below the waveforms. Wave V is marked for each set of waveforms recorded with an intensity level of 20 dB nHL (lower portion of figure), with the corresponding latencies also displayed in the table. The latency values for these stimuli (click and 4000 Hz tone burst), at these intensity levels, can then be compared to normal latency data displayed in Table 5–9. Once again, the ABR waveforms plotted in the figures were recorded using the same test protocols (refer back to Table 5–2 and Table 5–7) that were employed in the collection of the normative data. A similar comparison of analyzed waveforms for ABRs evoked by 1000 and 500 Hz tone burst stimuli (in Figure 5–7) relative to the normative data in Table 5–9 confirms that wave V latency values are well within normal limits for each of the intensity levels. Our interpretation, therefore, is that the ABR findings are normal, consistent with hearing sensitivity within normal limits within the speech frequency region. Based on these ABR results, hearing sensitivity is adequate for normal speech and language acquisition. Referral to a speech-language pathologist with expertise in the diagnostic assessment of language in children is clearly indicated.

For routine ABR assessment of a generally healthy child in an audiology clinic setting, body temperature rarely must be considered. However, for children who are undergoing ABR assessment in a NICU or pediatric intensive care unit (PICU) setting, or in an OR under general anesthesia, body temperature should be routinely documented. In these test settings, body temperature is generally monitored continuously along with other physiological parameters (e.g., heart rate, oxygen saturation, blood CO_2 levels, etc.). ABR latencies must be adjusted based on body temperature. Let's consider as an example a 3-year-old child who is undergoing ABR assessment in the operating room under anesthesia. Assume that ABR wave I to V latency interval was 4.8 ms. Three nonpathologic factors that might influence ABR findings must be taken into account in this case: (a) age, (b) anesthesia, and (c) body temperature. Because the child is older than 18 months, age can be ruled out as a factor, even if the child was born prematurely. The next necessary question is: "What anesthetic agent was used?" If the answer to this question is propofol, then we might expect a modest (0.1 to 0.2 ms) anesthesia-induced increase in latency. If monitored body temperature shows that the child is slightly hypothermic (e.g., 36°C versus normal 37°C), we must adjust the interwave latencies for the effect of the decrease in body temperature. As indicated in Table 5–10, and reviewed in detail in numerous articles and a recent textbook (Hall, 2007), a decrease in body temperature of 1 degree will on the average increase the wave I to V latency interval by 0.2 ms. Analysis of the child's ABR in the context of these three findings leads to the conclusion that the ABR wave I–V interval of 4.8 ms is within normal limits (≤4.5 ms), when "corrected" for the additive effects of the slight delays due to the anesthetic agent and reduced body temperature. Failure to take into account these two factors would have resulted in an incorrect interpretation of ABR findings, and misdiagnosis of auditory brainstem dysfunction. Of course, these three important nonpathologic factors—age, body temperature, and anesthetic agent—also affect the analysis and interpretation of wave V latency.

Pathologic Factors

Pathologic factors influencing pediatric ABR assessment can include various forms of auditory dysfunction and neural dysfunction involving the auditory pathways. The most common general types of auditory and neural abnormalities are summarized in Table 5–10. Of course, this small list of auditory abnormalities may be associated with literally hundreds of different diseases, pathologies, and pathophysiologic processes. Even a cursory discussion of these many and diverse diseases, or a review of the literature on ABR findings in varied patient populations, is far beyond the scope of this chapter. For more information, especially on ABR findings for a specific disease or clinical entity, the reader should consult textbooks devoted to auditory evoked responses (e.g., Hall, 2007) or perform a focused review of the literature with a professional search engine such as Medline (http://www.nlm.nih.gov). A fundamental objective of any pediatric ABR assessment is diagnostic differentiation among the few categories of disorders listed in Table 5–10. Among these disorders, auditory neuropathy is perhaps the most challenging to diagnose and to manage audiologically. This topic is addressed in the chapter on electrocochleography (Chapter 4).

Noise, Sedation, and Anesthesia

Accurate estimation of auditory thresholds with ABR or ASSR is directly dependent on detection of a signal (the ABR) in the presence of noise. Noise in ABR recordings is inevitable, and arises from multiple and highly varied sources, including:

- Airborne electrical or electromagnetic energy from, for example, lights, cell phones, and electrical devices (e.g., copy machines, x-ray machines, elevators, conveyer belts)
- Power-line electrical energy from, for example, outlets, power cords, and power strips
- Rectified RF noise
- Physiological electrical activity from, for example, the brain (e.g., EEG during awake and sleep states) and the heart (e.g., EKG)
- Myogenic activity, also referred to as muscle or movement artifact, from large muscles around the head and neck and from small muscles (e.g., extraocular muscles)

Electrical and physiological noise in conventional ABR recordings is best minimized by locating electrodes and electrode wires as far away as possible from the sources of the noise. Without doubt, some test settings are electrically noisier than others. If there is some latitude about where auditory evoked responses are recorded, for example, where a new audiology clinic will be built or which room in an audiology clinic will be used for auditory evoked response recording, then trial ABR recordings should be conducted to identify the electrically quiet areas. Unfortunately, ABR assessment must often be performed in hospital settings with multiple essential electrical devices, like monitors, equipment, security systems, that are sources of electrical artifact. In these electrically hostile environments, artifact is best minimized by modification of test parameters and by other simple techniques, such as the use of short electrode wires and braiding electrode wires, which are also helpful for reducing the negative impact of electrical noise.

Muscle or movement artifact is perhaps the most serious contaminant affecting pediatric ABR recording, and a source of noise that can often be controlled clinically. For over 30 years, a quiet state has been achieved in pediatric ABR measurement by one of three approaches: natural sleep, conscious sedation, or light anesthesia. Infants under the age of 3 to 4 months, and older children over the age of about 5 years, can often be successfully evaluated with ABR as they sleep naturally. The likelihood of successful ABR measurement is enhanced if it is conducted in a darkened room, immediately after feeding, and during a time of day when the child typically sleeps. The tendency of young infants (less than 4 months old) to spend considerable time in deep sleep argues strongly for the strategy of scheduling, after newborn hearing screening failure, follow-up diagnostic ABR assessment within this time frame.

Advantages and disadvantages associated with conscious sedation versus anesthesia are summarized in Table 5–11. Conscious sedation drugs, such as chloral hydrate or Versed, are controlled substances that must be dispensed by qualified medical personnel. Only medical personnel (such as a registered nurse or physician) should monitor physiological parameters (respiration, heart rate, blood oxygen saturation, blood pressure) of children who are given conscious sedatives according to well-defined protocols developed by medical specialties, including pediatrics and anesthesiology (e.g., American Academy of Pediatrics, American Academy of Dentistry, Coté, Wilson, the Work Group on Sedation, 2006). A wealth of information on conscious sedation is available on the Web site of the American Academy of Pediatrics (http://www.aap.org). Sedation and anesthesia in

Table 5–11. Advantages and disadvantages of conscious sedation in a clinical setting versus anesthesia in an OR for achieving adequate subject state when recording ABRs from infants and young children

Setting		
Sedation in clinic	• Relatively inexpensive • ABR performed near or within audiology clinic • Scheduling ease	• Limited sedation options • Limited medical support • Increased liability • Uncertain success (sometimes ineffective) • Uncertain test time • Discouraged by anesthesiologists
Anesthesia in OR	• Otolaryngology services at hand • Ideal patient state • Limited liability for audiologist • Controlled sedation • Always effective	• More expensive (>$4000 USD) • Location away from audiology clinic • Transportation of equipment • Noisier environment • Scheduling is more complicated

ABR recording is also reviewed in some detail in a recent textbook (Hall, 2007, pp. 306–312).

In recent years, physicians, especially anesthesiologists in the United States, have for pediatric ABR measurement discouraged the use of conscious sedation in a clinic setting and, instead, have recommended reliance on light anesthesia in an operating room or ambulatory surgery suite. Without question, muscle and movement interference is quickly and effectively eliminated by general anesthesia. As a result, test time for ABR assessment is reduced and consistently accurate estimation of auditory threshold is enhanced. Why not recommend ABR assessment under general anesthesia for all children who will not sleep naturally for the time required (e.g., about 45 minutes) needed for completion of threshold assessment with ABR? As noted in Table 5–11, general anesthesia poses some health risk, considerable financial cost, and often scheduling challenges. And, of course, the medical facilities and personnel required for general anesthesia are not available in all locations or to all persons with the responsibility of performing pediatric ABR assessments. Fortunately, there are several alternatives to ABR measurement with conscious sedation or general anesthesia.

ABR Measurement without Sedation or Anesthesia

There are currently three main approaches—two techniques and one technology—to ABR measurement without sedation or anesthesia: (a) natural sleep, (b) natural sleep induced by nonprescription substances, and (c) ABR recording with instrumentation designed to minimize the deleterious affects of electrical and myogenic noise. These are summarized in Table 5–12. The first option has already been noted, that is, conducting the assessment under conditions likely to encourage natural sleep. The authors report moderate success with ABR assessment of children between the ages of 4 months and about 5 years who were seriously sleep deprived (one mother kept her 4-year-old girl up almost all night), and then scheduled for the procedure early in the morning (e.g., 8:00 A.M.) before the child had a nap and immediately after feeding. Preparation for the ABR measurement, including electrode placement, is completed before the child is allowed to fall asleep. The ABR is recorded in a darkened room with the child in a comfortable position.

Table 5–12. Options (techniques and technology) for recording ABR from infants and young children without sedation or anesthesia

Nonmedical techniques

- Sleep deprivation
- Record ABR immediately after feeding
- Bean bag "bed" to minimize movement
- Benadryl (with pediatrician approval)
- Melatonin (e.g., Schmidt, Knief, Deuster, Matulat, & am Zehnhoff-Dinnesen)

Technology: Vivosonic Integrity auditory evoked response device

- Bluetooth technology
  - To limit cables and wires
  - Reduce the "antennae" effect of conventional electrode leads
  - Eliminate line noise
  - Permit distance from patient and test equipment
- Amplitrode in-situ amplifier designed to:
  - Filter before amplification
  - Optimize gain
  - Reduce electrode lead length
  - Minimize electrical artifact from multiple sources
  - Amplify signal but not noise
- Kalman weighted averaging:
  - Estimates noise in each raw response
  - Weights window based on inverse of noise estimate
  - No signal is discarded
  - Noisy signals contribute less

Note. See "Melatonin Is a Useful Alternative to Sedation in Children Undergoing Brainstem Audiometry with an Age-Dependent Success Rate: A Field Report of 250 Investigations," by C.-M. Schmidt, A. Knief, D. Deuster, P. Matulat, and A. G. am Zehnhoff-Dinnesen, 2007, *Neuropediatrics*, *38*, pp. 2–4. Reprinted with permission.

A recent clinical report describes the effective induction of natural sleep with melatonin (Schmidt, Knief, Deuster, Matulat, & am Zehnhoff-Dinnesen,

2007). Melatonin is a hormone naturally produced by the pineal gland (small gland in center of the brain) that controls circadian rhythms. The physiologic effects of melatonin are enhanced by darkness and inhibited by light. In addition to its influence on circadian rhythms, melatonin is associated with antioxidant activity, and chronic reduction in melatonin is linked to cancer risk. Ingestion of exogenous melatonin, that is, synthetic forms of the substance available over the counter (without prescription), facilitates rapid induction of sleep without sedation. Peak serum concentration of melatonin is reached within 60 minutes after ingestion, and concentration declines within 4 hours. There is a remarkably substantial literature describing clinical applications of melatonin for induction of sleep during neuroradiologic studies (e.g., MRI) and electrophysiological procedures (e.g., EEG), and many published papers confirming the safety of melatonin (such as Brzezinski, 1997).

Briefly, Schmidt and audiology colleagues in Muenster, Germany, conducted an investigation of the usefulness of melatonin as an alternative to sedation in a series of 250 children ranging in age from 1 month to 13.7 years. Melatonin was dissolved in water, with the dosage of the melatonin varying as a function of children. "Children up to one year received 5 mg, children between 1 and 6 years 10 mg and older children 20 mg." (Schmidt et al., 2007, p. 3). Among this series, 230 fell asleep in an average time of 32 minutes (standard deviation of 21 minutes), and a successful click-evoked ABR recording was completed in 216 children. The authors reported completion of frequency-specific ABR measurement in 115 children, although it was not attempted in all the children who were given melatonin. With the inclusion of melatonin induced sleep in their clinic protocol, the authors described an 80% decrease in the proportion of children who required general anesthesia for ABR measurement. Schmidt et al. (2007) conclude that: "melatonin-induced sleep offers a risk-free alternative to sedation and general anesthesia especially in younger children undergoing brainstem audiometry. Widely accepted by parents, it permits earlier diagnosis and treatment of hearing loss in children" (p. 4).

A clinical evoked response system now available permits pediatric ABR measurement without sedation or anesthesia. The Vivosonic Integrity device utilizes Bluetooth technology to (a) limit cables and wires, (b) reduce the "antennae" effect of conventional electrode leads, (c) eliminate line noise, and (d) increase the distance between the patient and test equipment. In addition, the Vivosonic device includes a unique electrode design, the Amplitrode, which is an "in situ amplifier" designed to Filter before amplification, optimize gain, reduce electrode lead length, minimize electrical artifact from multiple sources, and amplify the signal (the ABR) but not measurement noise. Finally, the device employs Kalman weighted averaging that (a) estimates noise in each raw response, (b) weights the analysis window based on an inverse of the noise estimate, (c) does not discard activity following any signal presentation, and (d) weights noisy post-signal activity less than quiet post-signal activity. As an aside, Dr. Rudolph Kalman is an award-winning electrical engineer who was for a number of years chair of the engineering department at the University of Florida.

Plotting Electrophysiologically Estimated Auditory Thresholds

The foregoing discussion summarized the steps, procedures, and protocols that are involved in electrophysiologically estimating auditory thresholds prior to audiologic management of children with hearing loss. To facilitate accurate interpretation of frequency-specific estimations of auditory thresholds, findings can be plotted in a form that resembles an audiogram. As shown in Figure 5–8, the lowest stimulus intensity level that produces a reliable ABR wave V is plotted on the graph for the appropriate stimulus, including air or bone conduction click stimuli and each tone burst frequency. Importantly, the value plotted here is intensity level in dB nHL derived from the normative data for stimulus intensity (as determined in this chapter), and not simply the number representing intensity level from the evoked response system screen. Correction factors to compensate for the slightly higher electrophysiological threshold in estimating behavioral thresholds is typically 10 to 15 dB for 1000, 2000, and

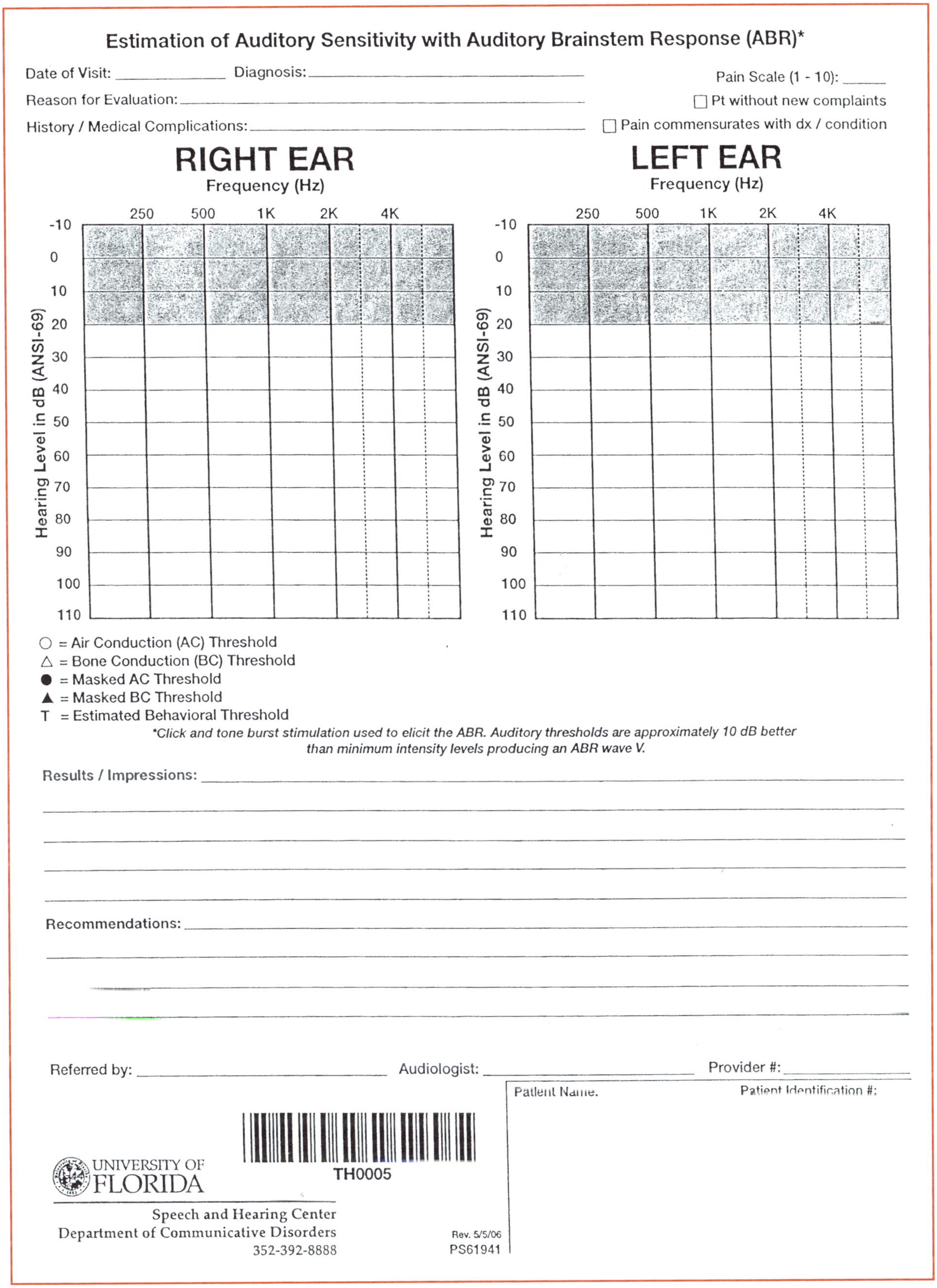

Estimation of Auditory Sensitivity with Auditory Brainstem Response (ABR)*

Date of Visit: ____________ Diagnosis: ______________________________ Pain Scale (1 - 10): _____

Reason for Evaluation: ______________________________ ☐ Pt without new complaints

History / Medical Complications: ______________________________ ☐ Pain commensurates with dx / condition

RIGHT EAR — Frequency (Hz): 250, 500, 1K, 2K, 4K — Hearing Level in dB (ANSI-69): -10, 0, 10, 20, 30, 40, 50, 60, 70, 80, 90, 100, 110

LEFT EAR — Frequency (Hz): 250, 500, 1K, 2K, 4K — Hearing Level in dB (ANSI-69): -10, 0, 10, 20, 30, 40, 50, 60, 70, 80, 90, 100, 110

○ = Air Conduction (AC) Threshold
△ = Bone Conduction (BC) Threshold
● = Masked AC Threshold
▲ = Masked BC Threshold
T = Estimated Behavioral Threshold

**Click and tone burst stimulation used to elicit the ABR. Auditory thresholds are approximately 10 dB better than minimum intensity levels producing an ABR wave V.*

Results / Impressions: ______________________________

Recommendations: ______________________________

Referred by: ____________ Audiologist: ____________ Provider #: ____________

Patient Name: Patient Identification #:

TH0005

UNIVERSITY OF FLORIDA
Speech and Hearing Center
Department of Communicative Disorders
352-392-8888

Rev. 5/5/06
PS61941

FIGURE 5–8. A form used to graph estimations of auditory threshold using frequency-specific ABR recordings with tone burst stimuli.

4000 Hz tone bursts and 15 to 20 dB for 500 Hz tone burst thresholds. These values may however vary with age (smaller corrections in infants) and is slightly less for sensory hearing loss compared to normal hearing (Stapells, 2000). The estimated auditory threshold (corresponding to the predicted behavioral threshold) is indicated with the vertical line ending with the short T-shaped horizontal line. The simple graph of auditory thresholds estimated with tone burst ABR recordings is useful for explaining findings to family members, physicians, and audiologists. It also offers a straightforward means of conveying the information required for the initial fitting of the hearing aid(s). The estimated thresholds, plotted in dB HL, can be converted to dB SPL and then incorporated into a prescriptive method for determining appropriate amplification for children, such as the Desired Sensation Level (DSL) technique.

6

Auditory Steady-State Response

HISTORICAL PERSPECTIVE ON THE AUDITORY STEADY-STATE RESPONSE

For several decades the auditory brainstem response (ABR) was the single method of choice for estimating hearing thresholds in patients who are unable or unwilling to provide behavioral responses to sound. It is only more recently that another auditory evoked response (AER) became available clinically for the same purpose, namely, the auditory steady-state response (ASSR). The first ASSR system became clinically available in 2001. The ASSR is, essentially, an auditory response evoked by continuous tones modulated in amplitude, and sometimes frequency, at specific rates or modulation frequencies.

Despite its relatively recent appearance in clinical test batteries, the ASSR was initially researched in the late 1970s and early 1980s. Several different terms were used to describe the response, as shown in Table 6–1. Over the years, papers described findings for the ASSR elicited by a wide variety of stimuli in both awake and sleeping adults. The earlier studies used lower modulation frequencies (between 35 and 55 Hz) to estimate hearing thresholds. Interest was greatly increased after the discovery that at a certain repetition (modulation) rate the response seemed quite strong, particularly at 40 Hz (Galambos, Makeig, & Talmachoff, 1981). Although the 40 Hz response resulted in good estimations of behavioral thresholds in normal and hearing impaired adults at low and high frequencies, the response was considerably affected by sleep and sedation and was unstable in infants and young children. The 40 Hz response, therefore, never translated into a viable technique.

In the early 1990s, alternative rates of stimulation (modulation frequencies) were introduced and investigated in an attempt to find optimal modulation frequencies. The aim was to identify stimulation rates that elicited responses which were resistant to state of consciousness and maturation, yet reliably recorded in children of all ages, including neonates. Higher rates of stimulation (70 to 110 Hz) produced such responses. After several studies in the mid- to late 1990s confirmed the

Table 6–1. Synonyms for the ASSR

SSEP	Steady-state evoked potential
SSER	Steady-state evoked response
ASSEP	Auditory steady-state evoked potential
AMFR	Amplitude modulation following response
FFR	Frequency following response

feasibility of higher rates of stimulation, the technique became available clinically in 2001 (Cohen, Rickards, & Clark, 1991; Rance, Rickards, Cohen, De Vidi, & Clark, 1995; Rickards et al., 1994). The clinical application of the high modulation stimulus technique has since been under continuous investigation for various applications, particularly estimation of frequency-specific hearing thresholds. The nature of the stimulus paradigms and response detection methods for ASSR recordings provide clinicians with an additional and unique tool in the test battery for objective assessment of auditory sensitivity in populations difficult to test using behavioral audiometry.

DEFINING THE AUDITORY STEADY-STATE RESPONSE

Introduction

It is important to remember that the term *ASSR* does not refer to a single response but, rather, ASSR encompasses a range of responses generated in different brain regions depending on the stimulus characteristics (Stapells, 2008). The ASSR is defined simply as an AER characterized by its periodic nature directly related to the periodic nature of the stimuli applied. The ASSR can be viewed as a demonstration of how the brain "follows" the periodic changes in a stimulus or how the stimulus "drives" the brain at a particular rate (Picton, John, Dimitrijevic, & Purcell, 2003). The most basic requirement for evoking an ASSR, therefore, is a stimulus that changes over time at a specific rate in amplitude and/or frequency. The most commonly used clinical stimulus is a tone modulated in amplitude as seen in Figure 6–1.

Response Generation

The tone, referred to as the carrier frequency or test frequency stimulus, translates to the area on the tonotopically arranged basilar membrane where stimulation of a group of hair cells and auditory nerve fibers takes place. The modulation frequency refers to the rate at which the tone is amplitude modulated, in other words, how many times the tone is modulated into distinct pockets of energy per second (Hz). Think of the acoustic stimulus as pockets of energy being presented to the cochlea. The carrier frequency determines

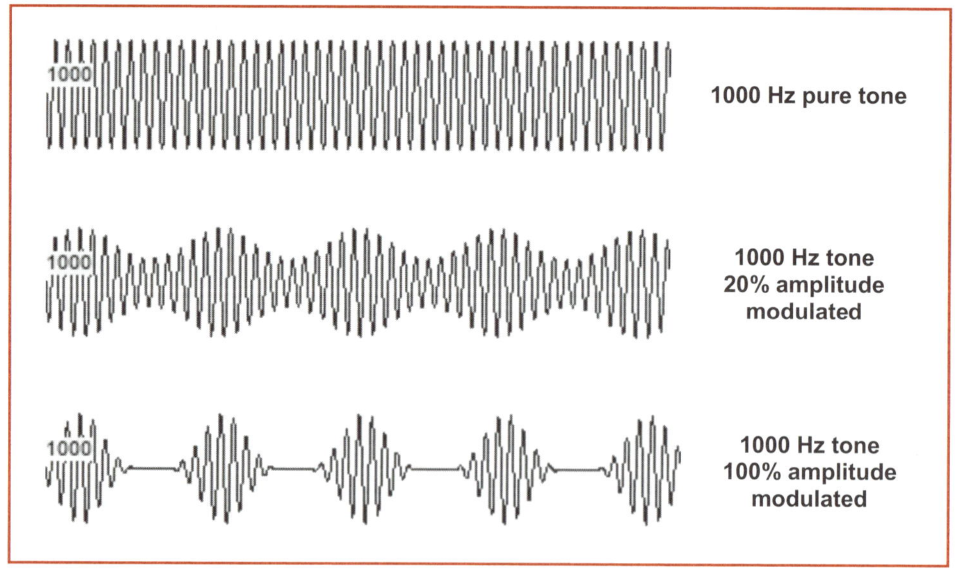

FIGURE 6–1. The top row illustrates a 1000 Hz pure tone, the middle row illustrates the 1000 Hz tone amplitude modulated at 20%, and the bottom row illustrates a 100% amplitude modulated tone (% refers to depth of amplitude modulation).

where these pockets will stimulate the basilar membrane, that is, it specifies the frequency region to be activated. The modulation frequency in turn determines how many pockets of energy will stimulate this region every second, or in other words the rate at which the cochlea is being stimulated. The rate of stimulation is transferred to the auditory system as a rate of neural firing. For example, a 1000 Hz tone modulated at a frequency of 80 Hz will stimulate the basilar membrane at the 1000 Hz region with 80 pockets of energy per second. This phenomenon is illustrated in Figure 6–2 where four frequencies are stimulating the cochlea simultaneously at different modulation rates.

The evoked response will result in a peak of neural activity at the rate of stimulation. The response is judged as present if there is a significant increase in neural activation at a rate corresponding to the modulation frequency of the acoustic stimulus. Therefore, the rate of modulation is the neural marker for determining if a response was present at the frequency region stimulated by the

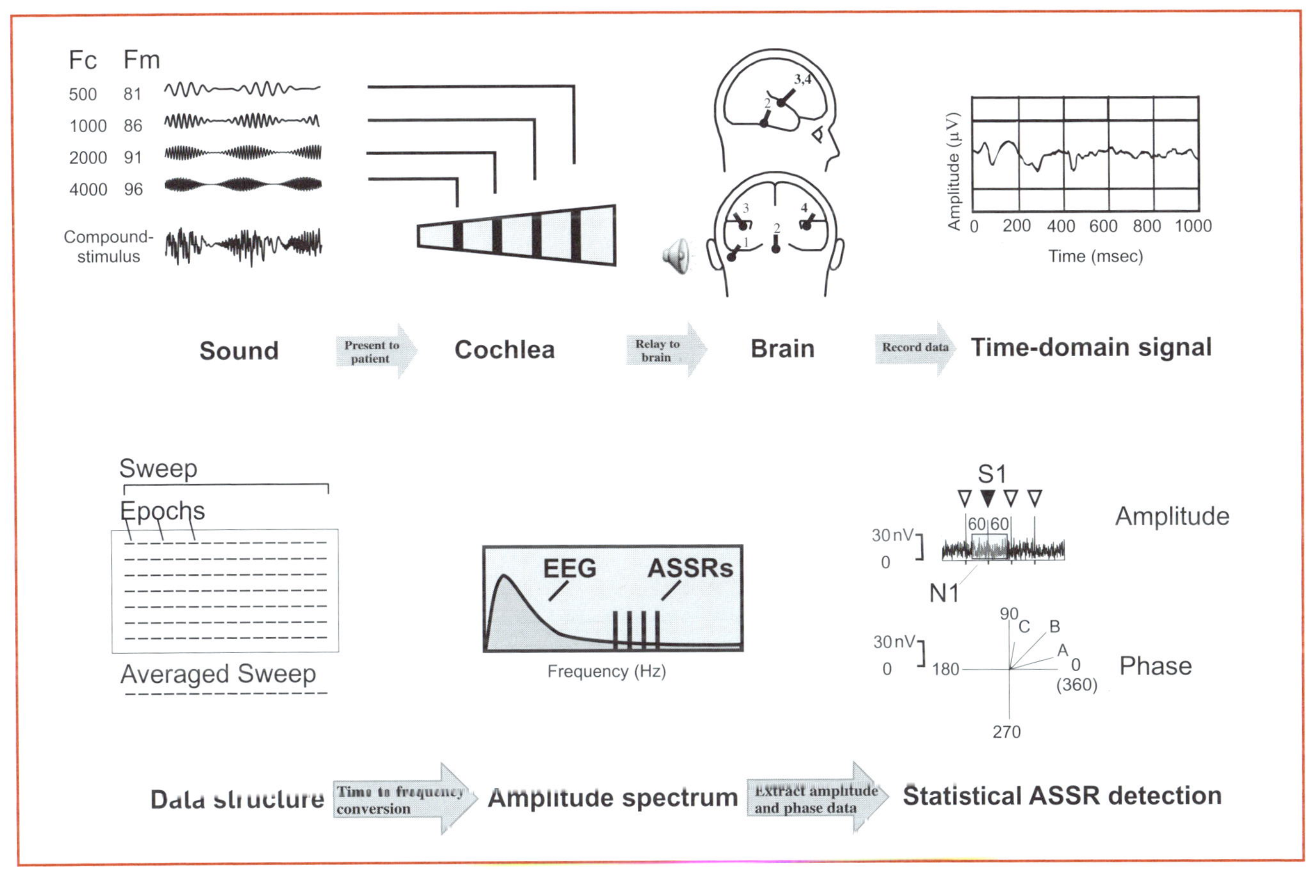

FIGURE 6–2. Overview of the major features of ASSR measurement. *Top row* illustrates four carrier frequencies (Fc) modulated at different rates (Fm), simultaneously stimulating the cochlea at different areas as determined by the carrier frequency. The response is recorded from the brain with scalp electrodes in the time-domain. *Bottom row* illustrates the epochs (usually ±1 sec), which together comprise a sweep (16 epochs) averaged together. The signal in the time-domain is converted to the frequency-domain, where signals are represented in the amplitude spectrum. Statistical analyses are either done by comparing the response amplitude at the modulation frequency with adjacent frequencies (amplitude-based analysis) or by assessing the phase of the response at the modulation frequency to determine if there is phase coherence (phase-based analysis). Because all four carrier frequencies were modulated at different rates they can be assessed by their signature modulation frequency, which allows simultaneous analysis of four frequencies per ear. *Source:* John, M. S., & Purcell, D. W. (2008). Introduction to technical principles of auditory steady-state response testing. In G. Rance (Ed.), *The auditory steady-state response* (pp. 11–54). San Diego, CA: Plural Publishing

carrier frequency. An ASSR is generated if the carrier frequency is presented at a rate (the modulation frequency) that is sufficient to cause an overlapping of transient responses resulting in a sustained response.

The physiology underlying ASSR measurement is based on cochlear mechanics, where sound waves cause polarization and depolarization of the inner hair cells. Only the depolarization of inner hair cells causes auditory nerve fibers to transmit action potentials. The transduction process of the hair cells and auditory nerve fibers involves rectification of the signal waveform, as illustrated by Figure 6–3. The compound electrical activity recorded from the cochlear nerve therefore contains a spectral component at the rate of modulation (rate of stimulation). Because the stimuli occur very rapidly, the brain's response to each stimulus is evoked before the response to the prior stimulus has terminated. Rather than being allowed to return to a baseline state, a steady-state or sustained response is elicited. The response can therefore be detected by assessing the amplitude and/or phase of the spectral component at the frequency of modulation as illustrated in Figure 6–2.

The nature of frequency-specific measurements with the ASSR and ABR techniques differs in three main areas: (a) stimulus type, (b) response measurement, and (c) response detection. A comparison of these differences has been summarized in Table 6–2.

Neural Generators

It is not simple to determine the neural generators of ASSRs because they reflect overlapping responses from different brain regions. Source analysis studies to determine the neural generators of the ASSR indicate that the whole auditory nervous system

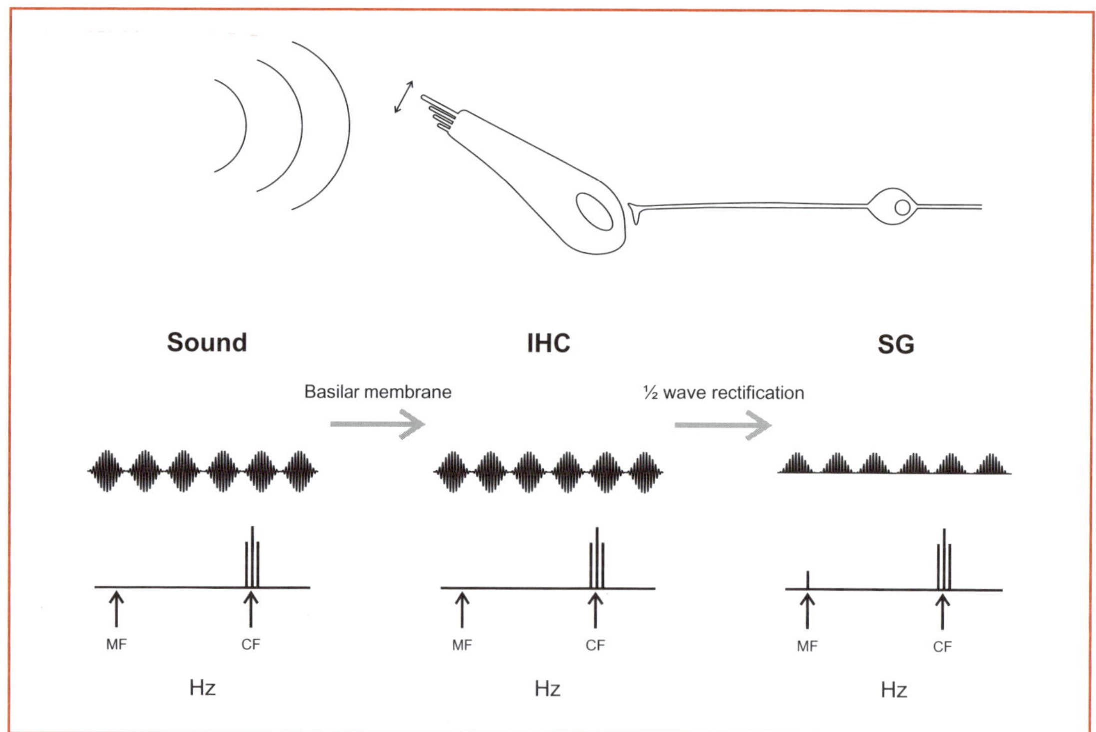

FIGURE 6–3. Transduction of amplitude-modulated sound by auditory nerve. As the sound enters the ear, stereocilia on inner hair cells are moved back and forth. Neurotransmitter release is initiated only on depolarization, so the signal undergoes half-wave rectification. This results in activity that can be recorded at the modulation frequency. CF = carrier frequency; IHC = inner hair cells; MF = modulation frequency; SG = spiral ganglion. *Source*: Dimitrijevic, A., & Ross, B. (2008). Neural generators of the auditory steady-state response. In G. Rance (Ed.), *The auditory steady-state response* (pp. 83–108). San Diego, CA: Plural Publishing

Table 6–2. Main differences between frequency-specific ASSR and ABR measures

Stimulus type	Transient stimuli *(distinct, separate stimuli)*	Continuous stimuli *(modulated in amplitude)*
	Frequency-specific tone bursts	Frequency-specific modulated tones
	Calibrated in dB nHL or dB peSPL	Calibrated in dB HL
Response measurement	Averaging time-locked to each stimulus	Averaging time-locked to a period of stimulation (e.g., 1 sec)
	Peaks of neural activity over time	Rate of sustained neural activity
Response detection	Amplitude and latency in time-domain	Amplitude and phase in frequency-domain
	Subjective response detection	Objective response detection

is activated by modulated tones with dominance by different regions of the auditory nervous system depending on the rate of modulation. For example, the cortex is more sensitive to slower modulation frequencies (below 20 Hz), and as the rate increases the central nervous system activity decreases until the brainstem becomes the dominant source at modulation rates greater than 50 Hz (Picton et al., 2003). Generation of the 40 Hz ASSR has been attributed primarily to the auditory cortices and thalamocortical circuits, with the cortex dominating in awake adults (Johnson, Weinberg, Ribary, Cheyne, & Ancill, 1988). Higher modulation rates (>70 Hz) evoke responses that are primarily generated in the brainstem. The general trend is, therefore, that faster modulation rates are mostly mediated by lower regions of the auditory system. Figure 6–4 provides an illustration of the response amplitude relationship to modulation frequency.

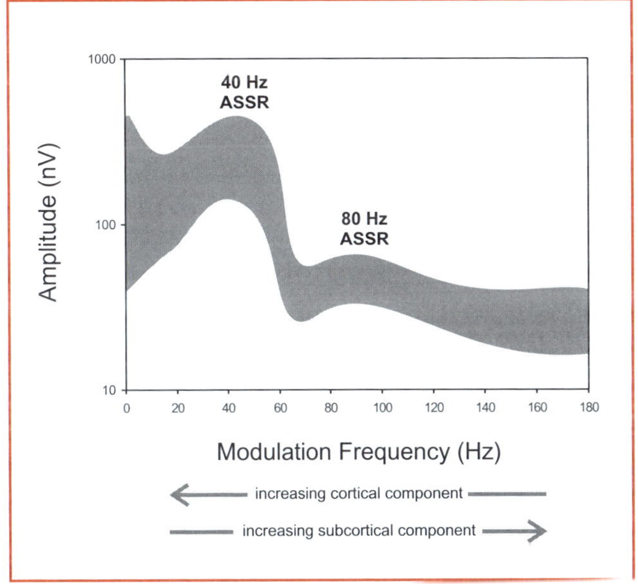

FIGURE 6–4. ASSR amplitude as a function of modulation frequency. The two major peaks in the function are at 40 and 80 Hz. 40 Hz ASSRs are generated predominantly by cortical generators, and 80 Hz ASSRs are generated predominantly by subcortical structures. *Source*: Dimitrijevic, A., & Ross, B. (2008). Neural generators of the auditory steady-state response. In G. Rance (Ed.), *The auditory steady-state response* (pp. 83–108). San Diego, CA: Plural Publishing

The primary neural generation sites dictated by the rate of modulation are clinically observable. For example, the 40 Hz response is significantly affected by sleep in adults and cannot be recorded reliably in young infants, probably because the auditory cortex and its connections are not yet fully developed. The response is, therefore, attenuated during sleep because it is primarily generated in the thalamocortical and cortical regions. Higher modulation rates produce responses that arise primarily in the brainstem, thus permitting assessment of patients while asleep or sedated. The ASSR to higher modulation rates is representative of similar neural generators as the ABR.

STIMULUS CHARACTERISTICS

Various types of stimuli are used to evoke ASSR. The defining characteristic of all the auditory stimuli used to elicit a steady-state response is the rate at which the stimuli are presented or the rate of change inherent in the stimulus. The rate of stimulus repetition or change is reproduced as neural activity in the auditory system that results in a steady-state or sustained response. The stimuli consist of a carrier frequency or stimulus, also called the test frequency or stimulus, that is modulated at a specific rate referred to as the rate of modulation or rate of stimulation. Commonly used terms related to stimuli employed in ASSR assessment are listed in Table 6–3, whereas clinical stimulus selection parameters are listed in Table 6–4. The effects of various stimulus variables on ASSR amplitude are summarized in Table 6–5.

Type of Stimuli

Examples of different stimuli used to evoke the ASSR include brief tones, modulated white noise, and modulated tones. The most common stimuli for estimating frequency-specific hearing thresholds are continuous tones with variations in amplitude and frequency modulation. Figure 6–5 illustrates the difference between amplitude and frequency modulation.

The amplitude modulated tone is the most basic stimulus used for evoking a frequency-specific ASSR. It consists of a carrier frequency, which is a pure tone, modulated in amplitude. The amplitude modulated tone in Figure 6–1 is a 1000 Hz pure tone completely modulated in amplitude (100% modulation depth) at a rate of 80 Hz. This means the 1000 Hz tone is modulated into distinct "pockets" of energy at a rate of 80 per second (Hertz = cycles per second). The result is a stimulus that is almost as frequency specific as a pure tone and, therefore, can be calibrated in dB HL, unlike stimuli used to evoke ABRs.

Frequency modulation is another possible variation in stimulus generation. Introducing frequency modulation changes the frequency spread of the carrier tone to adjacent frequency regions increasing the region stimulated on the basilar membrane. A 1000 Hz carrier stimulus with 50% frequency modulation, for example, means the spread of energy is 500 Hz, resulting in acoustic stimulation from 750 to 1250 Hz. The effect of frequency modulation is illustrated in Figure 6–5. Frequency modulation is most commonly applied to amplitude modulated tones in clinical practice. This combination is referred to as mixed modulation when the modulation frequency for both amplitude and frequency is the same. A variation of mixed modulation, referred to as *independent amplitude and frequency modulation* (IAFM), utilizes both amplitude and frequency modulation, but both are modulated at different rates. The response amplitude for this technique is slightly lower than for mixed modulation but allows for acquisition of two responses related to the two rates of change (in amplitude and frequency) applied to a single carrier (Dimitrijevic, John, van Roon, & Picton, 2001).

Other variations and advanced adaptations of these modulation paradigms have been developed with the aim of increasing the amplitude of the ASSR for easier recognition in noise, without compromising the desired frequency-specificity of the test stimuli. One such technique is exponential modulation of the amplitude modulation envelope (John, Dimitrijevic, & Picton, 2002). Another technique is the simultaneous use of two or more amplitude modulated carrier frequencies that differ by at least twice the modulation frequency, but which are all modulated at the same frequency and presented simultaneously (Stürzebecher, Cebulla, Elberling, & Berger, 2006). This produces larger amplitudes at the rate of modulation allowing for faster response detection. Another type of stimulus recently reported, a chirplike signal, compensates for the cochlear travel time by adjusting the phase of the stimulus components to achieve the maximum displacement of the basilar membrane simultaneously around the test frequency (Elberling, Don, Cebulla, & Stürzebecher, 2007).

Table 6–3. Common terminology related to ASSR stimuli, response recording, and analysis

Term		*Definition*
Related to stimuli		
Carrier frequency	Cf	Test stimulus that determines the site of stimulation on the basilar membrane
Modulation frequency	Mf	Refers to the rate at which the carrier or test frequency is being amplitude modulated into distinct pockets of energy
Amplitude modulation	AM	The test stimulus (or carrier frequency) is modulated in amplitude at a specific rate (modulation frequency)
40 Hz ASSR	40 Hz	ASSR technique with test stimuli modulated at a rate between 35 and 45 Hz
80 Hz ASSR	80 Hz	ASSR technique with test stimuli modulated at a rate between 70 and 110 Hz
Frequency modulation	FM	Modulation of the test signal in frequency (e.g., 10% FM of a 1000 Hz tone results in frequency energy between 950 and 1050 Hz)
Mixed modulation	MM	Combined amplitude and frequency modulation of a test (carrier) stimulus
Exponential Modulation	AM2	Amplitude modulation with a steep slope (exponential) for stimulus cycle
Modulation depth		The depth of the amplitude or frequency modulation (e.g., 20%)
Multiple stimuli technique		A presentation paradigm where multiple stimuli can be presented simultaneously to both ears (4 frequencies per ear)
Single stimuli technique		A presentation paradigm where only one stimulus is presented at a time
Related to response recording and analysis		
Fast Fourier transform	FFT	Transforms EEG activity in the time-domain (amplitude and latency) to the frequency-domain (frequency, amplitude, and phase information)
Phase analysis		Analysis of the response phase at the frequency of modulation to determine if a response is present (if present phases cluster together)
Phase coherence		Statistical test to determine if there is a significant difference between the distribution of phases in a recording compared to a random distribution
Spectral analysis		Considers response in frequency-domain to determine whether the response at the modulation frequency is significantly different from background EEG
F-test		Statistical test for spectral analysis, compares response amplitude at rate of stimulation to noise at adjacent frequencies for a significant difference
Physiologic recruitment		Abnormally rapid growth in ASSR amplitude due to cochlear damage; physiologic correlate to the perceptual phenomenon called recruitment

Table 6–4. Typical stimulus and response acquisition parameters for frequency-specific ASSR

Parameter	*Selection*	
Stimulus Parameters		
Carrier frequencies	500, 1000, 2000, 4000 Hz	
Modulation frequencies	70–100 Hz for infants and sleeping adults 40 Hz for awake adults Multiple simultaneous stimuli carrier tones modulated at distinct rates more than ½ octave apart	
Amplitude modulation (AM) depth	100%	
Frequency modulation (FM) depth	10–20%	
Advanced modulation options	Exponential modulation (AM2)—higher amplitudes Phase adjusted stimuli—higher amplitudes	
Stimulus intensity range	0–125 dB HL (depending on transducer and frequency)	
Transducers	Insert earphones, supra-aural earphones, sound-field speaker, bone oscillator	
Calibration reference	dB HL	
Recording Parameters		
Electrode montage	*Single-stimulus ASSR:*	
	Adults	**Infants**
	Noninverting = Cz or Fz	Noninverting = Cz or Fz
	Inverting = lower neck (inion in awake subject) or ipsilateral mastoid	Inverting = ipsilateral mastoid
	Ground = contralateral mastoid	Ground = contralateral mastoid
	Multiple-stimulus ASSR:	
	Adults	**Infants**
	Midline electrodes essential Cz or Fz for noninverting and lower neck or inion for inverting	2 channel ASSR; noninverting to ipsilateral side of each ear 1 channel ASSR test multiple frequencies in one ear at a time
Electrode impedance	<6 kOhms and interelectrode difference <3 kOhms	
Filter settings	40 Hz ASSR: 10–100 Hz* 80 Hz ASSR: 30–300 Hz* 6 dB/octave slope	
Amplification	10,000–50,000	
Averaging periods	40 seconds to 15 minutes	
Analysis time (epoch)	Usually ±1 second	
Epochs in sweep	16 (may vary)	
Sweeps	Variable	
Statistical tests	*F*-test for spectral analysis Phase coherence for phase analysis	

*Generic settings (system-specific filters).

Table 6–5. Stimulus effects on ASSR response amplitude

Carrier frequency			
Different effect for 40 & 80 Hz ASSR	Mixed modulation increases amplitude	Increase in modulation rate leads to decreasing amplitude (4–450 Hz)	Increase in amplitude with increased intensity
40 Hz ASSR: Amplitude decrease with increasing carrier frequency	Exponential AM increases amplitude	40 Hz region—amplitude increases significantly	Decrease in phase delay with increased intensity
80 Hz ASSR: Larger amplitude for mid-frequencies (1000–2000 Hz)	Increasing depth of AM and FM modulation increases amplitude	80 Hz region—amplitude increases but less than 40 Hz	Linear regression of amplitude and phase in dB for normal subjects

Source. "Auditory Steady-State Responses," by T. W. Picton, M. S. John, A. Dimitrijevic, & D. Purcell, 2003, *International Journal of Audiology*, *42*, pp. 177–219.

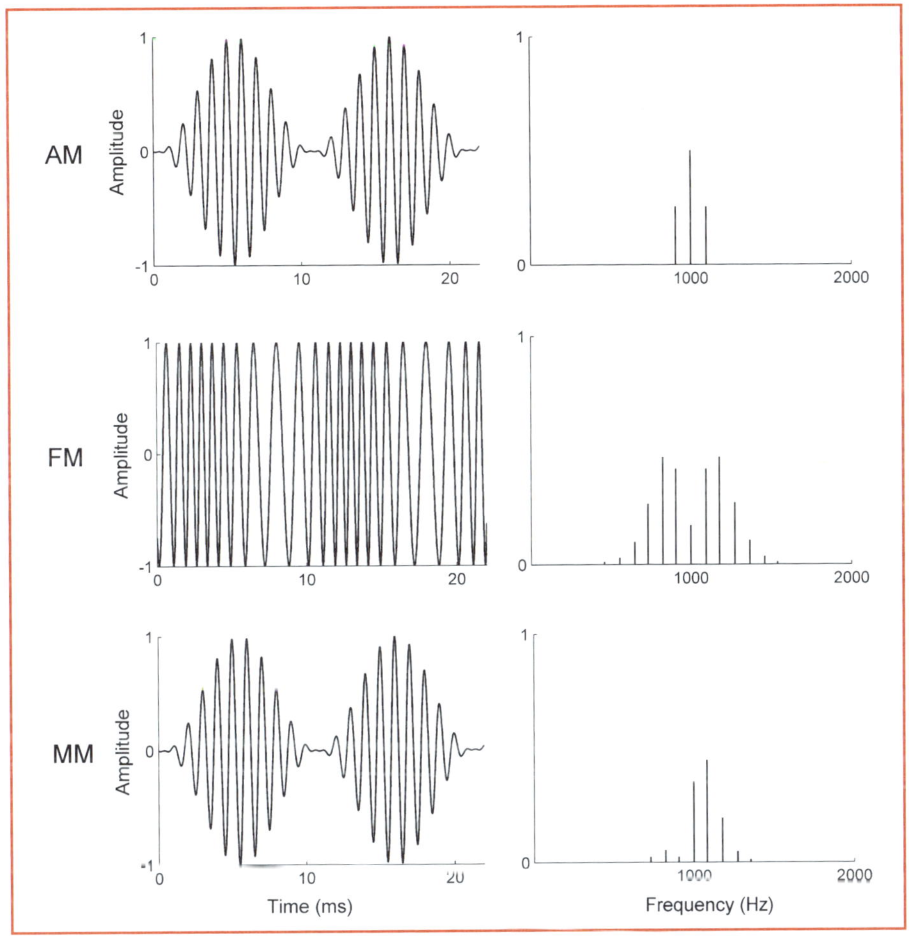

FIGURE 6–5. Amplitude, frequency, and mixed modulation illustrated in the time-and frequency-domain. The top row indicates a 1000 Hz pure tone 100% modulated at 90 Hz. The frequency component shows an energy band at 1000 Hz and at sidebands of energy to the left and right of 1000 Hz. The middle row indicates a 1000 Hz tone frequency modulated with a large spread of energy evident in the frequency-domain. The bottom row illustrates mixed modulation of a 1000 Hz tone combining amplitude and frequency modulation.

Presentation of Stimuli

The nature of the stimuli employed for evoking an ASSR allows for significant flexibility in presentation methods, in comparison to the ABR. The simplest presentation method is a single stimulus presented to one ear. Advanced techniques also allow multiple stimuli presented simultaneously to one or both ears at the same time, as illustrated in Figure 6–2. Because each carrier signal can be modulated at a different rate, several carrier signals, such as 500, 1000, 2000, and 4000 Hz, can be presented simultaneously to one ear provided that each is modulated at a distinctly different rate. These are referred to as the multiple simultaneous stimuli and can be used concurrently in both ears provided all stimuli in each ear and between each ear have a unique modulation frequency. The distinctive modulation frequency for each carrier allows recognition of responses by comparing the rate of neural activation to the specific modulation frequency.

The obvious advantage of the multiple simultaneous stimulus technique is the possibility of time savings. If responses for eight frequencies (four in each ear) are assessed simultaneously, the technique may offer significant savings in test time. The use of multiple stimuli may also offer a form of functional masking that deters regions of the basilar membrane adjacent to the stimulated region to respond, thereby ensuring more frequency specificity (John & Purcell, 2008). An intensity limitation inherent to the technique restricts its use to levels below 80 dB HL because stimulation at higher levels results in interactions between stimuli on the basilar membrane. Furthermore, amplitudes of the responses are smaller than for single-stimulus presentation. Another possible limitation may arise in steeply sloping and asymmetrical losses, where stimulation intensity level remains the same at all frequencies during the test period. This may lead to extended test time and excessively loud stimulation at certain frequencies while determining threshold at others. Simultaneous stimulus presentation could even become uncomfortable and wake up infants in natural sleep. At low intensities (e.g., ≤50 dB HL), response amplitudes for stimuli at 500 or 4000 Hz are often significantly lower than at 1000 and 2000 Hz. It may be more practical in some cases to record the three larger responses first and then return to assess the other frequency later if time permits (John & Purcell, 2008). Recently introduced versions of clinical ASSR systems have more flexible platforms, allowing for separate intensity selection for each of the stimuli comprising the multiple stimulus paradigms. The new algorithms may minimize measurement difficulties; however, the new stimulus techniques do require validation with clinical studies. Few reports are available describing the multiple simultaneous stimulation technique for hearing loss, especially in young infants, and essentially no data are available for the new flexible multiple simultaneous testing. A single study has, however, demonstrated in normal hearing subjects that the technique can be used with interstimulus intensity differences of 20 dB without causing interactions with adjacent frequencies (John, Purcell, Dimitrijevic, & Picton, 2002).

RESPONSE ACQUISITION

The stimuli employed clinically in ASSR measurement elicit a sustained auditory evoked response at the rate of stimulation represented by the modulation frequency. To record the response, far-field scalp electrodes are used to detect voltage changes on the scalp in response to, and time-locked with, the rate of stimulus presentation. Filters are used to ensure that only the desired bandwidth of brain activity is recorded. Because the response occurs at the frequency of modulation, the filter settings are set in such a way as to encompass this frequency region (e.g., a filter bandwidth of 30 to 300 Hz). The recorded brain activity is so small that it must be amplified to ensure the analog signal is converted to a digital signal (AD) without losing information. Once in digital format, the brain activity can be processed and manipulated electronically. Refer again to Table 6–3 for commonly used terms related to response recording and analysis and Table 6–4 for general response acquisition settings for recording ASSRs.

Improving the Signal-to-Noise Ratio

Like most clinically used AERs, the ASSR measured with scalp electrodes is very small compared to the continuous physiologic and myogenic background noise. Specialized techniques are required to improve the signal-to-noise ratio, where the signal is the steady-state response and the noise is the physiologic or myogenic background noise, so that the response can be confidently detected above the noise. Techniques used to improve the signal-to-noise ratio, that is, to increase the signal amplitude and to decrease the noise amplitude, are summarized in Table 6–6.

EEG activity is typically recorded from scalp electrodes using an appropriate filter bandwidth for the specific type of response, whereas excessively large recordings due to increased physiologic

Table 6–6. Improving the signal-to-noise ratio (SNR) in ASSR recordings

Increasing the Signal Amplitude
Stimulus adaptations: The signal amplitude is affected by the stimulus intensity, carrier frequency, and modulation frequency (type and depth of modulation). Increasing intensity results in higher amplitudes, but adaptations to the nature of the stimuli can also result in larger amplitude signals such as mixed modulation (MM) and exponential modulation (AM^2).
Electrode montage: The placement of scalp electrodes can affect the recorded signal amplitude and ideal positions differ for adults compared to infants. For adults best responses between vertex (or high forehead) and neck (or inion to avoid muscle artifacts) in midline or ipsilateral mastoid (earlobe). For infants best recorded from vertex (or high forehead) and ipsilateral mastoid.
Reducing the Noise Amplitude
Averaging: Process of reducing noise and maintaining signal amplitude. Signal time-locked to recording sweeps and noise is random. Averaging sweeps together results in cancellation of noise due to its random nature. Increased averaging leads to an improved SNR. Weighted averaging is an alternative method of averaging that allows for further improvement in the SNR.
Filtering: Process of recording desired range of frequencies while filtering out undesired frequencies that may contaminate recording. Filters set to be appropriate for response to be recorded. E.g., 40 Hz ASSR filter 10–100 Hz compared to 80 Hz ASSR filter 30–300 Hz.
Artifact rejection: Process of rejecting recording sections from averaging due to increased noise that may occur as a result of movement or swallowing. Removing these recordings with excessive noise avoids contamination of the averaged response due to sudden spikes in noise activity.
Patient adaptations: Aspects related to the patient state, positioning, movement, and muscle tension all have a significant impact on the amount of myogenic noise. Patients should preferably be asleep or as comfortable as possible.

noise are rejected from the averaged recording by the artifact-rejection function. Averaging is usually done in the time-domain over specific predetermined periods of time before the response activity is converted to the frequency-domain using a fast Fourier transform technique. The amount of averaging varies among clinical systems, but there are generally two types of averaging approaches.

The first approach utilizes a fixed averaging period, such as 90 seconds, for each stimulus intensity level. The Audera device includes this approach. The fixed amount of averaging may result in poorer signal detection at lower intensities because the short averaging duration does not allow for sufficient improvement in the signal-to-noise ratio. To compensate for the poorer signal detection at lower intensities, a predictive formula, based on group data, is used to estimate hearing thresholds from the ASSR threshold. The second approach is more flexible and allows for increasingly long averaging periods at lower intensities to compensate for the poorer signal-to-noise ratio at lower intensities. The variable averaging approach is incorporated into several ASSR systems (e.g., the MASTER device). This averaging strategy, however, requires longer test time as intensity is decreased (e.g., as much as 10 minutes for stimulus intensity levels close to threshold). With increased averaging for smaller signal-to-noise ratios, a consistent correction factor (e.g., 10 dB) may be applied to estimate the hearing threshold (behavioral threshold) from the ASSR threshold (physiologic threshold) across all intensities.

RESPONSE ANALYSIS

Although most auditory evoked responses are analyzed in the time-domain, ASSRs are usually analyzed in the frequency-domain. The 40 Hz ASSR response in waking adults can be visualized in the time-domain as repetitive peaks occurring over a recording period (e.g., 100 ms). The responses at higher modulation rates (>70 Hz) are significantly smaller in amplitude and, therefore, difficult to recognize in the time-domain. To assess these responses, the information in the time-domain is converted to the frequency-domain using a Fourier transform or Fourier analyzer. This conversion in essence takes the amplitude and latency information in the time-domain and transforms it to the frequency-domain, where the recorded neural activity is presented as spectral components visualized in frequency and amplitude. Each of these spectral components also contains phase information. Both the amplitude information in the frequency-domain and the phase information can be used to analyze and detect a response. Statistical techniques are employed to determine if the response is significantly different from the background EEG noise. The ASSR can be plotted either spectrally, showing response frequency and amplitude, or as a polar (vector) plot displaying response amplitude and phase.

Spectral Analysis Approach

With the spectral analysis approach, the ASSR is displayed in the frequency-domain. Statistical techniques confirm whether the response, measured at the signature frequency determined by the stimulus modulation frequency, is significantly different from the background EEG noise. The most commonly used statistical technique in ASSR analysis is the *F*-test. The *F*-test basically compares the power of the response, at the rate of stimulation (modulation frequency), to the power of the noise at adjacent frequencies. As the response and surrounding EEG noise is averaged over time, the response amplitude is continually compared to the amplitudes of surrounding frequencies. The technique uses a ratio, referred to as the *F*-ratio, to determine whether the response amplitude is significantly higher than adjacent frequencies above and below the response frequency. If a response is truly present, it should show up as a statistically significant response (e.g., $p < 0.05$). If the person does not have a response (e.g., the stimulus is below the threshold), the amplitude of the response measured at the rate of stimulation should not be detected as significantly different from the surrounding noise (e.g., $p > 0.05$). This is illustrated in Figure 6–6. The closer the statistical value is to zero, the more likely a response is present. Generally, an ASSR is usually present if statistical significance is at the level of $p < 0.05$ or $p < 0.03$.

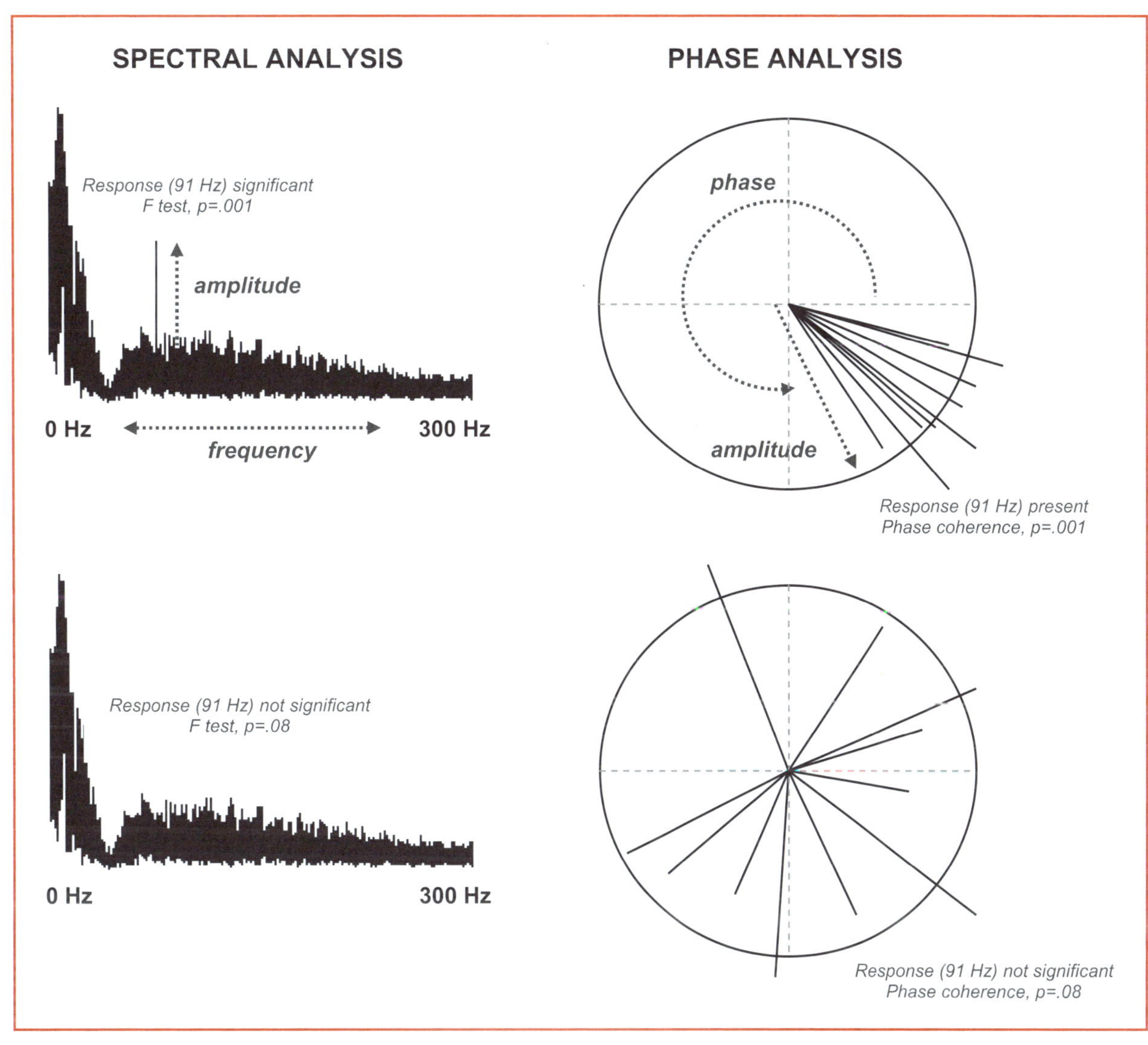

FIGURE 6–6. ASSR spectral and phase analysis approaches. The spectral analysis is done in the frequency-domain and the response amplitude at the modulation frequency (in this example at 91 Hz) is compared to adjacent frequency amplitudes. The phase analysis is illustrated on a polar plot with the response presented according to its phase deviation from 0° and amplitude represented by the length of the vector line. *Top row* illustrates significant responses with statistical values of $p < 0.01$. *Bottom row* illustrates responses that are not significant ($p > 0.01$) and therefore not considered as present in the spectral and phase analysis.

Phase Analysis Approach

Phase analysis for detecting an ASSR uses the phase information contained at the response and is usually illustrated on a polar or vector plot. The response is shown as a line projecting from the center of the polar plot with its length representing the amplitude and the phase represented by the angle between the line and the *x*-axis, measured counterclockwise from the axis (see Figure 6–6). A response is present when the recorded phases at the frequency of modulation cluster together, whereas a random representation of phases characterizes no significant response. A phase statistic, such as phase-coherence, can be used to determine whether there is a statistically significant difference (e.g., $p < 0.05$) between the distribution of phases in the recording and a random distribution as illustrated in Figure 6–6. As in the case of the spectral analysis, the closer the statistical value is to zero the more likely the response is present. A response is usually considered present if statistical significance reaches a level of $p < 0.05$ or $p < 0.03$.

Considerations in Response Detection

The question obviously arises, "Which statistical approach is best for detecting responses in the shortest possible time?" Studies all seem to show that statistical techniques considering phase and amplitude, and combinations of phase and amplitude (e.g., Hotelling's T^2 and magnitude squared coherence), have comparable detection rates (Valdes, Perez-Abalo, Martin, Savio, Sierra, et al. 1997). Recent adaptations using both phase and amplitude statistical techniques with inclusion of analyses of responses at harmonics of the response frequency, however, have demonstrated some promise for improving detection efficiency (Cebulla, Stürzebecher, & Elberling, 2006; Picton, Dimitrijevic, John, & van Roon, 2001).

Response detection is, however, more complex than just applying a statistical technique (Luts, Van Dun, Alaerts, & Wouters, 2008). Factors such as the number of sweeps (amount of averaging time) at a given intensity level and the number of times a statistical technique is applied may introduce detection errors. Typically, with clinical ASSR systems a statistical test is applied after each sweep. Each sweep requires up to 16 seconds, and then several sweeps are averaged together. A recording length of, for example, 32 sweeps compared to 16 sweeps may introduce statistical bias because the statistical test is being applied after each sweep. To cite an example, using a $p < 0.05$ statistical criterion introduces a 5% chance of a random significant response, and if this statistical technique is applied for 32 successive sweeps at the same intensity a greater chance of a response being considered significant by chance is possible.

The problem of faulty detection of a response may be avoided by ensuring that a significant response after a sweep must be repeated by at least one successive sweep before considering the response present. Another approach would be to record for a set period of time and to determine the significance of the response only after this period has passed. Unfortunately, this strategy is not commonly applied with clinically available systems (Luts et al., 2008). In addition, a specific period of time may be set for averaging (e.g., 10 minutes). However, the period of time allowed for averaging may need to be longer for lower intensities due to relatively small amplitude ASSRs. The amount of time allowed for each intensity level should be set according to normative data for adults and infants but, unfortunately, such data are not yet available (John & Purcell, 2008). As noted already, alternative clinical techniques employ a set recording period (e.g., 90 seconds) for all stimulus intensities. This approach minimizes statistical bias, but introduces poor response detection at lower intensities due to small ASSR amplitudes requiring increased averaging to reveal significance. The "fixed averaging" technique, therefore, requires predictive formulae based on normative data to compensate for elevated ASSR thresholds at lower levels of stimulation.

Another possible alternative detection strategy is to use a preset noise-level criterion for determining the presence of a response. Such an approach requires that the noise levels in the recording reach a fixed criterion (e.g., 15 nV) before recording is terminated and the statistical test is applied. Because the ASSR amplitudes are smaller at lower intensities, preset noise-level criteria will be lower at these levels compared to higher intensities. Normative data may be used to specify the required noise levels at different intensities, but these data are not yet available, especially for infants. A noise-level criterion of 10 to 15 nV has been suggested to determine the presence or absence of responses close to threshold (Vander Werff, Johnson, & Brown, 2008). It may make more sense to use a preset noise level than a preset time because some subjects may be noisier than others and therefore require longer periods of averaging. However, if subjects are restless, the averaging time may continue indefinitely. Therefore, a maximum time should be specified (John & Purcell, 2008).

Current clinical systems do not yet compensate for these limitations in response detection. Clinicians should be aware of the technical limitations when evaluating patients. Despite the fact that the ASSR uses "objective" detection methods, the audiologist must be aware of their limitations to ensure accountable interpretations of ASSR

Table 6–7. Limitation of current detection methods and clinical strategies to compensate

Limitations in Current Detection Methods	
Statistical bias	
Successive application of statistical criterion for consecutive sweeps introduces statistical bias, which may lead to false responses.	A sweep (e.g., 16 sec) with a significant response must be repeated at least once to confirm it. Confirm ASSR threshold by repeating it or 5 dB above.
Averaging criteria	
Population norms necessary for establishing preset noise-level criterion and/or averaging periods at different intensities for adults and infants.	Allow for increasing averaging time with decreasing intensity and actively monitor noise level (5–9 nV for infants near threshold).
Variability in noise levels	
Intersubject variability in noise levels characteristic and result in better thresholds for quiet subjects and elevated thresholds for noisy subjects.	Actively monitor noise level and interpret response or lack of response with caution when elevated, especially at low intensities (10–15 nV near threshold).
Preset averaging period	
A consistent averaging period (e.g., 90 sec) across all intensities produces elevated thresholds at lower intensities.	Requires predictive formulae based on population data (e.g., regression formulae for Audera) to estimate hearing thresholds from ASSR thresholds.

findings. Table 6–7 summarizes some of the current limitations in detection methods, and includes some proposed clinical strategies for overcoming the limitations.

SUBJECT FACTORS

There are a handful of important factors related to the subject or patient being tested that can have an important effect on the ASSR results. The factors, including maturation, age, and state of arousal, are considered in the following sections and are summarized in Table 6–8.

Age

In adults, the 40 Hz and 80 Hz ASSR do not seem to change significantly with increasing age. In a study of ASSRs for a group of adult subjects between the ages of 20 and 81 years of age, Picton and colleagues (2003) found no effect of age on amplitude or phase, although significant intersubject variability was characteristic of the sample.

In contrast to adults, infants do not have reliable and consistent responses with the 40 Hz ASSR. Response detection improves until around 14 years of age when the 40 Hz ASSR in awake children becomes more reliable than the 80 Hz ASSR (Aoyagi et al., 1994; Pethe et al., 2001). The age-related change in response detection is probably due to the immaturity of the infant auditory cortex. Because the 40 Hz response is primarily generated in the auditory cortex, which has a much longer developmental timeline than the brainstem, it is not adequate for assessing infants and young children.

In contrast, the 80 Hz ASSR, generated primarily in the brainstem region, can be recorded consistently in infants and young children. The fast modulation rate responses are, however, highly variable across subjects. In addition, the responses are significantly smaller in amplitude during the neonatal period, becoming progressively larger in the first 12 months of life (John,

Table 6–8. Summary of subject factors affecting 40 Hz and 80 Hz ASSR recordings in adults and infants

Subject Factors	*Effect*		*Clinical Implications*	
Age	Not significant	40 Hz unstable 80 Hz consistent Significant amplitude increase in neonatal period and in 1st year of life	40 Hz and 80 Hz reliable	80 Hz essential Test infants older than 4 weeks but be aware of variability through 1st year of life
Sleep	40 Hz and 80 Hz present in wakefulness 40 Hz has largest amplitude but is reduced by 50% during sleep In sleep 40 Hz amplitude larger at ≤1 kHz and 80 Hz amplitude larger at >1 kHz	40 Hz in asleep state is unstable 80 Hz in asleep state stable	For awake adults use 40 Hz For sleeping adults use 40 Hz for 0.5 and 1 kHz and 80 Hz for 2 and 4 kHz	80 Hz stable and reliable during sleep In awake subjects internal noise may mask response
Anesthesia	40 Hz reduced 80 Hz no effect	40 Hz ASSR unstable 80 Hz ASSR no effect	40 Hz to monitor effect on consciousness 80 Hz to monitor peripheral hearing	80 Hz reliably recorded
Attention	40 Hz demonstrate some effect	No data	No effect on threshold estimation	No data
Internal noise	80 Hz response smaller in awake state and more easily masked by internal noise close to threshold Less noise during sleep but smaller amplitude responses	Internal noise during awake state easily masks responses close to threshold In quiet sleep 80 Hz easily recorded	Awake subjects must be relaxed for reliable recordings Strategies to encourage sleep	Natural sleep, conscious sedation or anesthesia for reliable recordings

Brown, Muir, & Picton, 2004; Luts, Desloovere, & Wouters, 2006). It seems that the most significant increases in amplitude occur during the first few weeks of life. John et al. (2004) reported that ASSR thresholds may improve by as much as 10 dB after the first 3 weeks of life. This finding has implications for clinical application of ASSR, and may suggest that diagnostic ASSR assessments should be done only after the first 4 to 8 weeks of age (adjusted for prematurity). The relationship in young infants between ASSR and behavioral thresholds, however, is not well defined and remains variable through the first year of life (Rance, 2008).

Sleep

Subject state of arousal alters the electrical activity of the brain. Commonly, sleep affects auditory evoked responses that are generated in higher order regions of the auditory system such as the cortex. Because it is clear that ASSRs to faster stimulation rates (i.e., 80 Hz ASSR) are more representative of neural generators in the brainstem, these responses are less affected by sleep than the 40 Hz ASSR, which is primarily representative of cortical generators.

In awake adults, both 40 Hz and 80 Hz ASSR recordings can be performed with equal success. The 40 Hz ASSR does, however, have significantly larger amplitudes and is more easily distinguished from ongoing background EEG activity. The smaller amplitude 80 Hz ASSR, in contrast, is more difficult to detect close to threshold especially in awake adults who typically have higher levels of internal noise than when they are asleep. The 40 Hz ASSR is, therefore, the method of choice in awake adults. Nonetheless, a quiet subject state of wakefulness is still required for reliable estimates of threshold.

In sleeping adults, the 40 Hz ASSR is significantly reduced in amplitude, to approximately 50% of amplitude in the wakeful state. Several studies have indicated that the 40 Hz ASSR is larger in amplitude at 1000 Hz and lower frequencies, whereas the 80 Hz ASSR has larger amplitudes at frequencies of 1500 Hz and above (Aoyagi et al., 1994; Cohen et al., 1991; Dobie & Wilson, 1998). For clinical protocols in sleeping adults, therefore, the 40 Hz ASSR may be most appropriate for frequencies of 1000 Hz and below, whereas the 80 Hz ASSR is best recorded with frequencies of 1500 Hz and higher

Infants are almost always assessed with auditory evoked responses during sleep. This is especially true with small amplitude responses such as the ASSR that are easily masked by internal physiological noise associated with awake infants. Multiple studies have demonstrated that the 40 Hz ASSR is unstable and not consistently recorded in infants and young children, in contrast to the consistent and reliable recordings for higher rates, like 80 Hz ASSR (Aoyagi et al., 1994; Levi, Folsom, & Dobie, 1993; Rickards et al., 1994; Stapells, Galambos, Costello, & Makeig, 1988). The study by Rickards et al. (1994) indicated that for newborn infants the best modulation frequencies were between 65 and 100 Hz. Higher rates of stimulation for infants (80 Hz ASSR) are effective because the primary neural generation site is the brainstem, which is not affected during sleep and is mature long before higher order auditory regions. The 80 Hz ASSR is, therefore, the only reliable way to assess thresholds in infants and young children utilizing the ASSR technique.

Anesthesia

Anesthetic agents (including fentanyl, isoflurane, thiopental, enflurane, sufentanil, and propofol) are associated with significant reductions in amplitude of the 40 Hz ASSR in adults (Gilron, Plourde, Marcontoni & Varin, 1998; Plourde, 1996; Plourde & Picton, 1990; Plourde & Villemure, 1996). The amplitude reduction is probably due to anesthetic effects on thalamocortical activity underlying both consciousness and generation of the 40 Hz ASSR (Cone-Wesson, 2008; Plourde & Picton, 1990). Interestingly, Ketamine-induced anesthesia has the opposite effect on the 40 Hz ASSR; that is, it increases response amplitudes and, therefore, induces anesthesia through a different mechanism from other agents (Plourde, Baribeau, & Bonhomme, 1997). Clinically, the 40 Hz ASSR can be used to monitor the effect of anesthesia on patient consciousness. If hearing thresholds need to be monitored during surgery, the 80 Hz ASSR can be used. The 80 Hz response is especially useful because certain surgical techniques or prolonged anesthesia may affect hearing sensitivity by changing the middle ear pressure (Picton et al., 2003). The 80 Hz ASSR does not seem to be affected by anesthesia in adults or infants. A study by Rance et al. (1995) found no difference between 80 Hz ASSR thresholds in subjects assessed in natural sleep, under conscious sedation, or anesthetized. Because the 80 Hz ASSR is primarily generated in the brainstem, and is therefore not affected by the anesthetic agent, it is robust and reliable in patients undergoing anesthesia.

Attention

Attention does not seem to have a clinically significant effect on estimation of hearing thresholds in adults despite minor effects on the 40 Hz ASSR reported due to changes in attention. However, findings among studies are conflicting. Some studies suggest that a decrease in ASSR amplitude may be induced if attention is diverted to stimuli unrelated to the ASSR-evoking stimuli (Cone-Wesson, 2008; Makeig & Galambos, 1989). In contrast, other studies suggest that attending to the ASSR-evoking stimuli may increase response amplitude (40 Hz ASSR), which may reflect sensory perception and discrimination during an attention task (Ross, Picton, Herdman, Hillyard, & Pantev, 2004).

Internal Noise

Internal physiological noise due to background EEG, myogenic activity, and other physiological processes is inherent to all patients and particularly affect the recording of small amplitude auditory evoked responses, such as the ASSR. Internal noise is unique to each individual and his or her state of arousal. Subjects who are awake usually have higher levels of internal noise due to more muscle movements associated with activities such as swallowing, eye-blinking, and even muscle tension from stress. It may be difficult and even impossible to record accurate ASSR thresholds in awake adults who are tense and stressed due to high levels of internal noise. The 80 Hz ASSR amplitude is so small that with higher levels of internal noise associated with awake adults, it may be difficult to detect responses close to threshold especially for normal or near normal hearing subjects. The 40 Hz ASSR is larger in amplitude in awake adults and is, therefore, most appropriate for clear detection of the response from the background EEG. Despite the larger ASSR amplitudes, it may still be necessary to encourage sleep or quiet wakefulness. Also, the test should ensure that the subject is comfortable with a pillow to support the neck; instruct him or her to close the eyes and switch off bright lights.

Infants and young children must be assessed during either natural sleep or conscious sedation or anesthesia using the 80 Hz ASSR. The aim is to ensure the subject is as quiet and relaxed as possible to ensure ASSR thresholds are detected as close to behavioral thresholds as possible. Usually if a child sleeps restfully, conditions are sufficient for reliable estimation of ASSR thresholds. However, in a small number of cases, for example children with strained breathing, coughing, or snoring, the detection of responses close to threshold may be compromised. Due to its low amplitude, the 80 Hz ASSR is easily masked by internal noise that may elevate the physiologic response threshold. Quiet and restful sleep is invariably required throughout an assessment to ensure reliable estimations of behavioral thresholds are possible from ASSR recordings.

OBJECTIVE HEARING ASSESSMENT WITH THE AUDITORY STEADY-STATE RESPONSE

The main clinical application of ASSR is estimation of frequency-specific hearing thresholds, sometimes referred to as objective audiometry. An objective approach is necessary in difficult-to-test populations, such as infants and young children, multiply handicapped individuals, malingerers, or anyone unable or unwilling to provide reliable responses during behavioral audiometry. Like any other auditory evoked response techniques, the ASSR is not a true hearing test. However, physiological thresholds evoked by frequency-specific stimuli can be used to estimate behavioral hearing thresholds. Behavioral pure tone audiometry remains the gold standard for characterizing hearing sensitivity. Auditory evoked response techniques are used to estimate pure tone behavioral thresholds when behavioral techniques are not clinically feasible. Both air conduction and bone conduction testing may be utilized during auditory evoked response measurement. The sections below consider the utility of the ASSR for these measurements in infants and adults.

Hearing Screening

Objective response detection of the ASSR and the possibility of simultaneous bilateral stimulation with several stimuli makes it a very appealing tool for rapid, automated hearing screening. The challenge, however, is to identify stimuli that are efficient for evoking large amplitude responses in a brief period of time to ensure an effective screening technique. This is especially challenging because response amplitudes to conventional stimuli are small close to threshold, particularly for neonates and infants in the first few weeks of life. The use of clicks or chirplike stimuli, which compensate for cochlear delay by adjusting the phase for a more synchronous basilar membrane displacement, have been proposed as a way of rapidly detecting responses at high rates (several hundred per second) and harmonics of these rates (Stürzebecher et al., 2006). Other proposed techniques include amplitude modulated white noise that evokes a larger response in infants than modulated tones and the possibility of using low and high frequency stimuli to screen for hearing loss across the frequency spectrum (Picton, John, & Dimitrijevic, 2002). Future developments may permit the ASSR to become a viable screening tool, but at present more research is necessary to validate ASSR screening techniques alongside existing screening technologies, that is, automated OAE and ABR.

Estimating Behavioral Threshold

The term *threshold* in auditory evoked response measurements refers to the lowest stimulus level at which a response is present. Typically, stimulation begins at a moderately high intensity where a response may be clearly visible. The intensity is subsequently reduced until no response is present. A bracketing technique of 10 dB, or for greater accuracy but longer test duration 5 dB, may be used close to threshold. If no response is present at the initial stimulation level, then the intensity is increased until a response is recorded or until the maximum intensity is reached without a response.

The physiologic threshold recorded in this manner is typically higher than the actual behavioral threshold for the same stimulus because the physiologic response is extracted from background EEG that masks the small amplitude response close to or at threshold level. The physiologic threshold must, therefore, be used to estimate or predict the behavioral threshold at the specific frequency. Verifying how close the physiologic threshold is to the actual behavioral threshold is not an easy task, however. It is complicated by at least four factors related to ASSR testing: (a) At low levels of stimulation close to threshold, the amount of noise in the recording (due to muscle movements, physiological processes, etc.) may easily mask the small amplitude ASSR. (b) Intra- and intersubject differences in the amount of background noise in recordings introduce inherent variability in physiologic thresholds. (c) ASSR thresholds in cochlear hearing loss are closer to behavioral thresholds due to physiologic recruitment. (d) Smaller response amplitudes in neonates and infants result in elevated physiologic thresholds compared to older children and adults. These factors exert a significant influence on the relationship between physiologic and behavioral thresholds, and on how to best to quantify the difference (refer to the section on response detection for more information).

Commercial ASSR systems implement one of two general approaches to estimate behavioral thresholds from the physiologic thresholds. Table 6–9 summarizes the main differences between these approaches. The first approach, called the regression approach, is to record for a short period (e.g., 90 seconds) at a specified intensity to determine the presence or absence of relatively large amplitude responses. Smaller responses at lower intensities cannot be recorded due to the brief preset recording time (e.g., 90 seconds), which does not allow for sufficient averaging to improve the signal-to-noise ratio for response detection. To predict behavioral thresholds from physiologic thresholds with this approach requires formulae based on normative population data to correct for the physiologic-behavioral difference. The GSI Audera ASSR system, for example, employs the regression formulae by Rance and colleagues (1995), which were compiled from physiologic and behavioral threshold data for numerous subjects, including children and adults, with varying degrees of hearing loss. The formulae are characterized by correction factors of increasing magnitude with decreasing intensity that are specific to each frequency as determined by the normative data.

Table 6–9. Comparison of ASSR threshold estimation approaches

Correction Approach	*Regression Approach*
Recording characteristics	
• Recording time varies with intensity (e.g., 10 minutes at 40 dB HL vs. 3 minutes at 90 dB HL) • Longer averaging periods with decreasing intensity • Stop criterion either specified time (e.g., 10 minutes) or noise level (e.g., 9 nV)	• Consistent recording period (e.g. 90 seconds) • Recording time relatively brief • Stop criterion based on time (e.g., 90 seconds)
Threshold estimation	
• A consistent correction (e.g., 10 dB) independent of threshold intensity is used to estimate behavioral threshold • May differ across frequency (e.g., 15 dB for 0.5 kHz) • Physiologic recruitment is compensated for by increasing amount of averaging at lower intensities	• Regression formulae based on normative data used to estimate behavioral threshold • Correction magnitude increases with decreasing intensity • Regression formulae compensate for physiologic recruitment (e.g., 25 dB correction at 50 dB HL ASSR threshold vs. 5 dB correction at 90 dB HL)
Limitations	
• Extended recording time at low intensities may not be clinically feasible except if a multiple stimuli technique is used • Exact criteria based on normative data for the amount of averaging required at an intensity or the noise level to be reached is not yet available	• Large corrections at lower intensities result in significant variability • Cannot accurately differentiate between mild hearing loss and normal hearing

The alternative approach, called the correction approach, utilizes longer periods of averaging at lower intensities (e.g., Bio Logic MASTER). This approach compensates for the smaller amplitude responses at intensities close to normal hearing that require more averaging to detect a response from the background EEG. Recording time at higher intensities is shorter because response amplitudes are larger, and in cases of cochlear hearing loss, physiologic recruitment also results in higher amplitudes and therefore faster detection of responses. Because the effect of smaller amplitudes at lower intensities is compensated for with an extension of the time required for averaging, a consistent correction value (e.g., 10 dB) is used to estimate behavioral thresholds independent of the physiologic threshold level.

Threshold Accuracy

This section will consider the accuracy of ASSR thresholds in estimating behavioral thresholds. Because the vast majority of our current understanding is based on air conduction ASSR measurement, we will only consider thresholds determined through air conduction. Separate discussions in subsequent sections are devoted to bone conduction and free-field ASSR measurement. Table 6–10 summarizes the clinical implications for estimating air conduction behavioral thresholds.

Adults

The 40 Hz ASSR is most appropriate and accurate for estimating behavioral thresholds in awake

Table 6–10. Clinical implications of current knowledge on estimating air conduction behavioral thresholds with the ASSR

Adults
• 40 Hz ASSR in awake subjects most accurate (within 10 dB ± 10 dB)
• 80 Hz ASSR in subjects with normal hearing within 10–25 dB ± 7–15 dB
• 80 Hz ASSR in subjects with hearing loss within 5–20 dB ± 3–13 dB
• 500 Hz poorer correlation with behavioral thresholds
• 80 Hz ASSR and tone burst ABR present comparable thresholds
• Artifactual ASSRs may be present at high intensities, although software upgrades should alleviate the problem for higher frequencies (1–4 kHz)
Infants
• 80 Hz ASSR maturational effect on thresholds
• ASSR thresholds in normal hearing infants 10–15 dB higher in 1st year of life
• Should not use in first 6–8 weeks of life due to elevated thresholds
• Average range of normal thresholds for 500 Hz is 35–45 dB HL
• Average range of normal thresholds for 1000–4000 Hz is 25 to 40 dB HL
• More accurate in sensorineural hearing loss of moderate and greater degree
• Difficult to differentiate between normal hearing and mild losses without longer averaging
• Cannot identify or differentiate auditory neuropathy from sensorineural hearing loss

adults. The accuracy of ASSR measured in adults is commonly determined by looking at the difference between the ASSR thresholds and behavioral thresholds. The accuracy of the 40 Hz ASSR in awake adults suggests physiologic thresholds are within 10 dB of behavioral thresholds, with a standard deviation of approximately 10 dB (Picton et al., 2003). In sleeping adults, the amplitude of the 40 Hz ASSR decreases significantly and, therefore, the 80 Hz ASSR becomes more appropriate especially for higher frequencies (>1000 Hz).

Thresholds for the 80 Hz ASSR in adults have very good correlation with behavioral thresholds (correlation coefficients of 0.85 to 0.95). This is especially true for higher frequencies (1000, 2000, and 4000 Hz), whereas 500 Hz is generally associated with slightly poorer correlations. In normal hearing adults, ASSR threshold levels usually vary between 20 and 30 dB HL at low frequencies (500 Hz) and around 15 and 20 dB HL at higher frequencies (1000, 2000, and 4000 Hz). Differences between ASSR and behavioral thresholds are greater in normal hearing adults compared to adults with hearing loss. The average range of threshold differences reported in normal hearing adults is 10 to 25 dB with a standard deviation of between 7 and 15 dB (Herdman & Stapells, 2003; Picton et al., 2003; Vander Werff, Johnson, & Brown, 2008). ASSR thresholds in adults with hearing loss are recorded closer to behavioral thresholds as a result of physiologic recruitment. The average differences between thresholds vary between 5 and 20 dB with standard deviations from 3 to 13 dB (Herdman & Stapells, 2003; Picton et al., 2003; Vander Werff et al., 2008). The variability of results between studies is attributed to different presentation methods and differences in recording time. Typically, longer recording periods produce smaller differences between behavioral and physiological thresholds.

Comparisons between 80 Hz ASSR and tone burst ABR thresholds in adults are scarce, but the limited data available suggest that both techniques are comparable in their estimations of behavioral thresholds in subjects with hearing loss (Stapells, 2008).

Infants

The 80 Hz ASSR has been used effectively to predict hearing thresholds in infants and young children. A maturational effect on the ASSR thresholds throughout the first 12 months of life, and probably longer for lower frequencies (500 Hz), is clearly evident from current literature (Rance, 2008). Studies indicate that ASSR thresholds in presumably normal hearing neonates and infants, within the first year of life, are between 10 and

15 dB higher than those in normal hearing adults (Lins et al., 1996; Luts et al., 2006; Rance & Rickards, 2002). Most studies on ASSR thresholds in these normal hearing infants indicate average thresholds between 35 and 45 dB HL at low frequencies (500 Hz) and 25 and 40 dB HL at higher frequencies (1000, 2000, and 4000 Hz) with standard deviations of between 6 and 13 dB. Initial studies on premature babies suggest that ASSR thresholds are even more elevated in these very young babies, confirming the maturational effect on the ASSR in the neonatal and early infancy periods (Cone-Wesson, Parker, Swiderski, & Rickards, 2002; Luts et al., 2006). Normal hearing levels for infants beyond the first few weeks of life with air conduction ASSR are currently reported as 50 at 500 Hz, 45 at 1000 Hz, and 40 at 2000 and 4000 Hz. This means that for ASSR thresholds to be considered normal they have to be found at or below these intensity levels.

For neonates and infants with sensorineural hearing loss, current ASSR data are mostly limited to the single-stimulus recording technique with little data available for multiple-stimulus ASSR. Preliminary data suggest, however, that responses can be obtained significantly closer to behavioral threshold due to the physiologic recruitment phenomenon (Rance, 2008). ASSR thresholds in infants with hearing loss are detected closer to behavioral thresholds with increasing hearing loss severity (Luts et al., 2006; Rance et al., 2005;). The limited variability in the data indicates that ASSR thresholds in infants with sensorineural hearing loss can provide reasonably reliable estimations of behavioral thresholds for moderate to severe degrees of hearing loss (Rance et al., 2005). The small amplitude of the ASSR in early infancy, and especially the neonatal period, makes clear differentiation of normal hearing versus mild hearing loss difficult, if not impossible, with current clinical protocols. As a result, ASSR assessment approaches may not be the most appropriate for accurate estimations of behavioral thresholds during the first 6 weeks of life (Rance & Tomlin, 2006).

To establish the ASSR as a part of the electrophysiological test battery, it is necessary to compare thresholds with tone burst ABR in infants with and without hearing loss. Unfortunately comparisons between ASSR thresholds and tone burst ABR thresholds in infants are scarce. A study by Rance, Tomlin, and Rickards (2006) compared tone burst ABR and ASSR thresholds in newborns and infants for frequencies of 500 and 2000 Hz. The findings suggest that in normal hearing newborns, the ASSR is significantly more elevated and more variable than tone burst ABR thresholds. These differences are largely negated by 6 weeks of age, although the variability in the ASSR may still be slightly higher (Stapells, 2008). There are no comparisons of these techniques in infants with hearing loss, including no ASSR data for children with conductive or mixed hearing losses. However, case studies have indicated that tone burst ABR findings of subjects with steeply sloping hearing loss may underestimate the degree of high frequency hearing loss, whereas the ASSR may more accurately reflect the steeply sloping high frequency hearing loss (Rance, Luts, Cone-Wesson, Van Maanen, & King, 2008). Presumably, the modulated tones used to evoke the ASSR are more frequency specific than tone bursts and, therefore, provide a more accurate representation of the audiometric configuration. In contrast, at lower frequencies the tone burst ABR better predicts behavioral thresholds.

At present, the tone burst ABR with its long clinical history and established research foundation is still considered as an essential frequency-specific measure for determining hearing thresholds in infants. The ASSR can, however, be utilized to complement the test battery in unique ways that may offer important advantages for specific cases.

Auditory Neuropathy

This is an important clinical entity to consider with ASSR measurement, analysis, and interpretation. Auditory neuropathy, now referred to as auditory neuropathy spectrum disorder (ANSD), comprises approximately 10% of all cases of permanent hearing loss and is associated with atypical auditory evoked potential findings (Rance, 2005; Sinniger, 2002). The condition is characterized by absent or abnormal ABR waves with present otoacoustic emissions and/or a cochlear microphonic (CM) response. These diagnostic findings, attributed to dyssynchrony in neural firing of the auditory nerve, typically result in a loss in hearing sensitivity of varying degrees with perceptual difficulties related to temporal processing. ANSD was reviewed earlier in Chapter 4.

Abnormal auditory evoked response findings are usually found in ANSD because the responses, especially those generated in the brainstem, are dependent on synchronous neural firing and ANSD is characterized by a disruption of neural synchrony. The ABR, for example, is invariably absent or abnormal, yet this finding is not correlated with hearing sensitivity. Studies have reported a similar pattern of findings with the ASSR, that is, no correlation between ASSR thresholds and actual behavioral thresholds (Rance et al., 1999; Rance et al., 2008; Rance & Briggs, 2002). When ASSR thresholds are recorded, they are typically significantly elevated by 30 to 40 dB and cannot be used to predict behavioral thresholds.

A major disadvantage of ASSR versus ABR measurement in cases of auditory neuropathy is that the ASSR technique does not allow for differentiation between cochlear and retrocochlear pathologies. In ABR measurement the presence of a cochlear microphonic response can be used to establish whether there is cochlear functioning present, even with markedly abnormal neural auditory status. The ASSR cannot differentiate between auditory neuropathy and conventional sensorineural hearing loss without information from other procedures in the test battery such as OAE and ABR. It is therefore important to always conduct ASSR measurement in combination with at least a click-evoked ABR.

Artifactual Responses

Initial clinical investigations demonstrated that ASSR offers an advantage for determining thresholds in severe to profound hearing loss when ABRs are absent at high intensities. However, more recent reports of artifactual or spurious ASSRs in cochlear implant patients with no behavioral response to sound at high intensity air conducted stimulation have raised serious concerns regarding this proposed advantage (Gorga et al., 2004; Small & Stapells, 2004). Using a version of the MASTER device, Gorga and colleagues (2004) recorded ASSR thresholds at an average intensity level of 100 dB HL in adults with profound hearing loss even when no behavioral responses were present at maximum intensity outputs that were 18 to 22 dB higher. The findings clearly indicated that ASSRs recorded at these high intensities were not generated in the auditory system.

There are several possible reasons for these artifactual responses. The most prominent reason is related to the relatively slow analog-to-digital (A/D) rates (e.g., 500 and 1000 Hz) employed by many early research and clinical systems. Inadequate sampling rates may result in aliasing of stimulus artifact to the recording for carrier frequencies that are integers of the A/D rate. If a 500 Hz A/D rate is used, for example, aliasing can be expected at the modulation rates of carrier frequencies commonly used, that is, 500, 1000, 2000, and 4000 Hz. If a 1000 Hz A/D rate was used, stimulus artifact may be expected at integers of 1000, including the commonly used frequencies of 1000, 2000, and 4000 Hz. The application of higher A/D rates (e.g., 1250 Hz) that are not integers of commonly used carrier frequencies, with a steep anti-aliasing filter (such as 300 Hz low pass filter, 115 dB/octave slope), eliminates most of these responses (Small & Stapells, 2004; Picton & John, 2004). Single-polarity air conduction stimuli employing a 1250 Hz A/D rate appear to allow accurate threshold determination for all frequencies (except 1000 Hz, perhaps), up to at least 114 to 120 dB HL. These reports resulted in important modifications to the Biologic MASTER clinical ASSR system to avoid such artifactual responses. Other clinical systems probably do not use A/D rates that are likely to cause aliasing (e.g., GSI Audera), but the possibility of spurious responses has not yet been investigated (Small & Stapells, 2008a). Further practical techniques to minimize interference in recordings are to use insert earphones as opposed to supra-aural earphones, and to use braided electrode wires.

Another source of spurious responses has been reported for low frequencies (<1000 Hz) at higher levels of stimulation. These questionable ASSRs are differentiated from spurious responses due to stimulus artifact at higher frequencies because they do not change in phase with inverting polarity (Small & Stapells, 2004). The second type of spurious response, therefore, seems to be physiological but not from the auditory system. The vestibular system has been identified as the most likely source because vestibular responses can be evoked by high level low frequency auditory stimuli (Small & Stapells, 2008a). The vestibular evoked myogenic potential (VEMP) is, of course, an example of a vestibular response recorded with high intensity low frequency sound stimulation. High intensity ASSR thresholds at 500 Hz should be interpreted with caution and within the context of other findings to verify, or cross-check, whether they truly represent an auditory response.

Bone Conduction Auditory Steady-State Responses

Frequency-specific, bone conduction threshold estimation with auditory evoked responses allows for differentiation of conductive versus mixed or sensorineural hearing loss. In recent years, clinical investigations of bone conduction ASSR in adults and infants have been reported, but findings are still somewhat limited (Dimitrijevic et al., 2002; Jeng, Brown, Johnson, & Vander Werff, 2004; Lins et al., 1996; Small & Stapells, 2004, 2005, 2006, 2008b, 2008c, Small, Hatton, & Stapells, 2007). Average threshold levels for bone conduction ASSR in normal hearing adults are reported to be 28, 24, 16, and 17 dB HL at 500, 1000, 2000, and 4000 Hz, respectively (Small & Stapells, 2008a). For infants (0 to 11 months), average bone conduction ASSR thresholds are 15, 4, 25, and 15 dB HL at 500, 1000, 2000, and 4000 Hz, respectively (Small & Stapells, 2008a). Results indicate that high frequency bone conduction thresholds improve and low frequency bone conduction thresholds worsen with increasing age. This trend is the opposite of the maturational effect on air conduction ASSR. The normal hearing levels for bone conduction ASSR for different age groups are summarized in Table 6–11.

An important consideration in the measurement of ASSR evoked by bone conduction stimulation is the occurrence of spurious responses at higher intensities due to stimulus artifact and the possibility of vestibular responses for low frequency (<1000 Hz) stimulation. The mechanisms underlying nonauditory ASSRs were discussed in the previous section on artifactual ASSR responses. The interference of the bone-oscillator stimulus artifact, and other artifacts with low frequency stimuli, on ASSR recordings occurs at much lower

Table 6–11. Normal levels of bone conduction ASSR in dB HL

	500 Hz	1000 Hz	2000 Hz	4000 Hz
Preterm infants	≤30	≤30	≤50	≤50
Post-term infants (0–11 months)	≤30	≤20	≤40	≤30
Infants (12–24 months)	≤40	≤20	≤40	≤30
Adults	≤50	≤40	≤30	≤30

*More than 90% of subjects with normal hearing had response present at these levels.

Source. Recommendations from "Multiple Auditory Steady-State Responses to Bone-Conduction Stimuli in Adults with Normal Hearing," by S. A. Small and D. R. Stapells, 2005, *Journal of the American Academy of Audiology*, *16*, pp. 172–183; "Multiple Auditory Steady-State Response Thresholds to Bone-Conduction Stimuli in Young Infants with Normal Hearing," by S. A. Small and D. R. Stapells, 2006, *Ear and Hearing*, *27*, pp. 219–228; "Maturation of Bone-Conduction Multiple Auditory Steady-State Responses," by S. A. Small and D. R. Stapells, 2008, *International Journal of Audiology*, *47*, pp. 476–488.

intensities than for air conducted stimuli despite strategies to avoid problems, such as selecting a more appropriate A/D rate (e.g., 1250 Hz). We recently assessed 13 infants (average age of 2.2 years) with severe-to-profound sensorineural hearing loss using bone conduction ASSR (with the GSI Audera) to determine the levels at which spurious responses occur (D. Swanepoel, Ebrahim, Friedland, Pottas, & A. Swanepoel, 2008). Table 6–12 provides the effective range of stimulation for infants and adults (Small & Stapells, 2004; Swanepoel et al., 2008) before spurious ASSRs begin to occur with bone conduction stimulation. At low intensity levels, particularly for 250 Hz where artifactual responses occurred at intensities as low as 25 dB, the clinical utility of the technique is limited. It is not certain whether these low frequency spurious responses are due to a stimulus artifact or possibly are a result of a physiologic response from the vestibular system. Techniques to minimize the effect of the stimulus artifact include the selection of appropriate A/D conversion rates (clinical systems have adopted these), braided electrode wires, nonmastoid inverting (reference) electrode placement to avoid close proximity with the bone oscillator, and stimuli designed to alternate in polarity across different epochs (not yet implemented clinically).

An alternative method for determining bone conduction thresholds with ASSR to avoid stimulus artifacts is the use of the sensorineural acuity level (SAL) technique. The SAL technique determines bone conduction thresholds by delivering narrowband masking noise through the bone oscillator while assessing air conduction ASSR thresholds at this frequency. Once the ASSR threshold is masked, this is deemed as the bone conduction threshold. Cone-Wesson and colleagues (2002b) adapted the SAL technique for ASSR to distinguish between sensorineural and conductive hearing loss in young infants. The SAL ASSR technique has the advantage over a conventional bone conduction paradigm of avoiding the masking dilemma associated with interaural attenuation of stimuli, although in young infants interaural attenuation for the ASSR is less problematic than in adults. Because air conduction stimuli are used to evoke the response, the SAL technique also avoids the difficulties associated with electrical and mechanical artifacts generated by the bone oscillator. Limitations of this technique, however, include the possibility of bone conducted noise increasing the ASSR noise levels. Because bone conduction thresholds are derived from two estimated thresholds, they are also open to more variability.

Taking into consideration the upper limit for normal hearing levels in ASSR measurement, as presented in Table 6–12, the effective range of assessment for bone conduction ASSR in adults and children is rather constrained. The limited range for bone conduction ASSR is due to elevated normal hearing levels, especially in infants, and the possibility of spurious responses at reasonably low intensity levels. At this point, due to the possibility of spurious responses, sensorineural hearing loss of a moderate or greater degree in the high frequencies (1 to 4000 Hz), and of a mild or greater degree in the low frequencies (500 Hz),

Table 6–12. Effective range in dB HL for bone conduction ASSR testing before spurious responses begin to occur

	250 Hz	500 Hz	1000 Hz	2000 Hz	4000 Hz
Adults*		0–40	0–50	0–50	0–60
Infants and children†	0–20	0–35	0–55	0–55	0–55

*From "Artifactual Responses when Recording Auditory Steady-State Responses," by S. A. Small and D. R. Stapells, 2004, *Ear and Hearing*, *25*, pp. 611–623.

†From "Auditory Steady-State Responses to Bone Conduction Stimuli in Children with Hearing Loss," by D. Swanepoel, S. Ebrahim, P. Friedland, L. Pottas, and A. Swanepoel, 2008, *International Journal of Pediatric Otorhinolaryngology*, *72*, pp. 1861–1871.

cannot be confidently quantified using bone conduction ASSR. In cases of conductive hearing loss, bone conduction ASSR can effectively quantify sensory hearing between 500 and 4000 Hz, but mixed hearing losses may not be effectively identified due to the limited dynamic range associated with these technical problems.

Before bone conduction ASSR can be considered as a substitute for bone conduction tone burst ABR measurement, more studies are necessary to validate the feasibility of ear-specific findings and the accuracy of threshold estimations, especially for patients with mixed losses and conductive pathologies. Recent studies (Small et al., 2007; Small & Stapells, 2006, 2008b) have investigated procedural factors that may influence bone conduction ASSR measurements in infant populations. The clinical implications of these findings for bone conduction ASSR in infants are summarized as follows:

- *Coupling method:* Elastic band or handheld coupling of bone oscillator is appropriate (requires training).
- *Placement of bone oscillator:* Temporal or mastoid placement can be used and a forehead placement should be avoided.
- *Occlusion effect:* Testing may be done with ears occluded or unoccluded without significant effect on threshold estimation (unlike for adults where correction for the occlusion effect is necessary).
- *Calibration of stimuli:* dB HL calibration is appropriate, but be cognizant that normal hearing levels for bone conduction are different for infants.
- *Isolating the test cochlea:* Infants have greater interaural attenuation for bone conduction stimuli compared to adults making isolation of the test cochlea easier (at least 10 to 30 dB of interaural attenuation compared to no more than 10 dB in adults)

Two-channel recordings may be used to determine ear-specific findings, that is, which cochlea is generating a response. The channel containing the response with larger amplitude and shorter phase delay indicates the cochlea being evaluated (clinical systems do not currently offer this feature).

Sound-Field ASSR

The nature of ASSR stimuli allows for more effective presentation in a sound-field environment compared to the limitations associated with transient evoked potentials such as the ABR. The transient stimuli used with the ABR may be distorted by presentation in the sound field or by amplification. In contrast, the ASSR is evoked by continuous stimuli modulated in amplitude and/or frequency that are unlikely to be distorted by amplification in either the sound-field speaker or a hearing aid (Picton et al., 1998). This possibility has allowed for the validation of aided ASSR responses in adults and infants for whom behavioral responses are not possible (Picton et al., 1998; Stroebel, Swanepoel, & Groenewald, 2007). Figure 6–7 illustrates the aided sound-field ASSR thresholds for an infant with profound hearing loss.

Studies to date have indicated reasonable correlation between aided ASSR thresholds and behavioral thresholds, although unaided thresholds demonstrate even better correlation (Picton et al., 1998; Stroebel et al., 2007). The aided ASSR

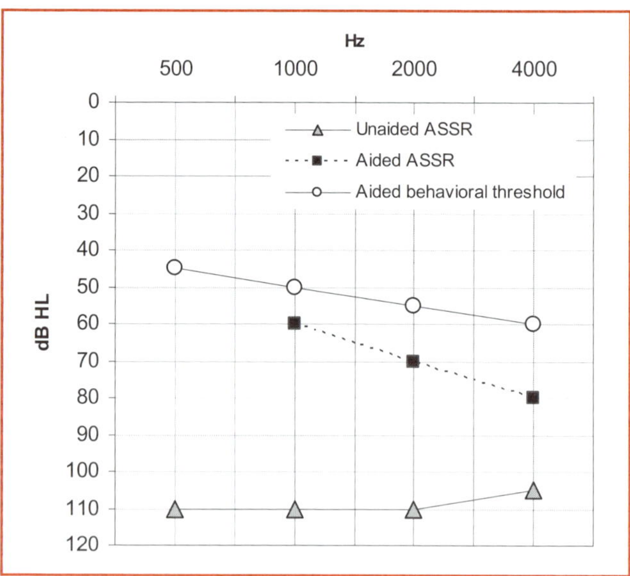

FIGURE 6–7. Aided ASSR thresholds for an infant with profound hearing loss. *Note.* Adapted from "Aided Auditory Steady-State Responses in Infants," by D. Stroebel, D. Swanepoel, and E. Groenewald, 2007, *International Journal of Audiology*, *46*, pp. 287–292.

threshold for 500 Hz signals showed the largest variability and could not be recorded in over half of infants assessed. Despite poorer correlations and variability, the aided ASSRs may provide the first robust evidence of hearing aid benefit in young infants who are commonly fitted with hearing aids before they are able to provide reliable behavioral responses to sounds. Information of this kind may be valuable in guiding initial case management decisions soon after diagnosis of the hearing loss when no other information is available (Stroebel et al., 2007). Future applications of sound-field ASSR may involve evaluating suprathreshold discrimination abilities with specialized stimuli in hearing aid users as well as determining the dynamic range across frequencies for accurate hearing aid fittings in infants (Picton et al., 2002; Zenker-Castro & Barajas, 2008).

CLINICAL PROTOCOLS AND EQUIPMENT

Current recommendations for employing ASSR in clinical practice require a combined approach with ABR measurement. Currently, there is not enough evidence to recommend reliance only on an ASSR approach for estimating hearing thresholds in infants. More research evidence is necessary, especially for multiple stimulus techniques and for infants with various types, degrees, and configurations of hearing loss. This caution regarding ASSR is reflected in the latest recommendation by the Joint Committee of Infant Hearing (JCIH, 2007) to use frequency-specific ABR as the primary diagnostic procedure to estimate hearing loss, type, degree and configuration. The current strengths and weaknesses of the ASSR technique are summarized in Table 6–13. The ASSR does, however, complement the current test battery for estimating hearing loss with auditory evoked responses in unique ways and provides an objective cross-check strategy to verify results. Table 6–14 summarizes the complementary roles of the ASSR and ABR. Figure 6–8 and Figure 6–9 illustrate how the single-frequency and multiple-frequency ASSR can be used in a combined ABR protocol.

Table 6–13. Summary of clinical strengths versus weaknesses of ASSR

Strengths

- Frequency-specific estimation of hearing thresholds
- Objective response detection by statistical techniques
- Multiple frequencies can be presented simultaneously to both ears
- Stimuli allow for processing in sound-field speakers
- Stimuli allow for processing by hearing aids for aided assessment
- Elevated intensity levels for stimulation (exceeding 100 dB HL)
- Very accurate in more severe degrees of sensorineural hearing loss
- Can provide information on auditory processing of amplitude modulation
- Can provide information on auditory processing of frequency modulation
- Mixed modulation stimuli are representative of speech stimuli

Weaknesses

- More normative data for infants with hearing loss required
- Exact neural generators not clearly defined
- Small amplitude responses sensitive to myogenic noise
- Measurement requires natural sleep, sedation, or anesthesia
- Cannot differentiate between cochlear and neural hearing loss
- Limited data on ASSR in conductive losses
- Difficult to differentiate between mild hearing loss and normal hearing
- Extended time for averaging necessary at low intensities
- Artifactual responses may occur at high intensities
- Bone conduction ASSR requires further validation

Note. All electroacoustic and electrophysiologic measures share a number of clinical advantages, as summarized in Chapter 1 and described in detail throughout the text.

Table 6–14. Complementary roles of the ASSR and ABR for testing infants and children

ABR	
• Neurological integrity can be evaluated • Cochlear microphonic response can be evaluated (preneural functioning) • ABR can differentially diagnose auditory neuropathy • ABR threshold accuracy better in first weeks of life (<6 to 8 weeks) • ABR more reliable (faster) for testing low to mid-intensity levels (<60 dB) especially at 500 Hz • Delayed latencies can provide indication of conductive loss • Bone conduction validated as reliable technique to differentiate conductive losses	• Stimuli more frequency-specific • Multiple frequencies may be assessed simultaneously in both ears (four per ear) • Frequency-specificity allows for better representation of steeply sloping high frequency losses • High intensity stimulation allows assessment in severe and profound range (ABR limited to <90 dB) • Stimuli presented in sound field without distortion • Stimuli processed without distortion by hearing aids • Objective response detection avoids interpretation bias

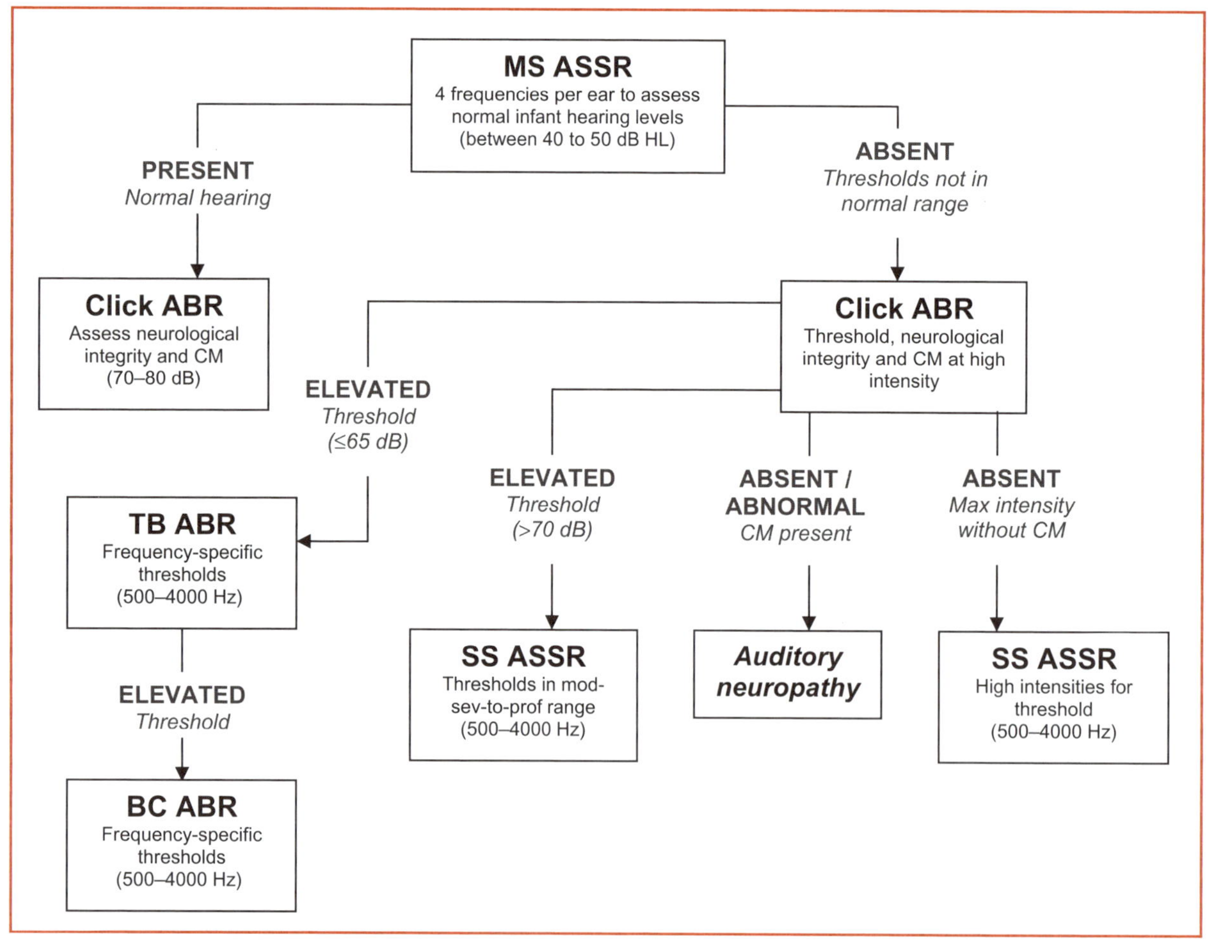

FIGURE 6–8. Combined protocol for multiple-frequency ASSR and ABR in infants. MS = multiple stimuli; SS = single stimuli; TB = tone burst; BC = bone conduction; CM = cochlear microphonic.

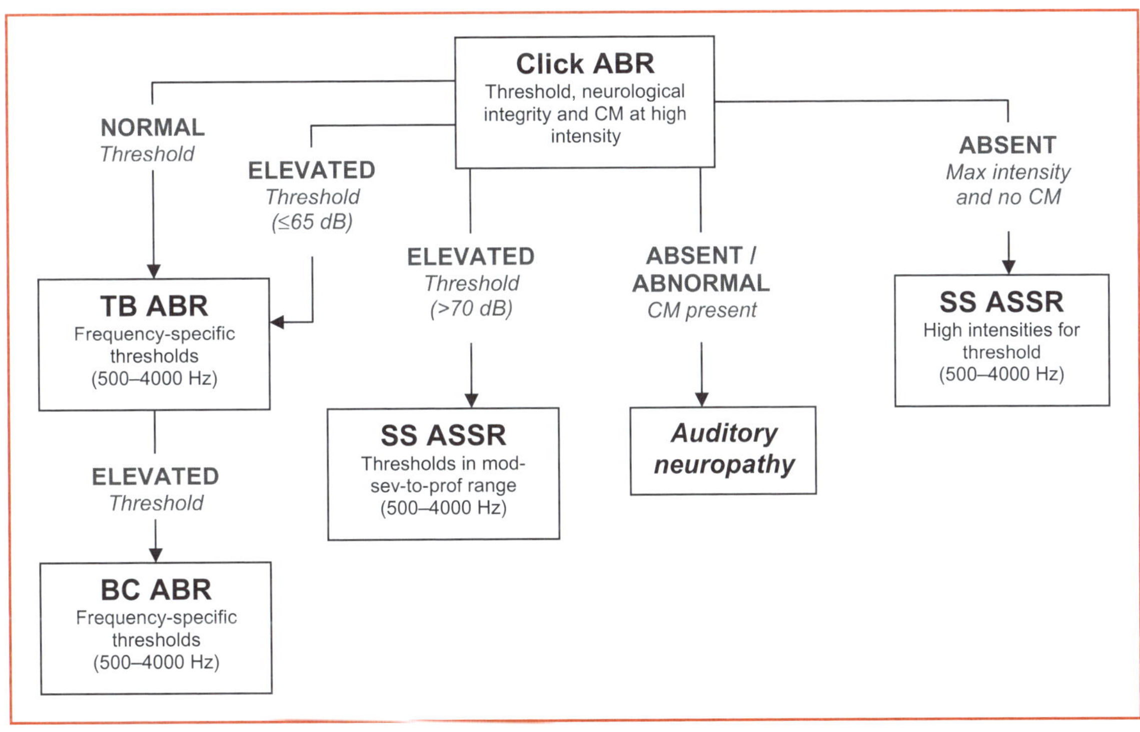

FIGURE 6–9. Combined protocol for single-frequency ASSR and ABR. SS = single stimuli; TB = tone burst; BC = bone conduction; CM = cochlear microphonic.

Commercial devices with ASSR capabilities have become increasingly available over the past several years. The first device to appear on the market was the AUDIX (Neuronic, SA) followed by the Audera (GSI-Viasys) and the MASTER (Bio-Logic-Natus). The majority of current research data has been conducted with these devices. Recent commercial releases of ASSR equipment by other manufacturers have introduced intriguing adaptations to stimuli, detection algorithms, and threshold seeking techniques, but these require independent research to validate the techniques. Table 6–15 provides a summary of currently available commercial ASSR equipment.

FUTURE APPLICATIONS OF THE AUDITORY STEADY-STATE RESPONSE

Research on the ASSR has seen a tremendous growth over the past decade, and findings have steadily contributed to the development of clinical systems with improved accuracy and efficiency in estimating hearing thresholds. This trend will no doubt continue with development of more efficient stimuli and response detection strategies validated on diverse populations with various types, degrees, and configurations of hearing loss to improve and validate the ASSR alongside existing techniques such as the ABR. There are, however, several other areas of current research that show promise for future application of the ASSR in clinical practice. The most prominent of these include the use of the ASSR for hearing screening, fitting of hearing aids, and assessing suprathreshold hearing.

As discussed in the section on hearing screening, the characteristics of the ASSR allowing for objective response detection and simultaneous bilateral stimulation with several stimuli hold promise for screening, specifically in the neonatal period. Several challenges remain, and much research must still be done to validate ASSR screening as a viable technique compared to existing technologies, like OAE and ABR. As noted already, another future application of the ASSR is

Table 6–15. Clinically available ASSR equipment

Company		
Neuronic S.A. *(Havana, Cuba)*	Audix	Multiple and single stimuli 1-channel ASSR
Viasys/Grason-Stadler *(Madison, WI, USA)*	Audera ASSR	Single stimuli 1-channel ASSR
Natus/Biologic *(Mundelein, IL, USA)*	MASTER	Multiple and single stimuli 1-channel ASSR
Intelligent Hearing Systems *(Miami, FL, USA)*	SmartEP ASSR	Multiple and single stimuli 2-channel ASSR
GN Otometrics *(Taastrup, Denmark)*	CHARTR EP ASSR	Multiple and single stimuli 1-channel ASSR
Interacoustics *(Assens, Denmark)*	Eclipse ASSR	Multiple and single stimuli 2-channel ASSR

fitting hearing aids with difficult-to-test populations, especially young infants who cannot provide feedback on the comfort and effectiveness of a hearing aid. Estimation of loudness growth, by analyzing the increase in ASSR amplitude for increasing intensities above threshold, has proven reasonably accurate (Zenker-Castro & Barajas, 2008). Utilizing these ASSR amplitude functions for various frequencies can provide an indication of the dynamic range for the individual, information that may be valuable in the initial adjustment of the hearing aid before valid measurement of behavioral responses is possible. Validation of the responses may also be done in the sound-field environment by recording aided ASSR thresholds. With the increasingly younger age of hearing aid fittings due to widespread newborn hearing screening, this line of research may prove beneficial in future clinical practice.

Finally, suprathreshold assessment for speech perception abilities is another exciting future application for the ASSR. As clinicians, we know that audiologic assessment is more than a description of hearing sensitivity across frequencies. Audiologic assessment should also include assessment of speech perception in quiet and in noise. In young infants and difficult-to-test populations, this has not been possible because conventional measures of speech perception rely on behavioral responses. However, a growing body of research evidence is showing that the use of novel stimuli, like independent amplitude and frequency modulated (IAFM) tones, vowel segments, or manipulation of stimuli modulation rate and depth, allow for evaluating suprathreshold discrimination abilities objectively with the ASSR. Suprathreshold evaluation with the ASSR may include determining physiological intensity-discrimination limens, frequency discrimination, and temporal resolution. Studies have demonstrated that such ASSRs contain representations of vowel pitch and formants, measures of sensitivity for amplitude and frequency modulation used in phoneme perception and speech in noise (Aiken & Picton, 2006; Dimitrijevic et al., 2001; Dimitrijevic, John, & Picton, 2004). This line of research holds great promise for clinical practice in the future and may allow assessment of speech discrimination abilities in young infants with and without amplification, a development that may guide intervention and hearing aid fitting.

7

Recommendations for Objective Identification and Diagnosis of Hearing Loss

INTRODUCTION

Objective measures only started to appear in audiology test batteries in the early 1970s. Initially, electroacoustic and electrophysiologic procedures were for the most part considered useful adjuncts to the range of behavioral tests. Since then, new discoveries and refinements of existing measures have made objective electroacoustic and electrophysiologic measures an integral and indispensible part of current audiological test batteries. In patients considered difficult to test, due to an inability or unwillingness to cooperate, objective measures are not only an integral component but are essential tools upon which accurate detection and diagnosis of hearing loss depend. Logically, then, guidelines for current audiological practice must include these measures as the standard of care for appropriate service delivery to patients of all ages for both the identification and diagnosis of hearing loss or auditory disorders.

RECOMMENDATIONS FOR DETECTION

Employing objective audiologic tests for detecting hearing loss has become increasingly popular with the development of technology and the expanding applications of these techniques. The following discussion highlights the current recommendations and peer-reviewed and evidence-based guidelines for the use of electroacoustic and electrophysiologic measurements in detection of hearing loss across various age groups.

Newborns and Infants

The influential, multidisciplinary Joint Committee of Infant Hearing (JCIH) in their 2007 position statement has recommended that no other screening procedures apart from automated OAE and ABR systems are to be used for newborns and infants. The recommendations for implementing these electroacoustic and electrophysiologic screening measures in a detection program are summarized in Table 7–1. Both techniques can detect sensory hearing loss, but only ABR can detect neural hearing loss. Even some sensory hearing losses will be missed by both OAE and ABR screening tests as a result of the stimuli and response detection criteria specified for each. The target hearing loss specified for detection by these screening techniques is 40 dB HL or greater, yet the OAE test stimuli are restricted to higher frequency regions and the ABR click stimuli detect hearing loss within a rather constrained frequency region (in the region of 3000 Hz). In other words, losses less than 40 dB HL in the high frequencies will be missed by click-evoked ABR screening, and low frequency hearing losses may also be missed by both click-evoked ABR and an OAE screening protocol. Recall that this limitation of hearing screening with 35 dB nHL click-evoked ABR technique was discussed in Chapter 5. The reason low frequency hearing losses are typically not the target of hearing screening is partly due to equipment limitations and partly due to the demographics of pediatric hearing loss. For OAEs activated with low frequency stimuli, background noise precludes fast and reliable screening, whereas the click-evoked ABR is representative of higher frequency regions in the cochlea. In addition, relatively few (<1/800 children) have isolated low frequency hearing loss in infancy. Milder losses are missed because of the preset criteria on the screening tests specified to identify losses of 35 to 40 dB and greater. If more sensitive ABR or OAE pass/fail criteria were employed for detection of milder hearing losses, the result would be too many referrals secondary to transient conductive problems (e.g., middle-ear effusion or vernix in the ear canal) and false failures that would undermine the efficacy and cost-efficiency of a screening program. The specified target disorder for a newborn screening program according to the JCIH (2007) is congenital permanent bilateral, unilateral sensory, permanent conductive hearing loss and neural hearing loss (e.g., auditory neuropathy) in infants admitted to the NICU.

Transient conductive disorders of the outer and middle ear are a significant contributor to false positive results on OAE and ABR screening tests. OAEs are particularly susceptible to such conditions because acoustic stimuli are affected with forward (to cochlea) and backward (from cochlea) propagation of acoustic signals. Although screening programs do not recommend detection of transient middle ear effusion, a useful electroacoustic technique for screening for this condition in infants younger than 7 months is tympanometry using a 1000 Hz probe tone. A simple screening criterion for the 1000 Hz probe tone tympanogram is whether a tympanogram with a discernible peak representing a normal middle ear system is recorded or a flat tympanometric shape without a clearly

Table 7–1. Current recommendations and guidelines for newborn and infant hearing screening (summarized from the JCIH, 2007)

Recommendation	
• Only ABR and OAE tests	• Only validated tests with adequate sensitivity and specificity rates
• Automated-response detection	• Avoid interpreter bias; allows non-specialist screeners
• OAE or ABR in well-baby nurseries	• Both can identify sensory hearing loss
• ABR for Neonatal Intensive Care Unit (NICU)	• Higher incidence of neural hearing loss which OAE cannot identify
• Avoid repeated testing	• Repeated testing introduces statistical bias
• If 1st screen ABR, OAE cannot be used as 2nd screen to pass baby	• Neural hearing loss may present an ABR fail and OAE pass

discernible peak indicating the presence middle ear effusion (Baldwin, 2006; Swanepoel 2007). The clinician may also need to consult more specific normative values for 1000 Hz tympanograms in neonates and infants (Kei et al., 2003; Margolis Bass-Ringdahl, Hanks, Holte, & Zapala, 2003; Swanepoel et al., 2007). The importance of tympanometry in hearing screening programs was cited in Chapter 2, and also Chapter 3.

Combined OAE/ABR Infant Hearing Screening

The multiple compelling clinical advantages of combining OAE and ABR technologies for infant hearing screening were reviewed in some detail in Chapter 3. A combined OAE/ABR hearing screening strategy is endorsed by the JCIH, and supported by clinical research evidence as effective in reducing failure rates, lowering the overall costs of a hearing screening program, reducing the proportion of infants who yield a refer outcome who are lost to follow up, and contributing to earlier and more precise intervention. A simple algorithm for applying the combined OAE/ABR hearing screening approach is illustrated in Figure 7–1. The technology used for the initial hearing screening is determined by the setting of the child, that is, intensive care unit or newborn intensive care unit (NICU) versus well baby nursery or home. ABR is the technology of choice for hearing screening in the NICU for two reasons. First, research evidence clearly documents a substantially increased

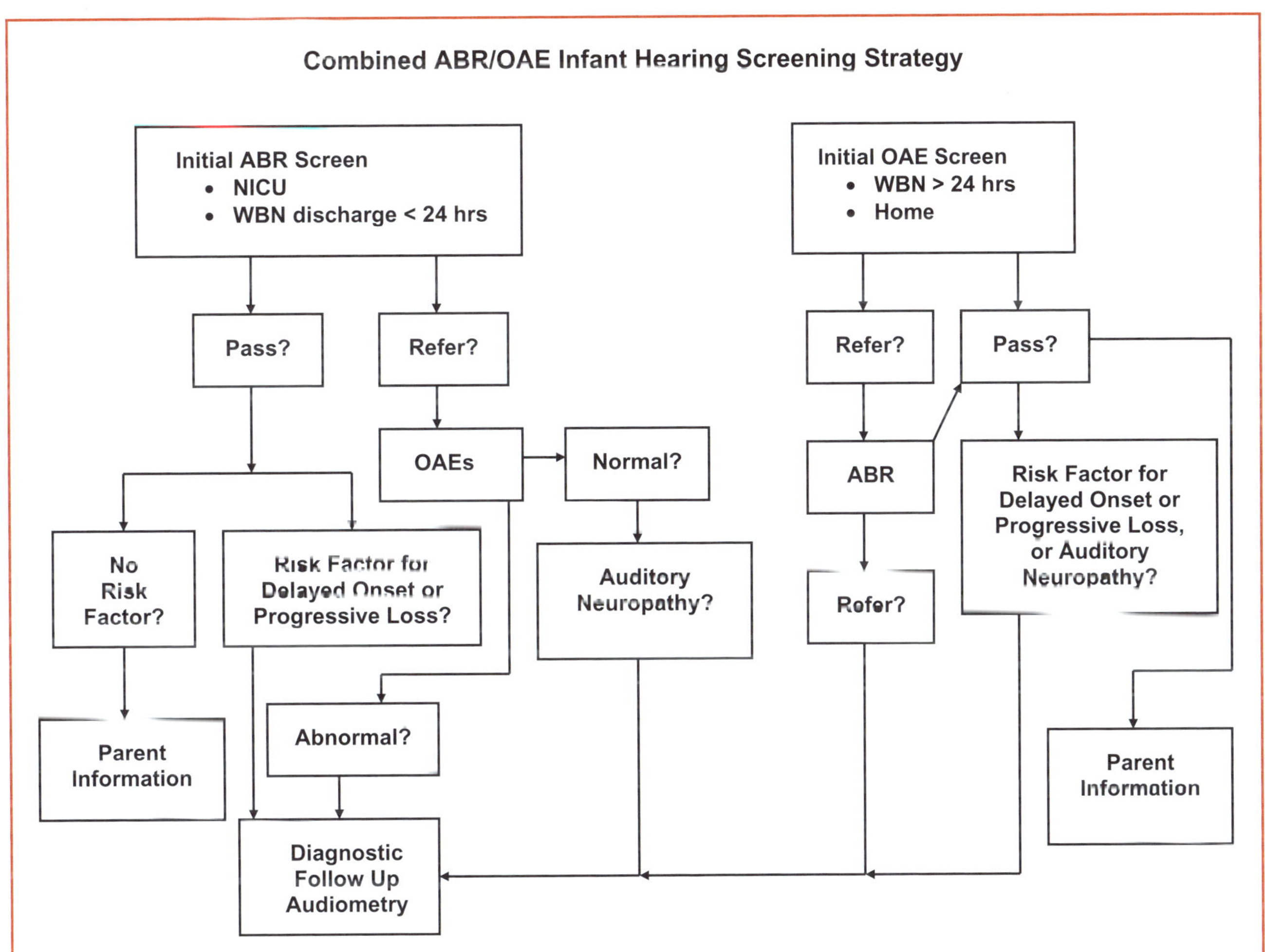

FIGURE 7–1. A simple algorithm for applying the combined OAE/ABR hearing screening approach in an infant hearing loss detection program.

likelihood of auditory neuropathy among infants admitted to the NICU. The presence of OAEs in newborn infants who fail an ABR screening is an early sign of possible auditory neuropathy. Also, due to extended hospital stay and measurement variables related to medical care (e.g., ventilation), middle ear disorders are more common in the NICU population. Detection of OAEs is adversely affected by even minimal disruption in middle ear function. ABR is relatively unaffected by minor and probably transient middle ear dysfunction.

ABR is also recommended at the primary hearing screening technology for healthy infants admitted to a well baby nursery when discharge within 24 hours is anticipated. Vernix caseosa in the external ear canal contributes to a high failure rate for OAE technology within the first day after birth. This common problem can be solved by either screening initially with ABR or (as shown in the right portion of Figure 7–1) screening first with OAE but then, in cases of a refer outcome, immediately screening with ABR. Keep in mind that up to 15% of all babies who eventually have hearing loss will pass a screening at birth. This group consists predominately of children with risk factors for delayed onset or progressive hearing loss, as detailed by the 2007 (JCIH).

Risk factors for various etiologies of congenital, delayed onset or progressive hearing identified by the 2007 JCIH are summarized in Table 7–2. The list of etiologies is obviously quite long and diverse. Even in the era of universal newborn hearing screening, a detailed and focused medical history is still an important part of a successful

Table 7–2. Risk indicators summarized by the JCIH (2007) to be associated with permanent congenital, delayed-onset or progressive hearing loss in children

1. Caregiver concern regarding hearing, speech, language, or developmental delay
2. Family history of permanent childhood hearing loss
3. Neonatal intensive care of more than 5 days or any of the following regardless of length of stay: ECMO assisted ventilation, exposure to ototoxic medications (gentimycin and tobramycin) or loop diuretics (furosemide/ Lasix), and hyperbilirubinemia that requires exchange transfusion
4. In utero infections, such as CMV, herpes, rubella, syphilis, and toxoplasmosis
5. Craniofacial anomalies, including those that involve the pinna, ear canal, ear tags, ear pits, and temporal bone anomalies
6. Physical findings, such as white forelock, that are associated with a syndrome known to include a sensorineural or permanent conductive hearing loss
7. Syndromes associated with hearing loss or progressive or late-onset hearing loss, such as neurofibromatosis, osteopetrosis, and Usher syndrome; other frequently identified syndromes include Waardenburg, Alport, Pendred, and Jervell and Lange-Nielson
8. Neurodegenerative disorders, such as Hunter syndrome, or sensory motor neuropathies, such as Friedreich ataxia and Charcot-Marie-Tooth syndrome
9. Culture-positive postnatal infections associated with sensorineural hearing loss, including confirmed bacterial and viral (especially herpes viruses and varicella) meningitis
10. Head trauma, especially basal skull/temporal bone fracture that requires hospitalization
11. Chemotherapy

early identification program. Of course, the task of identifying infants at risk for congenital permanent, delayed onset, or progressive hearing loss is not quite as daunting as suggested by the lengthy list in Table 7–2. With the likely exception of the first two risk factors, that is, (a) caregiver concern regarding hearing, speech, language, or developmental delay and (b) family history of permanent childhood hearing loss, infants with the risk indicators in Table 7–2 usually comprise less than 10% of the general population of newborn babies and in developed countries are almost always admitted to the NICU.

Preschool and School-Age Children

For years the screening tool of choice to identify children with possible hearing loss has remained pure tone behavioral audiometry. Despite limitations that can seriously influence the test outcome such as background noise, poor motivation, and cooperation from a child, audiologists have rarely veered from using this technique since its implementation as far back as the 1920s (Downs, 2000). With the advantages of objective measures such as rapid response detection independent of behavioral responses and automated response detection and interpretation, it is surprising that these have not been incorporated more readily into screening programs for preschool and school-age children. It is only in recent years that the use of OAE screening has been incorporated for testing these age groups. OAE screening in children offer several possible advantages to conventional pure tone audiometry which include:

- Recording responses quickly without the active cooperation of the child apart from sitting quietly for a minute or two
- Reliable measure of cochlear integrity, which can be used as a screen for sensory and conductive hearing loss
- Objective response detection avoiding any bias and allowing nonspecialist personnel to screen
- Handheld battery operated units offer portability

OAE screening will detect most types of peripheral hearing loss, even at an early stage when auditory dysfunction is modest and hearing sensitivity as screened with pure tone techniques remains within normal limits. The rather remarkable sensitivity of OAEs to auditory dysfunction can also be viewed as a disadvantage. The problem with OAEs in pediatric hearing screening is associated with middle ear dysfunction secondary to otitis media, the most common cause of hearing loss in young children. That is, OAEs cannot differentiate between sensory and conductive hearing loss. To address this limitation, OAE screening should be supplemented with tympanometry. The application of OAEs and tympanometry in these pediatric populations is illustrated in Figure 7–2. In combination, OAEs and tympanometry offer a powerful approach for efficient and effective hearing screening of preschool and school-age children. The OAE/tympanometry approach is efficient because it is quick, automated, and easily performed by nonaudiology personnel, such as nurses, teachers, and volunteers, using handheld battery operated devices. Combining the two technologies is also highly effective in the early detection of even subtle auditory dysfunction, and sometimes differentiates between medically manageable middle ear dysfunction versus permanent sensory hearing loss. The sequence of steps shown in Figure 7–2 is based on two assumptions. We assume that OAEs are at least as sensitive as pure tone screening methods for detecting hearing impairment. The literature includes plenty of evidence in support of this assumption (see Chapter 3). We also assume that the goal of the screening program is detection of any hearing loss (≥15 dB HL) that might interfere with communication and academic performance of a young child. This can be done in one of two ways.

Referring again to Figure 7–2, the hearing screening process begins with a simple otoscopic inspection of the external ear canal. A wide variety of natural and foreign objects and substances may be found in the external ear canals of young children. The otoscopic inspection serves one immediate purpose and one more far-reaching objective. The immediate purpose is to verify that the ear canal is clear and clean before a probe is inserted. Naturally, we do not want to put the child at risk for iatrogenic injury during the hearing screening process. The longer term objective

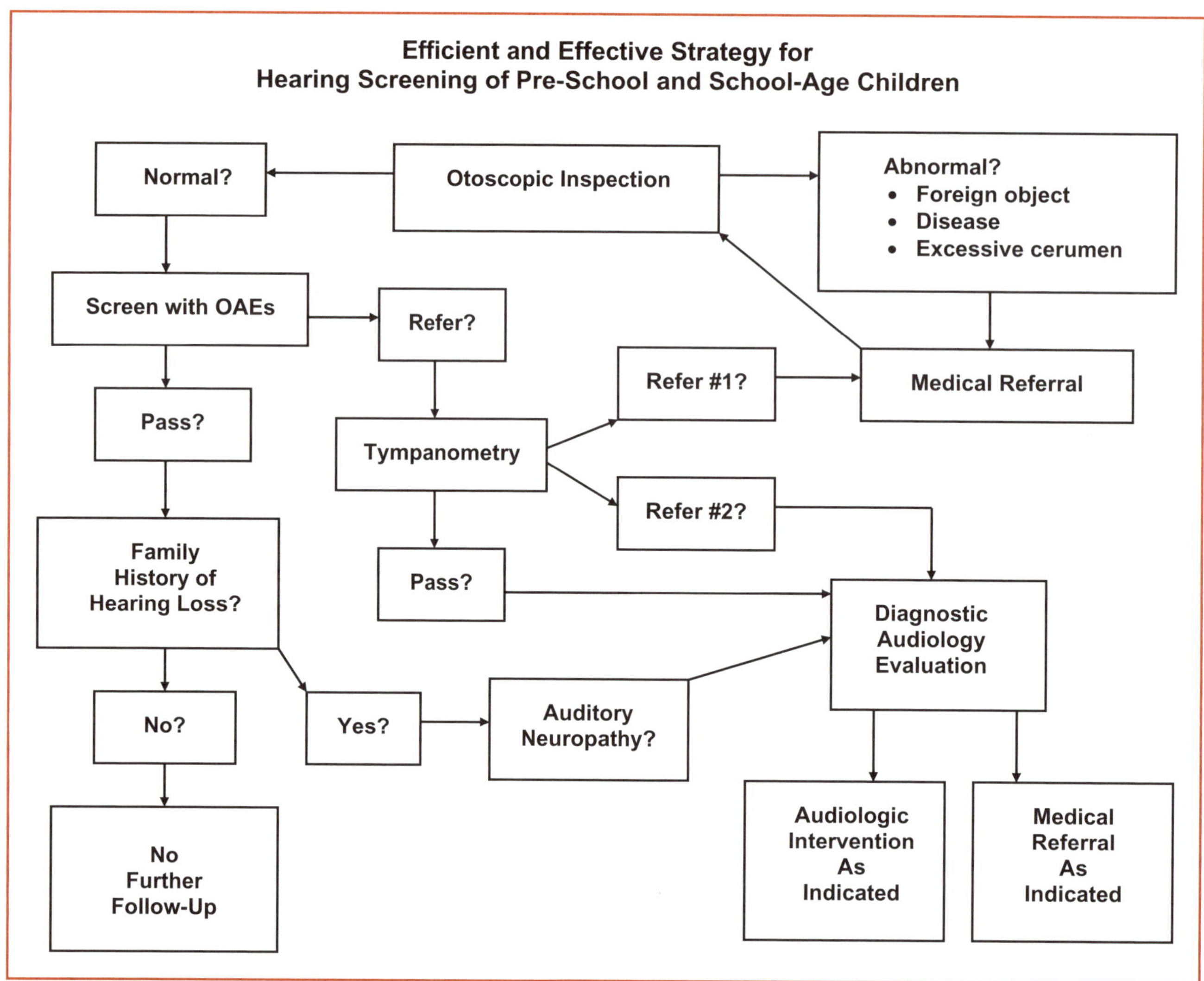

FIGURE 7–2. Algorithm for the application of otoacoustic emissions (OAEs) and tympanometry in an efficient and effective strategy for hearing screening in preschool and school-age children.

is to identify a disorder or pathology that requires medical management. Following otoscopy, and presuming the external ear canal is clear, all children are screened with OAE. OAE hearing screening is remarkably fast, usually taking no more than 30 seconds per ear with a reasonably cooperative preschool or school-age child. Children who meet criteria for the presence of OAEs (e.g., OAE amplitude 6 dB or greater above the noise floor for the majority of test frequencies) and who have no family history of hearing loss are viewed as a pass outcome and no follow-up is required. Children who fail OAE screening for one or both ears are then screened immediately with tympanometry. If a normal type A tympanogram and/or a normal gradient value (see Chapter 2) is recorded, the child should be referred for a diagnostic audiologic evaluation because middle ear dysfunction is unlikely, and the child is at risk for sensory hearing loss. If a type B or C tympanogram (or abnormal gradient value) is recorded, then the child may have middle ear dysfunction and possible conductive pathology. Referral to a primary care physician or clinic is recommended. Alternatively at this stage in the process, the presence of a sensory component could be ruled out by a diagnostic audiologic assessment if equipment, personnel, and other resources are available. As a measure of outer hair cell integrity, OAEs do not, of course, detect auditory neuropathy. Children with a family history of childhood hearing loss, or with hearing impaired siblings, should be considered at risk for neural auditory dysfunction, even if the OAE screening outcome is a pass. A conservative next step would be comprehensive diagnostic evaluation of auditory function, including measures of speech perception and retrocochlear auditory dysfunction (e.g., acoustic reflexes).

RECOMMENDATIONS FOR DIAGNOSIS

Diagnosis of hearing loss can be defined across several dimensions (as discussed in Chapter 1), but the primary focus aimed at audiological management includes a description of the type, degree, configuration, and symmetry (one or both ears) of the hearing loss. The implementation of objective measures for diagnosis of hearing loss and auditory disorders is assuming a growing prominence as new tests are developed and existing procedures refined. Current recommendations for the battery of tests to include in diagnostic audiologic evaluations across all age groups provide evidence for the importance of objective measures.

Infants Younger than 6 Months

Widespread newborn hearing screening has led to the clinical demand for audiologists to provide accurate diagnostic services to the youngest of populations, neonates and infants. Diagnostic evaluations for these very young infants rely almost exclusively on electroacoustic and electrophysiologic tests of auditory functioning to guide intervention decisions. Current recommendations and guidelines for assessing infants younger than 6 months as prescribed by the JCIH (2007) are also listed in Table 7–3. Two clinical objective tests omitted from these guidelines are acoustic reflex measurements and the auditory steady-state response (ASSR). Acoustic reflex measurements for newborn and young infants have demonstrated some inconsistency, especially with low probe tone frequencies. More recent evidence has suggested that acoustic reflexes in young infants are

Table 7–3. Recommended audiological test-battery for evaluating infants from birth to 6 months of age (compiled from the JCIH, 2007). The rationale for the specified procedures is provided and when it is indicated to include in the test-battery.

Procedures		
• **Child & family history**	Determine risk profile	Always
• **Frequency specific ABR**		
—*Air conduction*	Configuration of hearing sensitivity	Always
—*Bone conduction*	Determine presence of conductive loss	Abnormal tympanogram Elevated ABR thresholds
• **Click-evoked ABR** (condensation and rarefaction)	Determine presence of cochlear microphonic	Risk factor for auditory neuropathy No response on tone-burst ABR
• **DPOAE/TEOAE**	Evaluate integrity of cochlear outer hair cells	Always
• **Tympanometry** (1000Hz probe tone)	Evaluate middle-ear	Always
• **Observation of behavioral responses**	Cross-check for objective measures	Always

more consistently present when a 1000 Hz probe tone is employed, but more normative data would be helpful for high frequency tympanometry to be considered as a routine procedure for this population (Swanepoel et al., 2007). The ASSR is also not recommended by the JCIH (2007) as a stand-alone procedure for determining hearing thresholds in infants and children at this stage but, rather, as a complementary test for estimating hearing thresholds alongside the ABR. This is primarily due to a shortage of current research to validate its use in infants with hearing loss compared to the wealth of research that has validated the ABR for this purpose. The ABR is specified as the main tool for determining air and bone conduction thresholds across the frequency range and also has the very important function of differentiating sensory from neural (auditory neuropathy) based hearing loss with the use of opposite polarity click stimuli to reveal the presence or absence of a cochlear microphonic response. Table 7–4 provides an indication of the typical objective test findings for the various types of hearing loss and auditory disorders. The only subjective test recommended for these very young infants is the observation of behavioral responses to sounds, and this is only as a cross-check to confirm electro-acoustic and electrophysiologic test results.

Table 7–4. Typical findings for electro-acoustic and electro-physiologic measures across categories of hearing loss or auditory disorder

	Type of Hearing Loss or Auditory Disorder			
Test				
Immittance				
Tymp	Abnormal	Normal	Normal	Normal
AR	Absent or abnormal	Abnormal or absent	Absent or abnormal	Normal *(contralateral may be abnormal)*
OAE	Absent or abnormal	Abnormal or absent	Normal or absent	Normal
ECochG				
SP	Abnormal	Abnormal or absent	Present	Normal
CM	Abnormal or absent	Abnormal or absent	Present	Normal
AP	Abnormal	Present or abnormal	Absent	Normal
ABR	Abnormal *(i.e. elevated threshold delayed latency)*	Abnormal *(i.e. elevated threshold)*	Absent or abnormal	Normal *(speech evoked ABR may be abnormal)*
ASSR	Abnormal *(i.e. elevated threshold)*	Abnormal *(i.e. elevated threshold)*	Absent or abnormal *(i.e. elevated threshold)*	Normal

TESTS: Tymp = Tympanometry; AR = Acoustic reflex; OAE = Otoacoustic emissions; ECochG = Electrocochleography; SP = Summating potential; CM = Cochlear microphonic; AP = Action potential; ABR = Auditory Brainstem Response; ASSR = Auditory steady-state response.

CATEGORY: Abnormal = findings noticeable different than person with no hearing loss or auditory dysfunction; Absent = response not present at maximum intensities; Normal = typical finding in person with no hearing loss or auditory dysfunction; Present = Response present but not necessarily normal.

ORDER: The most common or typical finding is listed first.

Infants 6 to 36 Months

As infants begin to develop head control at around 6 months of age, behavioral audiometry becomes possible. The baby is conditioned to respond with a head turn to the presentation of stimuli, a technique known as visual reinforcement audiometry. With this technique, estimations of behavioral thresholds, more commonly called *minimum response levels*, are used to define the configuration of hearing across frequencies. Behavioral audiologic assessment may not, however, be possible in all infants at very young ages due to differences in development, attention, activity levels, and also due to the presence of disabilities such as cerebral palsy or visual impairment. In such cases, the use of an electrophysiologic procedure, that is, the ABR, should be applied to accurately estimate hearing thresholds. Again, the recommended test battery and the indications for using different procedures as prescribed by the JCIH (2007) were summarized in Table 7–5. Note that the guidelines require an ABR to be performed even when behavioral thresholds are obtained, if no ABR was done previously. The rationale for performing ABR assessment, including separate recordings with condensation and rarefaction stimuli, is to rule out a neural hearing loss (auditory neuropathy). For children within the age range of 6 months to 3 years, cross-checking behavioral and objective test results with each other makes diagnoses stronger and more reliable. As the children develop, the

Table 7–5. Recommended audiological test-battery for evaluating infants from 6 to 36 months of age (compiled from the JCIH, 2007). The rationale for the specified procedures is provided and when it is indicated to include in the test-battery.

Procedures		
• **Child & family history**	Determine risk profile	Always
• **Parental report**	Probe concerns regarding auditory and visual behaviors and communication milestones	Always
• **Behavioral audiometry**		
—*Pure tone thresholds*	Characterize hearing loss with visual reinforcement or conditioned-play audiometry	Always
—*Speech audiometry* (detection & recognition)	Describe hearing ability	Always
• **DPOAE/TEOAE**	Evaluate integrity of cochlear outer hair cells	Always
• **Immittance** (tympanometry & reflexes)	Evaluate middle-ear and assess neural acoustic reflex arc	Always
• **Frequency specific ABR**		
—*Air conduction*	Configuration of hearing sensitivity	Pure tone audiometry not possible
—*Bone conduction*	Determine presence of conductive loss	Pure tone audiometry not possible and bone conduction is indicated
• **Click-evoked ABR** (condensation and rarefaction)	Determine presence of cochlear microphonic	ABR not performed previously

behavioral measures of hearing sensitivity usually become more reliable and assume a more prominent role in the test battery.

Children and Adults

In the vast majority of children and adults, behavioral audiometry can be completed relatively easily and hearing sensitivity estimated rather accurately. Rarely is it necessary to rely on an electrophysiologic technique such as the ABR or ASSR to estimate auditory thresholds. Audiologic diagnosis, however, encompass much more than a description of hearing thresholds by behavioral audiometry. Diagnosis requires the evaluation of the auditory system at various levels. In some instances, objective measures provide the only means of adequately describing peripheral and central auditory function. OAEs are a good example of a procedure providing very important and precise information about the functioning of one component of auditory functioning, that is, the outer hair cells of the cochlea. No other auditory procedure offers such site specificity. OAEs should therefore be included as part of the basic test battery and should not be seen as an "advanced" or "specialized" test procedure reserved only for certain special cases. Aural immittance measures (tympanometry and acoustic reflexes) are another example of electroacoustic procedures that are critical components within the basic test battery. Aural immittance measurement provides objective assessment of middle ear integrity and functioning as well as information on the neural pathways within the acoustic reflex arc (e.g., the 8th and 7th cranial nerves and nuclei in the brainstem). Depending on the case history indications and initial test results, inclusion of the ABR may also be necessary to ascertain the risk of a neural disorder involving the 8th cranial nerve or auditory regions of the brainstem. Even in cooperative adults, objective electroacoustic and electrophysiologic test procedures remain indispensable components of the test battery to confirm and cross-check behavioral findings, or to assess the integrity and functioning of specific structures or processes of the auditory system.

In a small subgroup of children and adults who are either not willing or not capable of cooperating, the role of objective measures assume prominence as the sole measures for determining the presence of a hearing loss and characterizing the type, degree, configuration, and symmetry thereof. In such cases, electrophysiologic procedures like the ABR, ASSR, or cortical auditory evoked responses may be used. Frequency-specific ABR measurements, and the ASSR for fast stimulus modulation rates, have proven effective in estimating hearing thresholds in asleep adults and in awake adults who are in a quiet and restful state. In awake adults, however, the 40 Hz and other slow modulation rate ASSRs and cortical auditory evoked response may, in fact, provide better and more efficient frequency-specific estimations of behavioral pure tone thresholds. Audiologists today have an array of behavioral and objective tests to accurately diagnose hearing loss in patients of all age groups, independent of patient cooperation.

TEST BATTERY APPROACH

The proper selection of audiologic procedures combined into a test battery is the single most important step toward accurate diagnosis and, ultimately, effective intervention for auditory dysfunction in children and adults. Electroacoustic and electrophysiologic procedures play a critical role in the diagnostic process, particularly in infants and young children, as behavioral audiometry options are limited. As summarized in Table 7–4, different auditory disorders are associated with unique patterns of findings for an array of electroacoustic and electrophysiologic procedures. Analysis of the matrix of test results for commonly available objective auditory procedures leads predictably to the identification or diagnosis of specific types and sites of auditory dysfunction. Put simply, none of the major types of auditory disorders cited in Table 7–4 have the same pattern of findings for aural immittance, OAE, ECochG, and ABR measurements. The diagnostic power of the battery of electroacoustic and electrophysiologic tests is, of course, predicated on the assumption that each of the procedures is administered, and administered properly. There is a tendency to make faulty assumptions at the very beginning of the diagnostic process. For example, the assumption that "OAEs do not need to be recorded because it's clear the patient has a sensorineural hearing loss," or conversely, "OAEs do not need to be recorded because the patient's audiogram is normal," will inevitably lead to diagnostic errors. The errors will include failure to diagnose (for example, the assumption of normal auditory function when indeed there is auditory dysfunction) and misdiagnosis (e.g., classification of a hearing loss as sensory when it is really neural). Furthermore, the audiologist must have the clinical experience and knowledge necessary to analyze the constellation of test findings (e.g., recognize normal versus abnormal results) and then interpret them in combination, rather than in isolation. Overwhelming evidence from clinical research supports the routine application of a variety of independent electroacoustic and electrophysiologic procedures. In other words, the "cross-check principle" lives on. The minimal extra time required to perform a few extra procedures will yield valuable diagnostic dividends.

NEW DIRECTIONS FOR RESEARCH

The development of audiology has always been closely linked with the tremendous gains made in technological innovation over the past few decades. As the rapidly expanding body of hearing science increasingly embraces the potential of technological advances, audiologists will see new and improved electroacoustic and electrophysiologic techniques to allow more precise, accurate, and perhaps also more comprehensive detection and diagnosis of hearing loss.

Detection of Hearing Loss

The detection of hearing loss in newborns and young infants has revolutionized the practice of audiology, with over 90% of all newborns in selected developed countries already being screened within the first month of life. These are enormous numbers of infants and any improvements in the efficiency of screening methods will have far-reaching effects globally. Currently, ABR screeners use broadband click stimuli to evoke a response for detection. Recently, an improved stimulus, called a chirp, was proposed as a substitute to click stimuli for ABR and perhaps ASSR screening. The chirp stimulus is a broadband stimulus but its phase is adjusted to compensate for the cochlear delay along the basilar membrane to the apex when a conventional click stimulus is used. By doing this, the chirp stimulus is able to provide a more synchronous discharge of neurons from a larger portion of the basilar membrane, resulting in a larger amplitude response, which can be detected more easily and in a shorter period of time (Elberling, Don, Cebulla, & Stürzebecher, 2007). Future research into optimal stimuli for screening also entails the use of high and low frequency stimuli to ensure that hearing losses sloping in the high or toward the low frequencies will be identified. The currently used click-evoked ABR screenings will miss low frequency hearing loss. The ASSR technique, which allows for multiple stimuli to be presented simultaneously, may offer a unique advantage in the implementation of such stimuli for screening purposes in the future. All these measures, however, will have to produce comparable levels of efficiency compared to the current standard set by click-evoked ABR screening before they can be considered for mainstream clinical practice.

Clinical devices combining OAE and ABR technology, as well as devices permitting OAE measurement and tympanometry, are now available. The inclusion of a high frequency tympanogram (1000 Hz probe tone) or a wideband reflectance measurement as part of an OAE screening device may facilitate determination of the reason for an OAE fail outcome at the initial screen. Information from each technology at the time of screening may affect the care pathway for an infant and speed up the referral of infants at greatest risk for a permanent hearing loss (such as a baby with an OAE fail result and no indication of a middle ear problem with high frequency tympanometry or wideband reflectance measurements). Future developments and research in hearing screening are likely to be primarily focused on more efficient technologies that provide faster results identifying all types of permanent hearing loss (e.g., low and high frequency) as well as technologies that permit differentiation of types of hearing loss (conductive versus sensory versus neural).

Diagnosis of Hearing Loss

Accurate diagnosis of the type and extent of a conductive hearing loss in very young infants remains somewhat challenging in clinical practice. The recommended implementation of 1000 Hz probe tone tympanometry into diagnostic protocols has certainly improved diagnostic specificity for infants younger than 7 months, for whom conventional probe tone (226 Hz) tympanometry is not reliable. As more normative data and tympanometric results for specific types of pathology become available, tympanometry may also assist in more precise differential diagnosis of the conductive pathology as opposed to only assessing whether middle ear effusion may be present, as it is primarily used at present. An additional procedure that may assist in differentially diagnosing conductive pathologies in young infants, children, and adults is wideband reflectance (WBR) measurements. WBR assesses the efficiency of the middle ear system in conducting sound across the frequency range of 60 to 10,000 Hz. Initial findings point to improved prediction of hearing status and type of pathology when wideband reflectance measurements are included in a test battery (Keefe et al., 2000; Keefe, Gorga, Neely, Zhao & Vohr, 2003). As more research is accumulated and clinical systems become more widely available, WBR may well become a very useful tool in the audiologist's test battery.

Another important and exciting area of research in electrophysiologic procedures is the use of auditory evoked responses to assess suprathreshold auditory processing abilities. These measures may allow audiologists to move beyond describing simply the type, degree, configuration, and symmetry of a hearing loss with electroacoustic and electrophysiologic measures. In the near future, audiologists may actually make deductions regarding the impact of the hearing loss on speech perception. ASSRs evoked with stimuli modulated in both amplitude and frequency, closely resembling speech stimuli, can be employed to evaluate suprathreshold discrimination abilities objectively. Advanced ASSR technology and techniques may be used to determine frequency discrimination and temporal resolution, abilities that are essential for speech perception. ASSRs evoked by such novel stimuli, modulated in amplitude and frequency at suprathreshold levels, appear to be significantly correlated with the ability to recognize words correctly by normal hearing and hearing impaired subjects (Dimitirijevic, John, van Roon, & Picton, 2001). Other investigators have reported that ASSRs to novel stimuli may contain representations of vowel pitch and formants, measures of sensitivity for amplitude and frequency modulation used in phoneme perception and speech in noise (Aiken & Picton, 2006; Dimitrijevic et al., 2001; Dimitrijevic, John, & Picton, 2004). This research direction is very promising and may allow insight into the impact of a hearing loss on speech discrimination abilities in young infants and other difficult-to-test populations. Such information, obtained with and without amplification, can also be very valuable to evaluate the effectiveness of personal amplification and for adjusting fittings for optimal speech perception. A related development in ABR evaluations has been the use of speech stimuli to evoke responses in which abnormalities have demonstrated significant correlations to central auditory dysfunction associated with learning disabilities (e.g., King, Warrier, Hayes & Kraus, 2002). Audiologists can expect more research in these areas with clinical tools becoming available in the near future.

The clinical entity described as auditory neuropathy, recently termed auditory neuropathy spectrum disorder (ANSD), is an area of continued and fervent research. Many fundamental questions regarding mechanisms, diagnosis, and management of ANSD still need to be answered. The range and variability of clinical findings in this broad category or spectrum of auditory dysfunction have always called for more diagnostic specificity to isolate the site of lesion or dysfunction for a specific patient. The typical findings comprising the diagnosis of auditory neuropathy, including absent or abnormal neural components on the ABR in the presence of a cochlear microphonic response and/or present OAEs, leave open the possibility of a site of lesion anywhere from the inner hair cells, to the inner hair cell synapse, the spiral ganglion, the 8th cranial nerve, and even the brainstem. Recently, however, reports of ECochG measurements, specifically transtympanic recordings, in patients with auditory neuropathy have demonstrated promise for more accurate differentiation of the site of lesion (Lu et al., 2008; McMahon, Patuzzi, Gibson, & Sanli, 2008; Santarelli, Starr, Michalewski, & Arlsan, 2008). Analysis of the summating potentials (SP) and compound action potentials (CAP) recorded with ECochG show promise for identifying pre- and postsynaptic disorders of inner hair cells and auditory nerves (Santarelli et al., 2008). Increased diagnostic specificity of ANSD can have far-reaching implications for intervention options. For example, postsynaptic conditions may not provide optimal or comparable outcomes with cochlear implantation as opposed to presynaptic dysfunction. However, more research is necessary to describe and standardize these distinctions in infants and children and to investigate the effectiveness of less invasive recording techniques such as extratympanic methods for ECochG.

As the specificity of our test battery is enhanced with the development and new applications of objective test procedures, we as audiologists are able to provide increasingly accurate diagnoses of hearing loss. New technological developments are allowing us to isolate precise sites of lesions and to go beyond a description of basic hearing loss characteristics (e.g., degree and configuration) or types (e.g., sensory versus neural) in infants and other difficult-to-test populations. There is now a distinct possibility for audiologists to estimate the impact a hearing loss and prescribed amplification may have on speech perception abilities. The field of audiology is vibrant with new and exciting future possibilities for better diagnosis that ultimately will lead to improved outcomes for all the patients we serve.

8

Case Reports Illustrating Application of Objective Measures of Auditory Function

INTRODUCTION

The cases reported in this final chapter are patients evaluated by the authors using the electroacoustic and electrophysiologic procedures described throughout the book. To be honest, we practice in our daily clinics what we preach about in this book. Our clinical experience confirms that there are almost as many variations in electroacoustic and electrophysiologic test findings as there are children evaluated audiologically. We have included herein a small and not necessarily representative sample of patients—all children—to illustrate the application, analysis, and interpretation of electroacoustic and electrophysiologic procedures. We also highlight with the case reports some related new technologies or techniques, such as the use of melatonin to induce natural sleep or ABRs recorded with instrumentation designed to be used in children who are not sedated. Indeed, with this instrumentation children may undergo a valid ABR assessment when they are not sleeping but, rather, physically active. For each of the cases, the audiologic diagnosis would not have been made, at least not in a timely fashion, with exclusive reliance on behavioral test procedures. In other words, electroacoustic and electrophysiologic procedures were essential for early identification and diagnosis of auditory dysfunction. Perhaps most importantly, without the availability and the conscientious administration of a test battery of electroacoustic and electrophysiologic procedures, intervention for hearing loss in these, and most, young children would have been unacceptably delayed and patient outcome far from optimal.

CASE: FREQUENCY-SPECIFIC ABR FOR AN INFANT UNDER MELATONIN-INDUCED SLEEP

Patient

The patient, NM, was a female age 8.5 months at time of assessment.

History

NM was born at full-term birth. She spent 4 days in the NICU after birth. Before hospital discharge, she failed OAE hearing screening twice. Diagnostic audiological assessment was recommended.

Sleep/Sedation

The ABR was carried out following sleep deprivation and the ingestion of 9 mg of melatonin. Feeding was scheduled right before assessment. The assessment was conducted in a sound treated room while the infant's heart rate and oxygen saturation were monitored with a pulse oximeter.

Otoscopic Examination and Immittance Measurements

Neither the right nor the left tympanic membrane could be clearly visualized by otoscopic examination. The external ear canal was clear bilaterally.

Using a 226 Hz probe tone a type C tympanogram was recorded for the right ear, whereas a type B tympanogram was recorded in the left ear. Using a high frequency 1000 Hz probe tone, no discernible peaks were identified on the tympanograms for either ear.

Acoustic reflex measurements were made in the ipsilateral stimulus condition with a broadband noise (BBN) stimulus. No acoustic reflex was recorded in the right ear at the maximum intensity (95 dB). In the left ear, an acoustic reflex was only elicited at the maximum intensity of 95 dB.

DPOAE Measurement

The DPOAE recordings were very noisy as they were attempted before the patient fell asleep. Bodily movements and physiologic sounds (produced by the infant) resulted in unacceptably high noise floor levels (Figure 8–1). Despite the raised noise floors, some DPOAE activity was observed in the right ear at reduced amplitude in the higher frequency regions (4000 to 8000 Hz).

ABR Evaluation

The stimuli used for the ABR recordings were calibrated and adjusted for dB nHL a priori based on a group of normal hearing adult subjects. Therefore, values are reported in dB nHL and no further adjustment to compensate for normal hearing

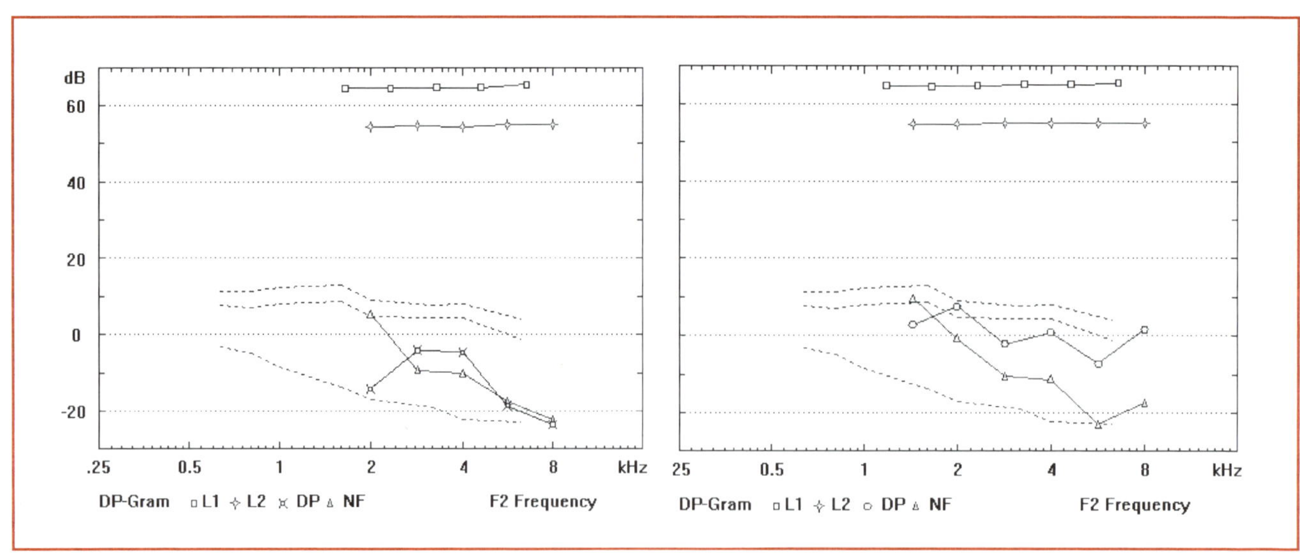

FIGURE 8–1. Distortion product otoacoustic emission (DPOAE) recordings for the left and right ears (Case NM).

levels is required in the examples presented for this case (Figure 8–2, Figure 8–3, and Figure 8–4).

The air conduction ABR recordings in the right ear revealed an electrophysiological threshold of 40 dB nHL for the click stimulus. This threshold is representative of a hearing threshold of approximately 30 dB HL (considering a 10 dB correction to convert the electrophysiological threshold to an estimated hearing threshold) in the high frequency region between 2 and 4 kHz. The 4000 Hz tone burst ABR recording revealed an electrophysiological threshold at 30 dB nHL, suggesting a hearing threshold at 20 dB HL (again, a 10 dB subtraction was applied to the electrophysiological

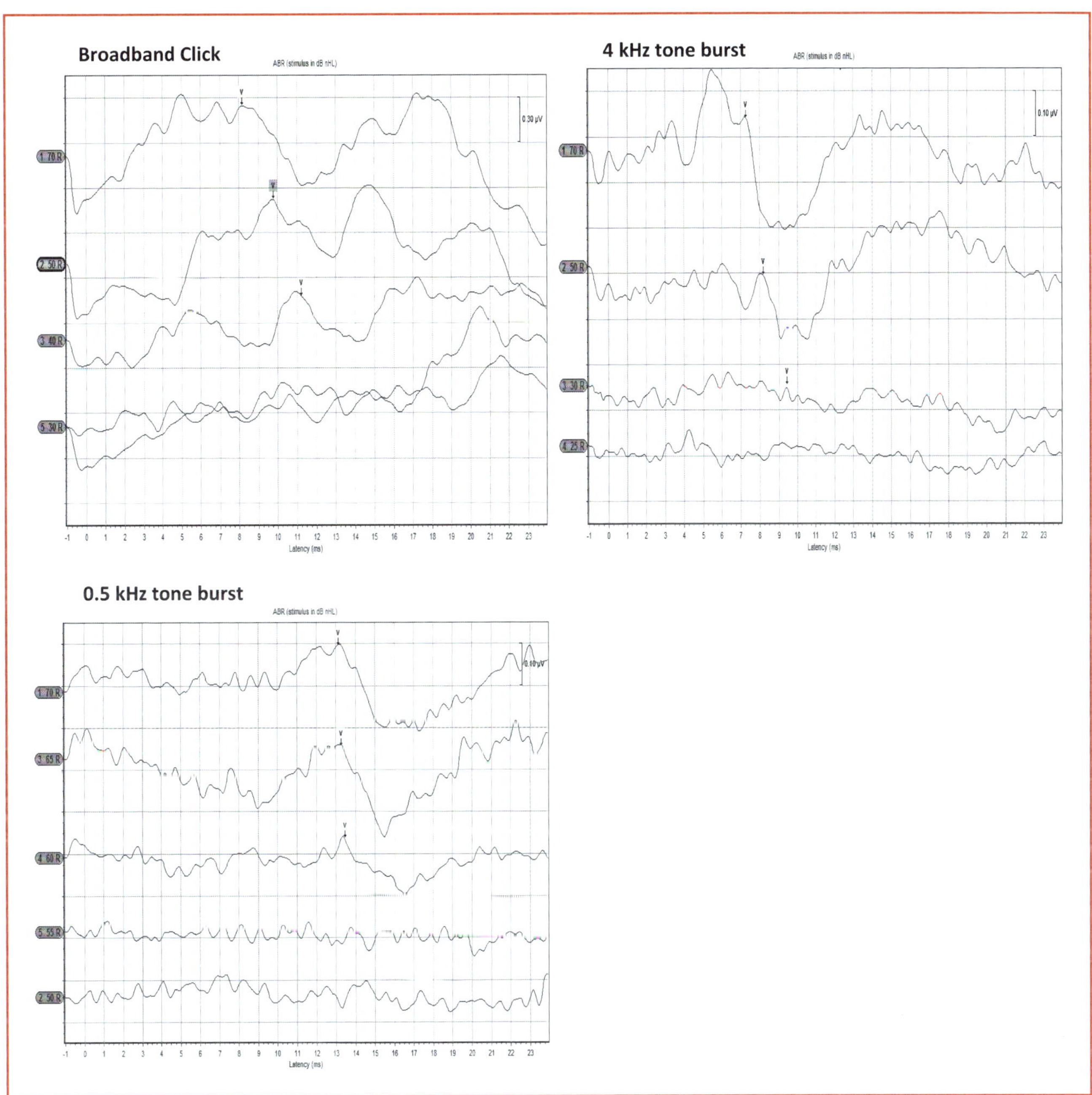

FIGURE 8–2. Air conduction auditory brainstem response (ABR) recordings for the right ear (Case NM).

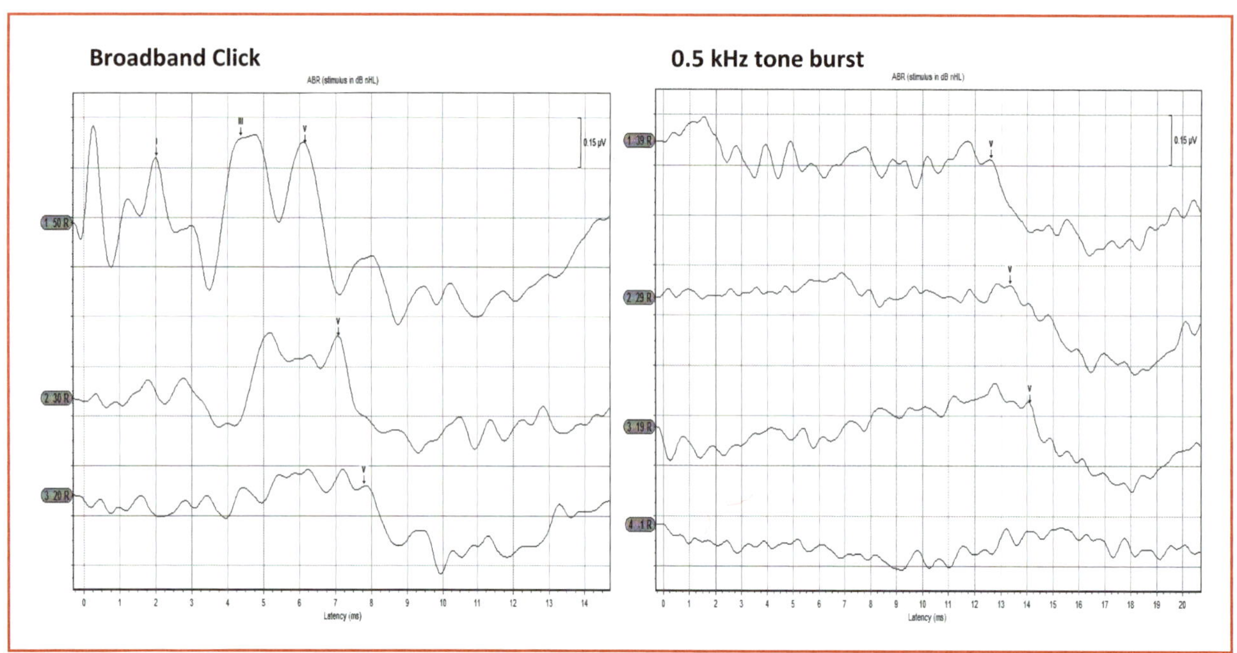

FIGURE 8–3. Bone conduction ABR recordings for the right ear (Case NM).

threshold to reach an estimated hearing threshold). For the 500 Hz tone burst stimulus, an electrophysiological threshold was identified at 60 dB nHL indicating an estimated hearing threshold of approximately 40 to 45 dB HL (using a 15 to 20 dB correction at 500 Hz to convert the electrophysiological threshold to an estimated hearing threshold).

For the left ear, air conduction electrophysiological thresholds for the click and 4000 Hz tone burst stimuli were at an intensity level 20 dB nHL, consistent with hearing thresholds at around 10 dB HL (see Figure 8–4). For the 0.5 kHz tone burst stimulus an electrophysiological threshold was however recorded at 45 dB nHL, which suggests a hearing threshold of approximately 25 to 30 dB HL (using a 15 to 20 dB correction to convert the electrophysiological threshold to an estimated hearing threshold).

Bone conduction ABR recordings could only be obtained before the patient awoke in the right ear for a click and 500 Hz tone burst stimulus. No further testing could be conducted (see Figure 8–3). The ABR threshold levels for the bone conducted click and 500 Hz ABR were at 20 dB nHL, suggesting hearing thresholds of 10 dB HL or better (within normal limits).

Diagnosis and Recommendations

In combination, the electroacoustic and electrophysiologic findings indicate a conductive hearing loss in both ears. In the left ear, auditory thresholds are significantly more affected for the low frequencies than the higher frequencies. In the right ear, auditory thresholds across the frequencies are elevated, although most significantly at 500 Hz. These findings were confirmed by the tympanometric evidence of abnormal middle ear functioning. Although bone conduction ABR thresholds could only be obtained for the right ear before the patient awoke, they indicated normal sensory hearing status, at least in the low and high frequencies. The estimated hearing levels, based on the findings from the ABR assessment, are presented in an audiogram-type format in Figure 8–5.

Recommendations included: (a) an assessment by an otolaryngologist for the conductive hearing loss and (b) follow-up audiological appointment to ascertain bone conduction ABR thresholds in the left ear (e.g., to rule out any sensory hearing loss component) and to obtain more frequency-specific thresholds in both the left and right ears.

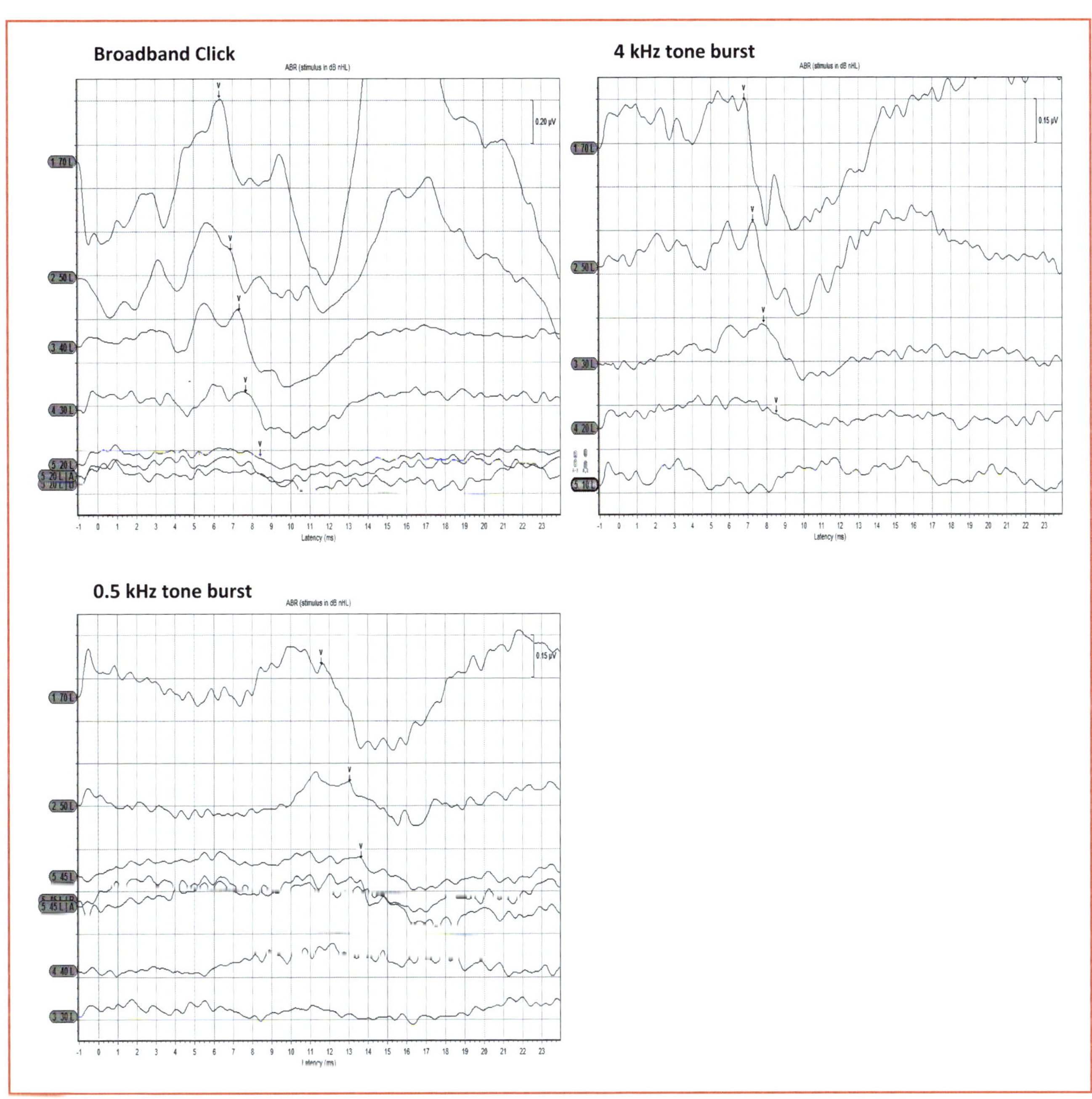

FIGURE 8–4. Air conduction ABR recordings for the left ear (Case NM).

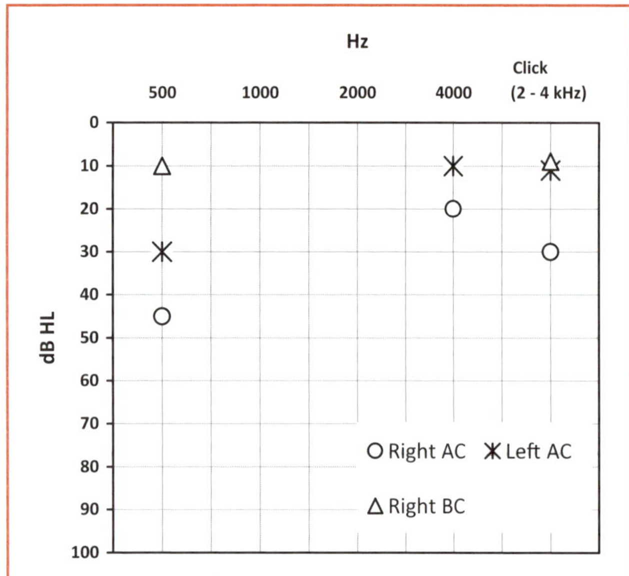

FIGURE 8–5. Hearing thresholds estimated from electrophysiological ABR thresholds (Case NM).

CASE: ABR EVALUATION OF AN AWAKE CHILD

Patient

Case IP was a male who was 4 years and 5 months of age at the time of the audiologic assessment.

History

Case IP was hospitalized for jaundice for a period of 6 weeks as an infant. His parents reported no history of otitis media. His speech consists of single words that are difficult to understand, even by parents.

IP was referred to the university clinic for a diagnostic electrophysiological assessment to determine his hearing abilities because reliable auditory thresholds could not be established in several behavioral assessments at other clinics.

Sedation

IP underwent the electroacoustic and electrophysiologic assessment following sleep deprivation and ingestion of 9 mg of melatonin. Although he did not fall asleep, he was reasonably cooperative during the assessment.

Otoscopic Examination and Immittance Measurement

Otoscopic inspection revealed a normal ear canal and normal tympanic membranes in both ears.

Using a 226 Hz probe tone, type A tympanograms were obtained bilaterally.

Acoustic reflex measurements were made in the ipsilateral condition with a BBN stimulus. Reliable acoustic reflexes were only elicited at the maximum intensity of 95 dB.

DPOAE Measurement

The DPOAE recordings were quite noisy because the patient was awake and moving somewhat throughout the recording session (Figure 8–6). Despite the slightly higher noise levels, robust DPOAEs with noise-floor and OAE amplitude differences exceeding 10 dB across the frequency range were recorded bilaterally.

ABR Evaluation

The stimuli used for the ABR recordings were calibrated and adjusted for dB nHL based on a group of normal hearing subjects and therefore do not require an adjustment to compensate for normal hearing levels in the examples presented for this case (Figure 8–7 and Figure 8–8).

Unfortunately, the patient did not fall asleep following ingestion of melatonin. He was playing and moving around on the floor throughout the assessment (see Figure 8–7). The wireless Vivosonic Integrity ABR device was strapped to his back, electrodes fixed to his scalp, and insert earphones were positioned in his ear canals. ABR recordings, illustrated in Figure 8–7, were made while the patient was moving about and playing quietly. ABR thresholds were estimated with click and 500 Hz tone burst stimuli under these measurement conditions for both ears, as illustrated in Figure 8–8. The ABR threshold for the left ear was

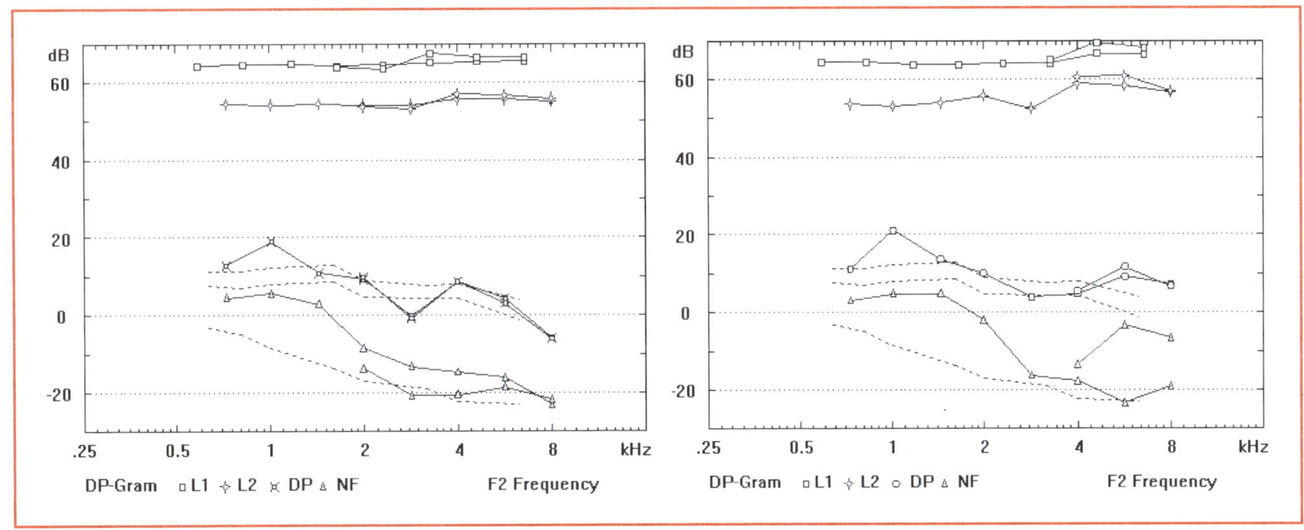

FIGURE 8–6. DPOAE recordings for the left and right ears (Case IP).

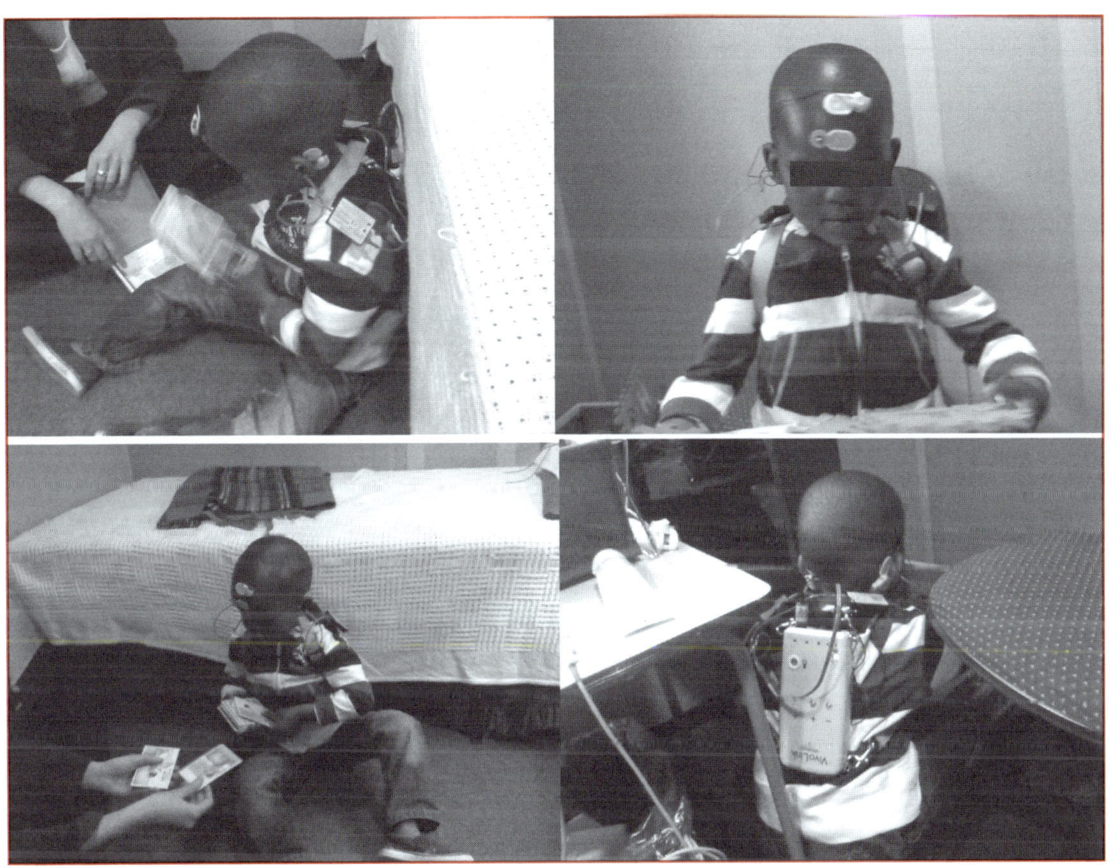

FIGURE 8–7. ABR recordings made from an awake patient (Case IP) with a new system designed to minimize the effects of movement and electrical artifact. The patient was playing quietly on the floor or standing up and moving around at times.

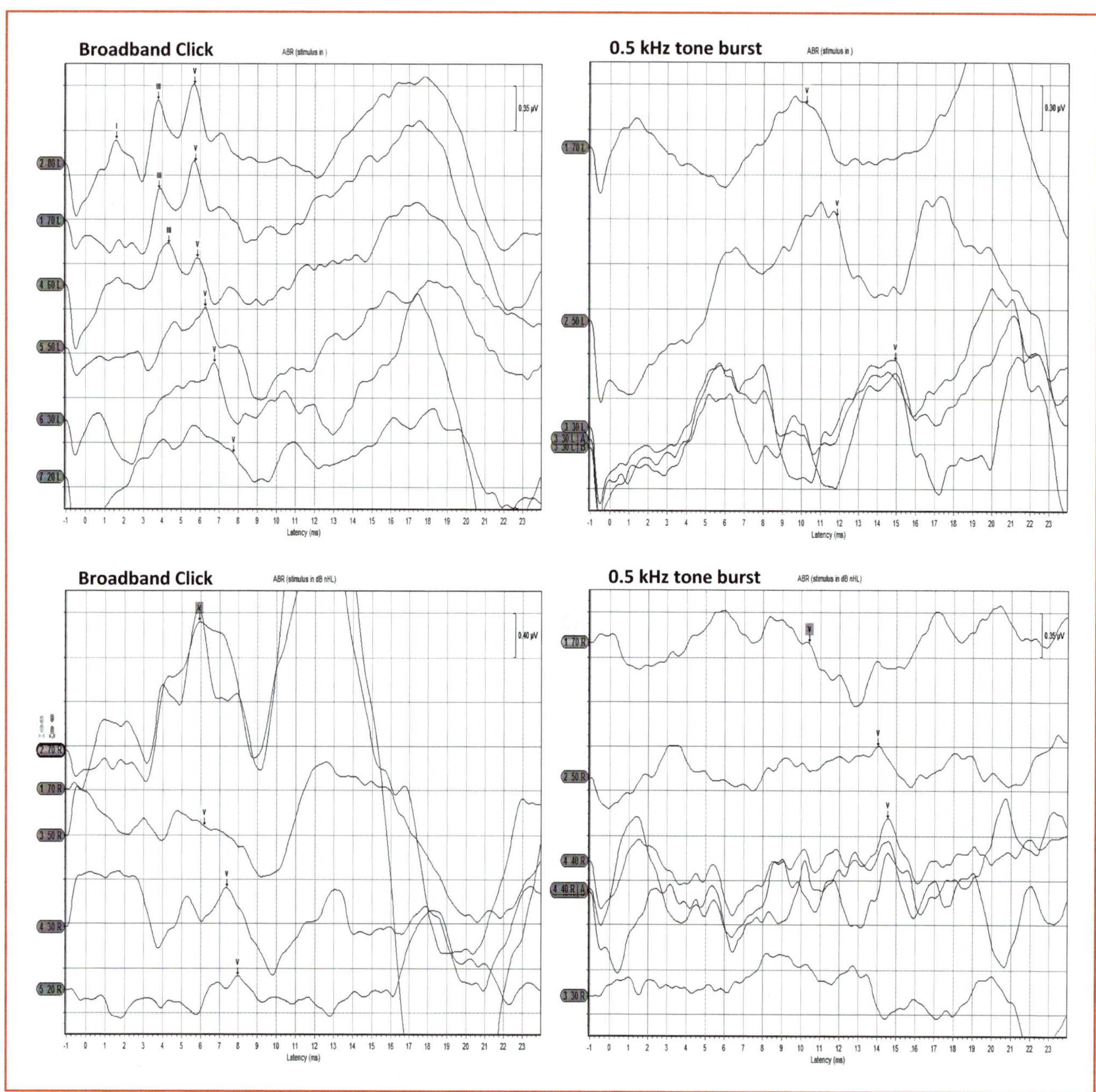

FIGURE 8–8. Air conduction ABR recordings for the left and right ear of Case IP.

20 dB nHL for the click stimulus and 30 dB nHL for the 500 Hz tone burst stimulus, indicating low frequency (500 Hz region) hearing thresholds of 15 dB HL or better (using a 15 to 20 dB correction to convert the electrophysiological threshold to an estimated hearing threshold) and high frequency hearing, as determined by the click stimulus, of 10 dB HL or better (using a 10 dB correction). For the right ear, a click ABR threshold was also found at 20 dB nHL indicating high frequency hearing thresholds of 10 dB HL or better. The 500 Hz tone burst ABR threshold for the right ear was recorded at 40 dB nHL. By this time, the patient became very restless and lower thresholds could not be obtained. Therefore, the patient's ABR threshold is probably only indicative of a minimum response

level at 20 dB HL for 500 Hz (using a 20 dB correction to convert the electrophysiological threshold to an estimated hearing threshold). The actual 500 Hz hearing threshold is at least 20 dB HL, but thresholds are probably even better.

Diagnosis and Recommendations

Despite the awake and sometimes restless state of the patient, reliable electroacoustic and electrophysiologic measurements were possible. Tympanometry and the otoscopic examination indicated normal middle ear functioning, and OAE findings were consistent with normal cochlear (outer hair cell) functioning. The Vivosonic Integrity device permits ABR recording under less than ideal circumstances by means of pre-amplifiers on the electrodes, wireless transmission, and the Kalman averaging technique. The device proved adequate to reliably characterize the patient's hearing in both ears at a high and low stimulus frequency.

A referral was made to a speech-language therapist for assessment of language and speech development as the first step towards a comprehensive intervention program.

CASE: AUDITORY NEUROPATHY AND CONDUCTIVE HEARING LOSS

Patient

CS was a male who was 1 year and 9 months of age at time of the audiologic assessment.

History

CS was born at 32 weeks gestational age and had severe asphyxia at birth. He stayed in the neonatal intensive care unit for several days. At the time of the audiologic assessment, CS only vocalized with no meaningful words and he responded poorly and inconsistently to sound. His parents had scheduled a speech and language evaluation due to his poor communication abilities. CS was referred to the university clinic for a diagnostic electrophysiological assessment to determine his hearing abilities because behavioral assessments at other clinics could not establish reliable thresholds.

Sedation

CS was sedated with chloral hydrate prior to the ABR assessment. Heart rate and oxygen saturation were monitored with a pulse oximeter for the duration of the assessment.

Otoscopic Examination and Immittance Measurement

An otoscopic examination indicated red inflamed tympanic membranes with fluid visible in the middle ear space.

Using a 226 Hz probe tone, type B tympanograms were recorded bilaterally.

DPOAE Measurement

The DPOAE recordings had slightly elevated noise levels within the low frequency region. For the right ear, DPOAEs were not detected in the low frequencies up to 2000 Hz and, for the left ear, up to 1000 Hz (Figure 8–9). Robust OAE amplitudes were recorded at 3000 and 4000 Hz in the right ear and at 2000, 3000, and 4000 Hz in the left ear. DPOAEs for higher test frequencies of 6000 and 8000 Hz were reduced in amplitude, or absent, in both ears.

ABR Evaluation

Click evoked ABR recordings are shown in Figure 8–10. No repeatable neural components of the ABR (e.g., waves III or V) were visible in either ear, but a clear cochlear microphonic (CM) response was present at 95 and 85 dB nHL in the left and right ear, persisting for several milliseconds (approximately 4 ms at 95 dB nHL). Rarefaction and condensation polarity recordings confirmed the presence of cochlear microphonic that inverted

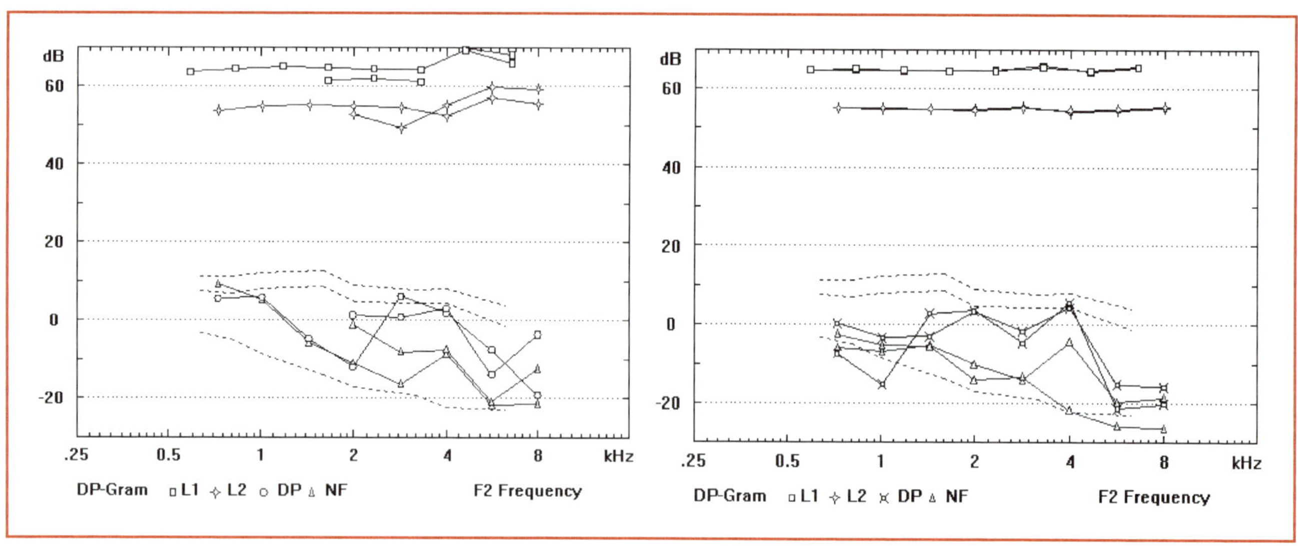

FIGURE 8–9. DPOAE recordings for the right ear (left graph) and the left ear (right graph) for Case CS.

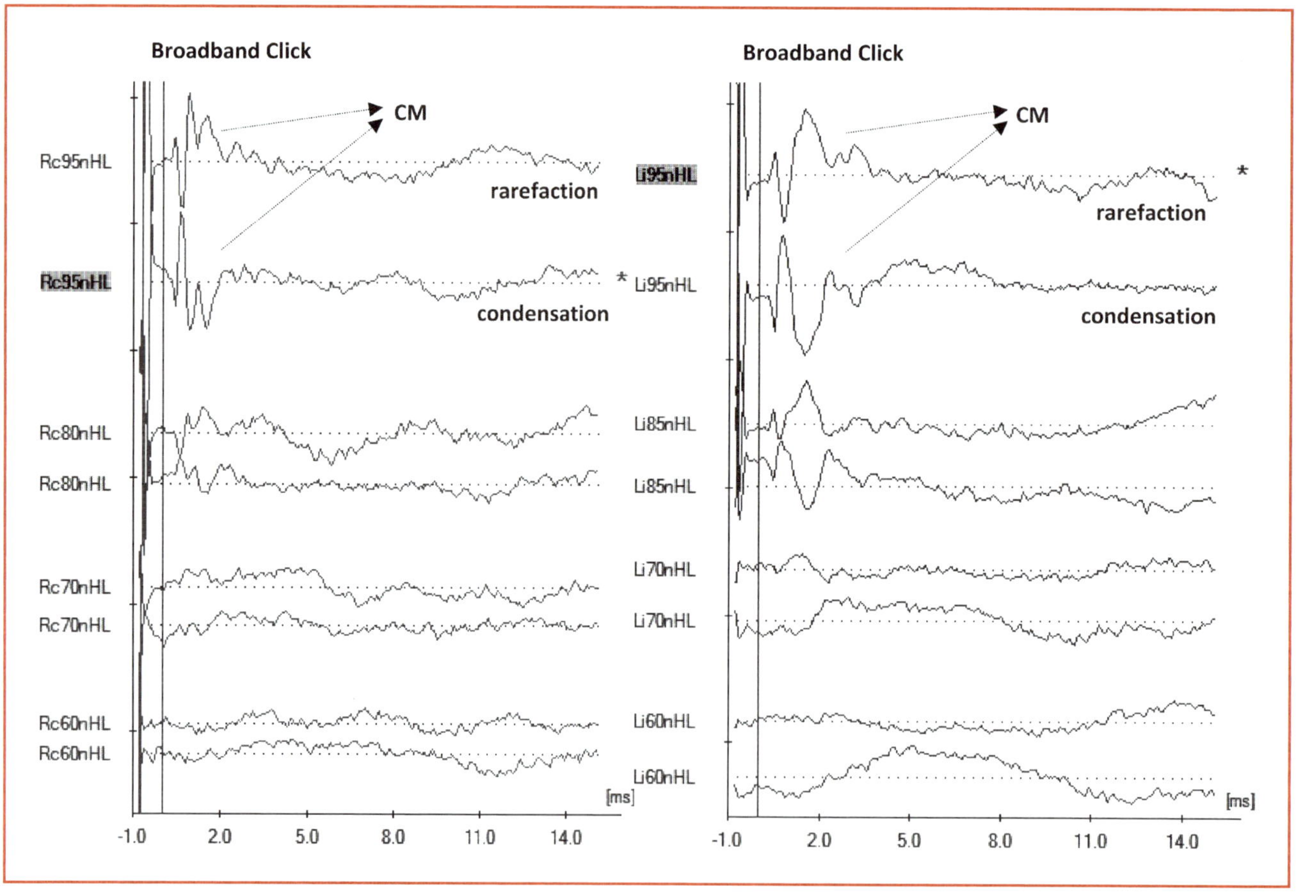

FIGURE 8–10. Air conduction ABR recordings for the right ear (left graph) and the left ear (right graph) for Case CS. CM = cochlear microphonic.

with changing stimulus polarity. This is in contrast to an ABR waveform that remains consistent (does not invert) for rarefaction and condensation polarity stimulation.

Diagnosis and Recommendations

Despite the presence of bilateral middle ear effusion, revealed through otoscopic examination and type B tympanograms, cochlear responses were obtained (i.e., OAEs in the high frequency regions and cochlear microphonic responses). These findings, in combination with the absence of any neural ABR components at maximum intensities of 95 dB nHL, clearly point toward a diagnosis of bilateral auditory neuropathy. The middle ear effusion also produced a slight low-frequency conductive hearing loss in addition to the auditory neuropathy.

Recommendations included referrals for an otolaryngology (ENT) evaluation to assess the middle ear disorder. CT scans were also recommended to investigate the integrity of the auditory structures from the 8th cranial nerve and auditory brainstem as part of an auditory neuropathy diagnostic workup. A follow-up audiological appointment to ascertain behavioral hearing thresholds was scheduled to provide information necessary for the initial fitting of hearing aids and/or consideration for possible cochlear implantation. The family was also referred to early intervention and speech-language therapy services for speech pathology services to facilitate language development.

CASE: BILATERAL CONDUCTIVE LOSS

Patient

CU was a male who was 3 years and 2 months of age at time of the audiologic assessment.

History

CU was born at term (40 weeks gestational age) with cleft palate. Subsequently, the diagnosis of VATER syndrome was made. The initials in the term *VATER syndrome* refer to five different areas of abnormalities, including vertebrae, anus, trachea, esophagus, and renal (kidneys). Hearing problems may be found in children with VATER syndrome, although the type of auditory dysfunction is dependent on which structures are involved.

Previous audiologic assessment had shown evidence of middle ear dysfunction by tympanometry and probable conductive hearing loss. Behavioral audiometry, however, had not produced ear- and frequency-specific information on auditory thresholds for air and bone conduction stimulation.

Sedation

ABR measurement was conducted in the operating room immediately following examination of the ears under microscope by a pediatric otolaryngologist. CU was anesthetized lightly with propofol during the ABR assessment.

Otoscopic Examination and Immittance Measurement

Otoscopic examination showed ventilation tubes in place from prior surgery. Immittance measurements were not made in the operating room.

DPOAE Measurement

In view of the long-standing history and clinical evidence of middle ear disorder, DPOAEs were not recorded in the operating room prior to the ABR assessment.

ABR and ASSR Evaluation

A reliable neurodiagnostic ABR was recorded using a conventional clinical protocol in both ears at a high click stimulus intensity level. Wave I was delayed, consistent with a conductive hearing loss bilaterally. ABR interwave latencies were within normal limits, suggesting auditory brainstem integrity.

A bone conduction ABR was observed bilaterally with threshold estimations consistent with no more than a 20 dB HL hearing loss for the right ear and 10 dB HL hearing loss for the left ear (at least for higher frequencies).

Due to the apparent severity of the hearing loss and the inability to precisely define auditory thresholds with an ABR elicited with tone burst stimuli, auditory steady-state response (ASSR) was performed to estimate hearing thresholds. The ASSR was recorded with the GSI Audera device.

Threshold estimations with ABR and ASSR are plotted in Figure 8–11. There was a substantial discrepancy in auditory thresholds estimated with ABR versus ASSR, although both techniques provided evidence of serious air conduction hearing loss bilaterally within the speech frequency region. It is possible that the conductive hearing loss affected the phase properties of the modulated pure tone stimuli used to elicit the ASSR and adversely influenced accurate estimation of auditory thresholds. Conductive hearing loss would not be expected to affect click-evoked ABR findings.

Diagnosis and Recommendations

Even though CU had ventilation tubes in place, ABR and ASSR findings confirmed a significant conductive hearing loss component. It is likely that the conductive hearing loss is secondary to structural abnormality of the middle ear system (e.g., fixation of the ossicular chain), perhaps related to the diagnosis of VATER syndrome. In any event, CU requires amplification to enhance speech and language development. He was scheduled for an audiological and otological consultation to consider candidacy for a bone-anchored

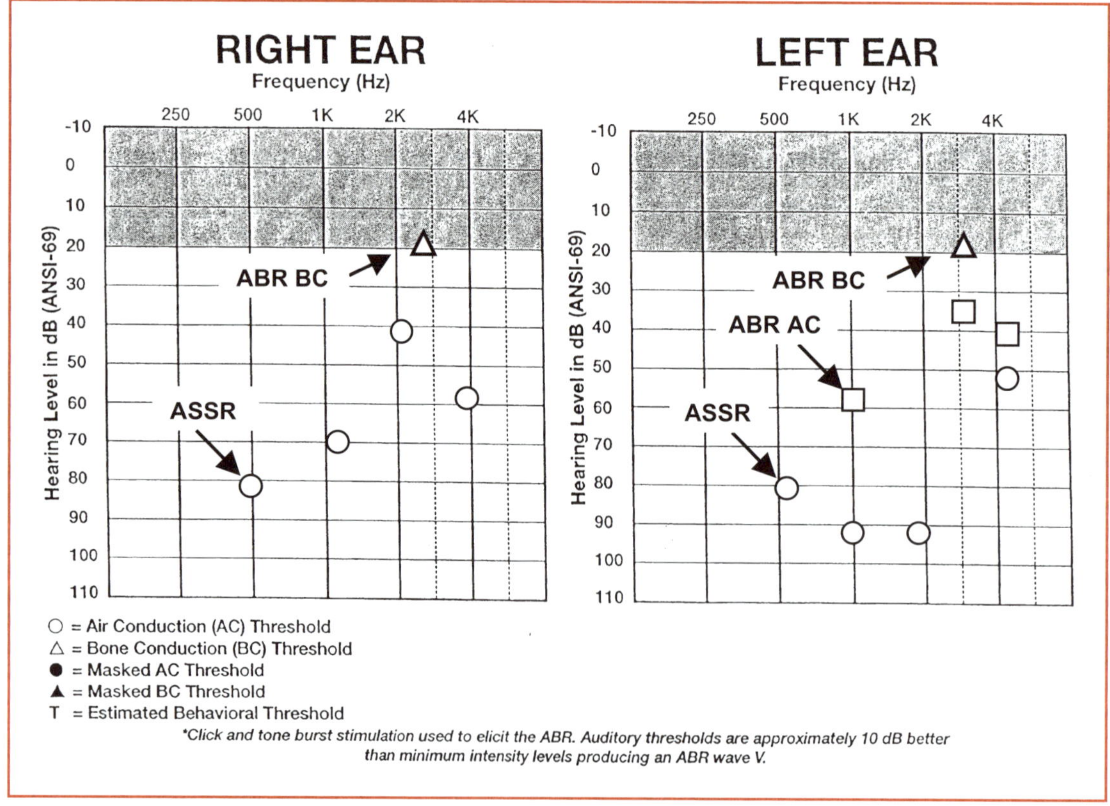

FIGURE 8–11. Graph showing auditory thresholds for CU estimated with ABR (click stimuli) and ASSR (modulated pure tone stimuli). For the ABR, estimated auditory threshold is 10 dB better than measured ABR threshold (minimum response level).

hearing aid (BAHA). The patient was also referred to speech pathology for a comprehensive evaluation and for intensive language therapy, as indicated by the findings. As an aside, given the apparently normal bone conduction hearing (by ABR) and the recommendation for management with a BAHA, the discrepancy in air conduction thresholds for ABR versus ASSR (just noted) poses no problem for effective audiologic management. Further investigation of the possible influence of conductive hearing loss, and maybe even different etiologies and mechanisms for middle ear dysfunction, on various ASSR analysis algorithms is warranted.

CASE: UNILATERAL SENSORY HEARING LOSS

Patient

Case AS was a female who was 5 months of age at the time of the audiologic assessment.

History

AS was born at term (40 weeks gestational age) with no obvious health problems. On a routine newborn hearing screening in the well baby nursery, she yielded a pass outcome for the right ear but a refer outcome for the left ear.

Sedation

Parents refused to consider sedation of their daughter for the purpose of an ABR assessment.

Otoscopic Examination and Immittance Measurement

Otoscopic examination revealed clear ear canals and normal tympanic membranes.

Immittance measurements made in the audiology clinic prior to an ABR evaluation showed type A tympanograms bilaterally (Figure 8–12).

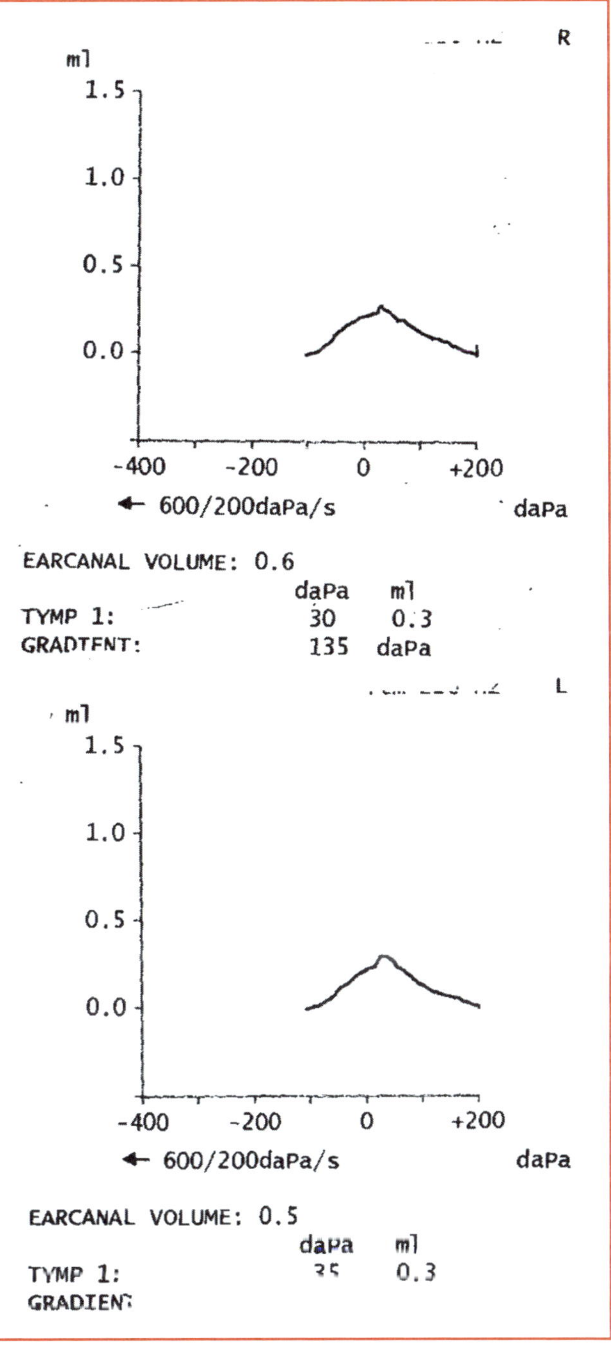

FIGURE 8–12. Tympanograms recorded in the audiology clinic for Case AS. Findings were consistent with normal middle ear function.

Acoustic reflexes for a BBN signal were present at 80 dB in the ipsilateral condition for the right. No acoustic reflex activity was observed with BBN stimulation of the left ear.

DPOAE Measurement

DPOAEs were recorded in clinic room prior to the ABR assessment. As shown in Figure 8–13, a DPOAE screening protocol (2000 to 4000 Hz) showed evidence of reliable DPOAEs for the right ear, with most amplitudes within normal limits. However, no DPOAEs were detected in the left ear.

ABR Evaluation

ABR recording was initially attempted with a conventional clinical protocol and evoked response device. The child was physically active and never slept during the ABR assessment. An ABR may have been present at the highest intensity level for right ear stimulation, whereas there was no appar-

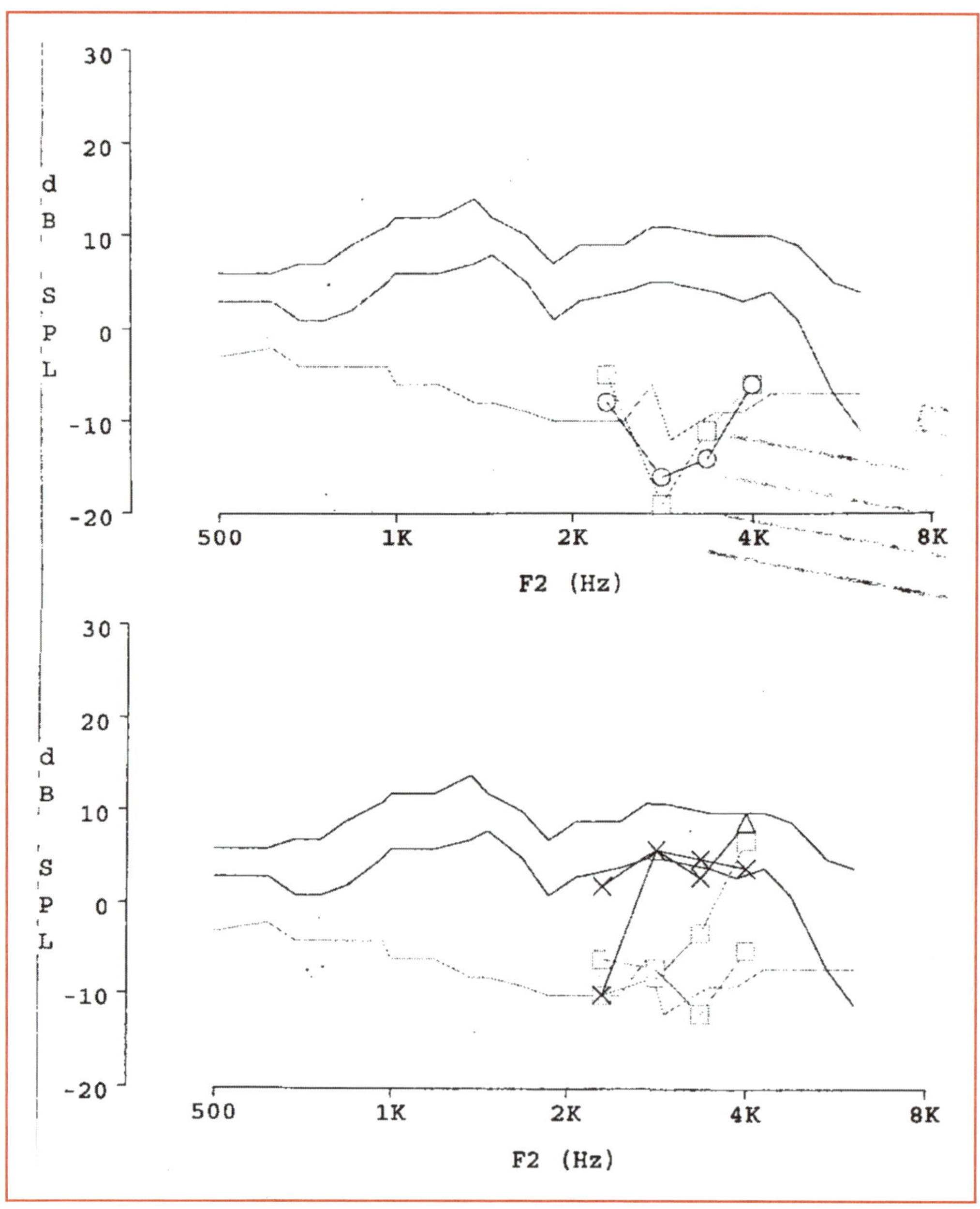

FIGURE 8–13. DPOAE recordings made in the audiology clinic for AS prior to ABR evaluation showing evidence of cochlear integrity on the left and absent DPOAEs on the right ear.

ent ABR with stimulus of the left ear maximum click intensity levels. Although these rather limited ABR findings, in combination with the aural immittance and OAE findings, suggested a unilateral (left ear) hearing loss, measurement conditions were extremely poor and frequency-specific recordings were not possible. The patient was scheduled for a follow-up visit to the audiology clinic for further ABR measurement following sleep deprivation.

Upon return to the University of Florida audiology clinic, AS underwent ABR assessment with the Vivosonic Integrity device. The parents had sleep deprived their daughter the night before. Although she was not sleeping during the ABR evaluation, she was reasonably quiet. An ABR evoked with click stimulation confirmed a severe sensory hearing loss for the right ear (Figure 8–14).

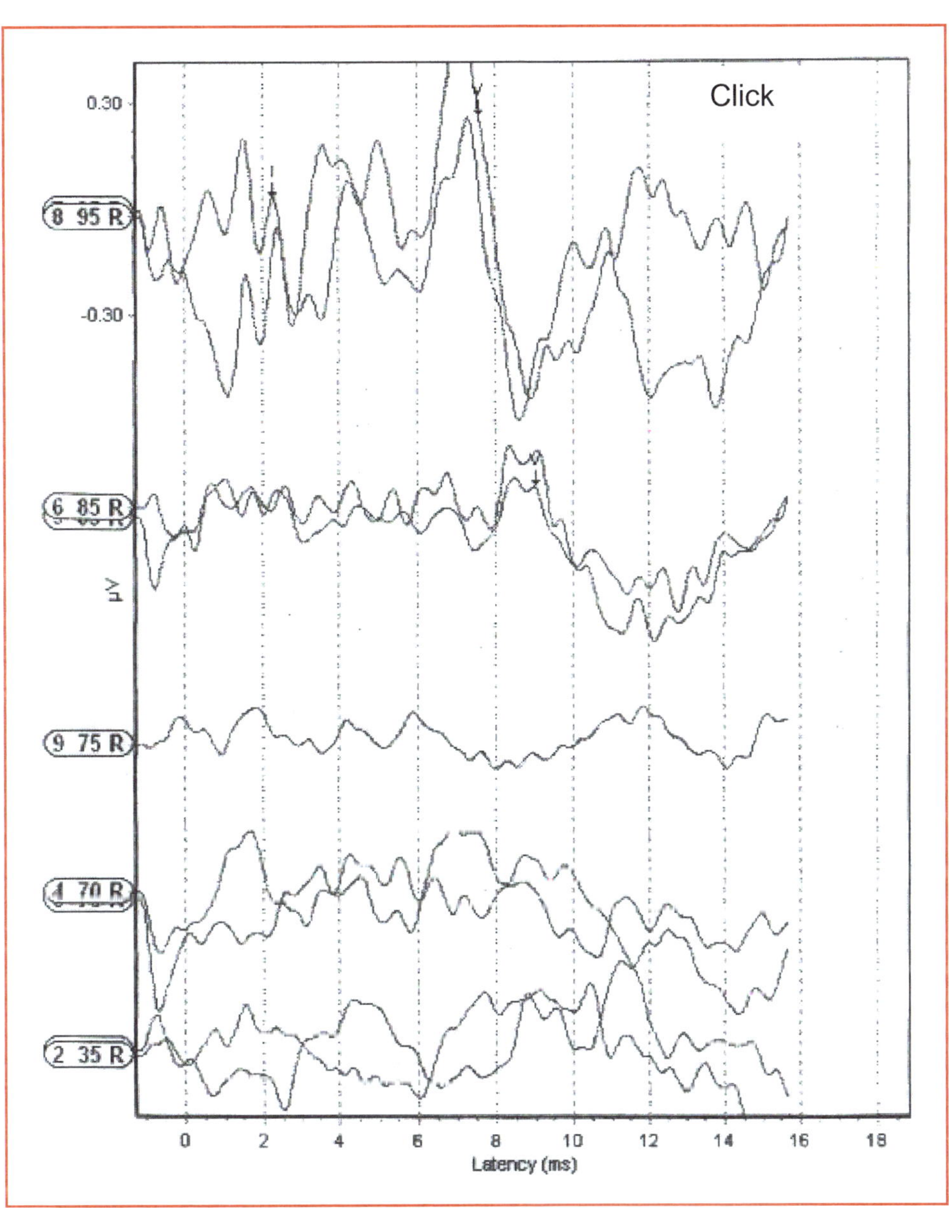

FIGURE 8–14. Click-evoked ABR recordings with right ear stimulation for AS made with the Vivosonic Integrity device on the second visit to the clinic. Findings confirmed severe sensory hearing loss. The patient was not sleeping and was restless throughout the assessment.

Tone burst evoked ABR recordings for the right ear confirmed a severe auditory sensitivity deficit for the the mid- to high speech frequency region (Figure 8–15) and also for the low frequency speech region (Figure 8–16). For the left ear, there was a well-formed and reliable ABR with click stimulation (not shown) and with tone burst stimulation of 4000 Hz (Figure 8–17), 1000 Hz (Figure 8–18), and 500 Hz (Figure 8–19) confirming hearing sensitivity within normal limits through the speech frequency region. In addition, previous aural immittance and DPOAE findings were verified on this clinic visit, confirming a unilateral (right ear) sensory auditory impairment.

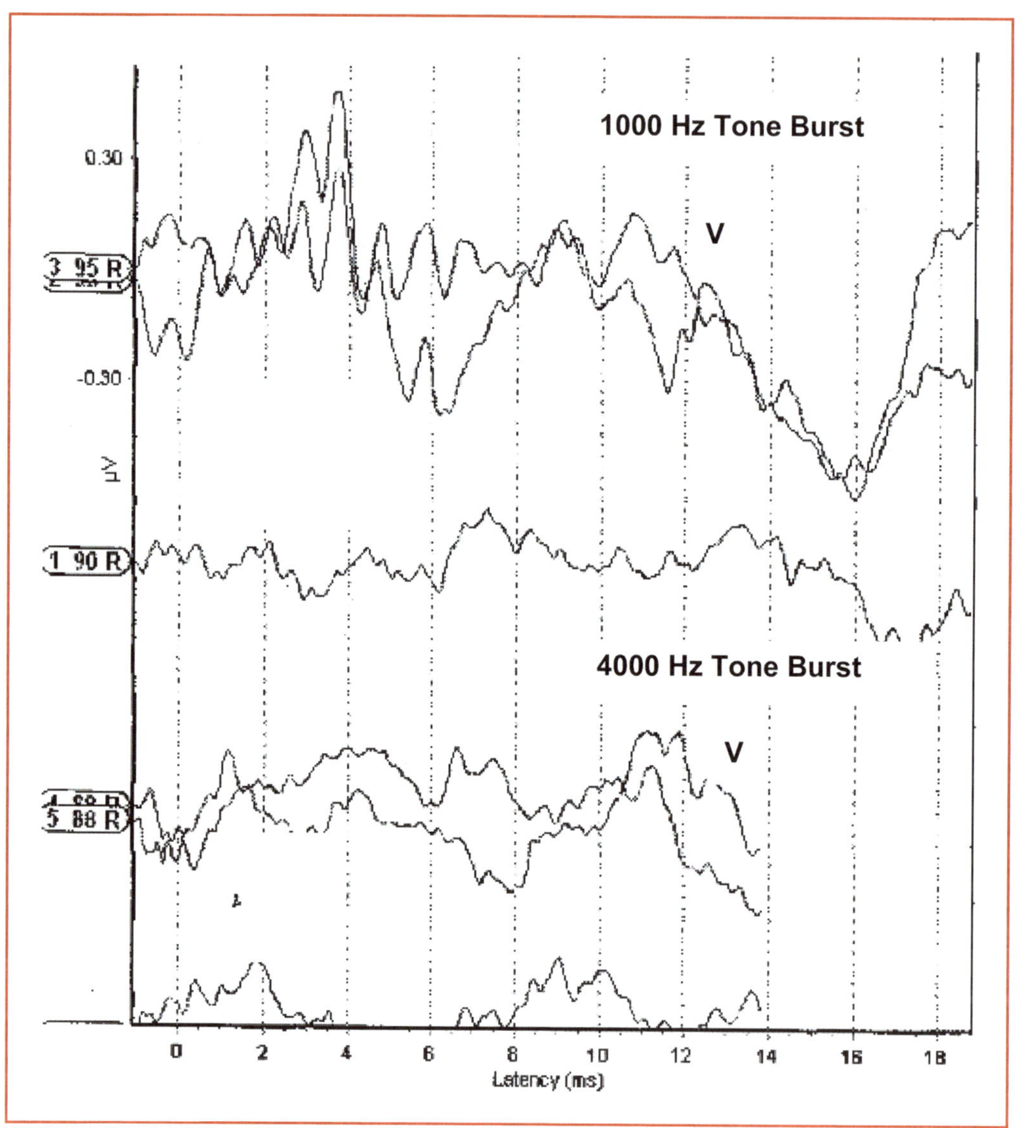

FIGURE 8–15. ABR recordings evoked with 1000 Hz and 4000 Hz tone burst stimuli presented to the right ear for AS with the Vivosonic Integrity device on the follow-up visit to the audiology clinic, confirming severe sensory hearing loss through much of the speech frequency region.

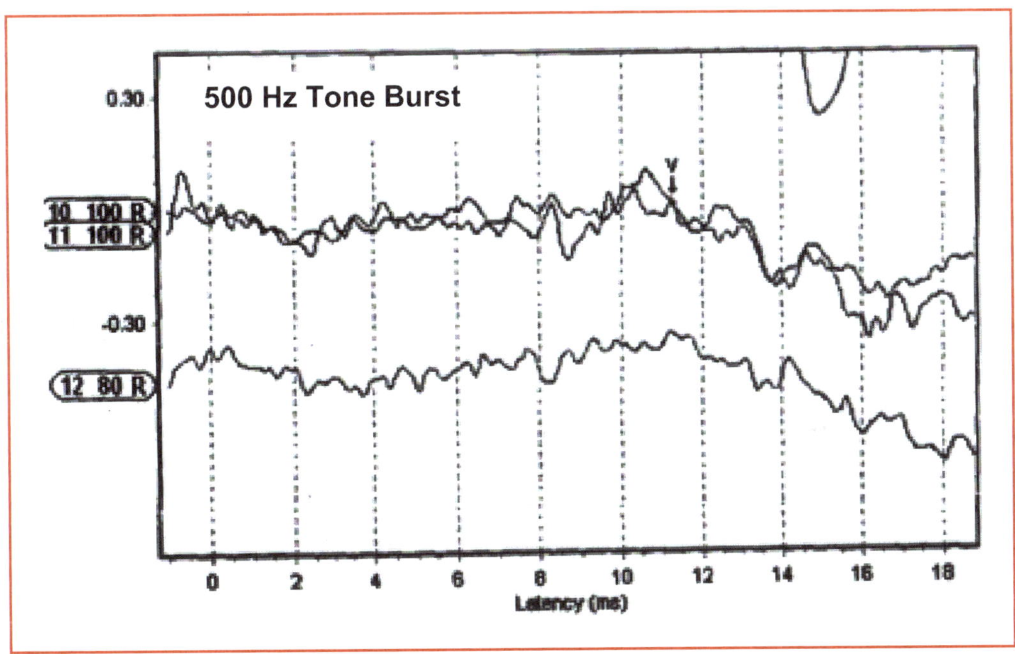

FIGURE 8–16. ABR recordings evoked with 500 Hz tone burst stimulus presented to the right ear for AS with the Vivosonic Integrity device on the follow-up visit to the audiology clinic, confirming severe sensory hearing loss in the low frequency region.

Diagnosis and Recommendations

AS was Hispanic and neither her father nor her mother spoke the English language. At each test session, all communication with the parents, including instructions about the test procedures, information about the findings and recommendations, and counseling, was done via telephone connection with a professional translator (Spanish language speaker). Siblings, who were not living in the United States, reportedly had normal hearing. There was no family history of a hearing loss. Parents were upset to hear that their daughter had a hearing loss in one ear. Counseling included information on the risk posed by unilateral hearing loss to communication, and the likelihood that AS would develop speech and language and later progress academically with normal hearing in one ear. Regular follow-up visits are scheduled to better define auditory status, especially speech perception in quiet and noisy listening conditions.

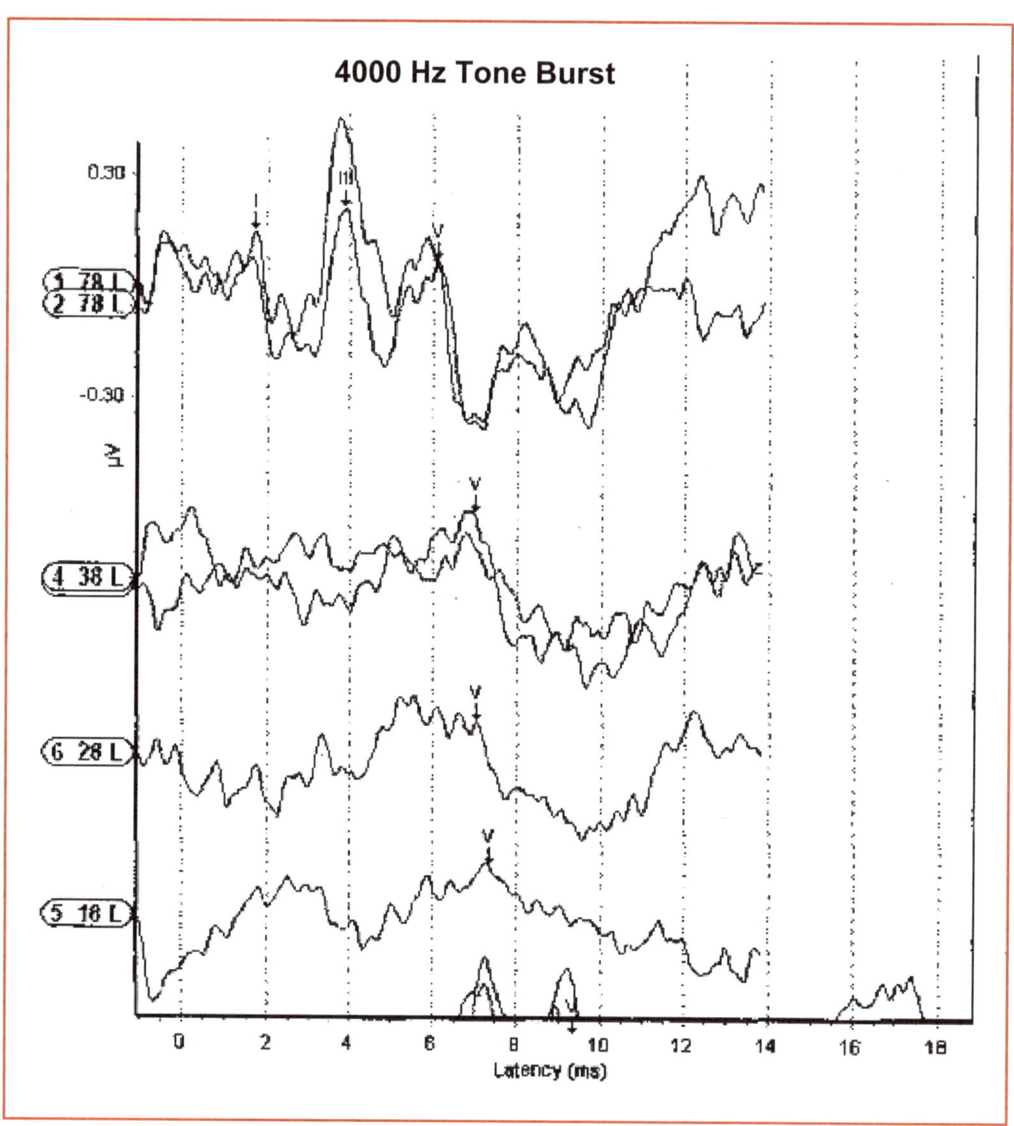

FIGURE 8–17. ABR recordings evoked with 4000 Hz tone burst stimulus presented to the left ear for AS with the Vivosonic Integrity device on the follow-up visit to the audiology clinic, confirming hearing within normal limits in the high frequency region.

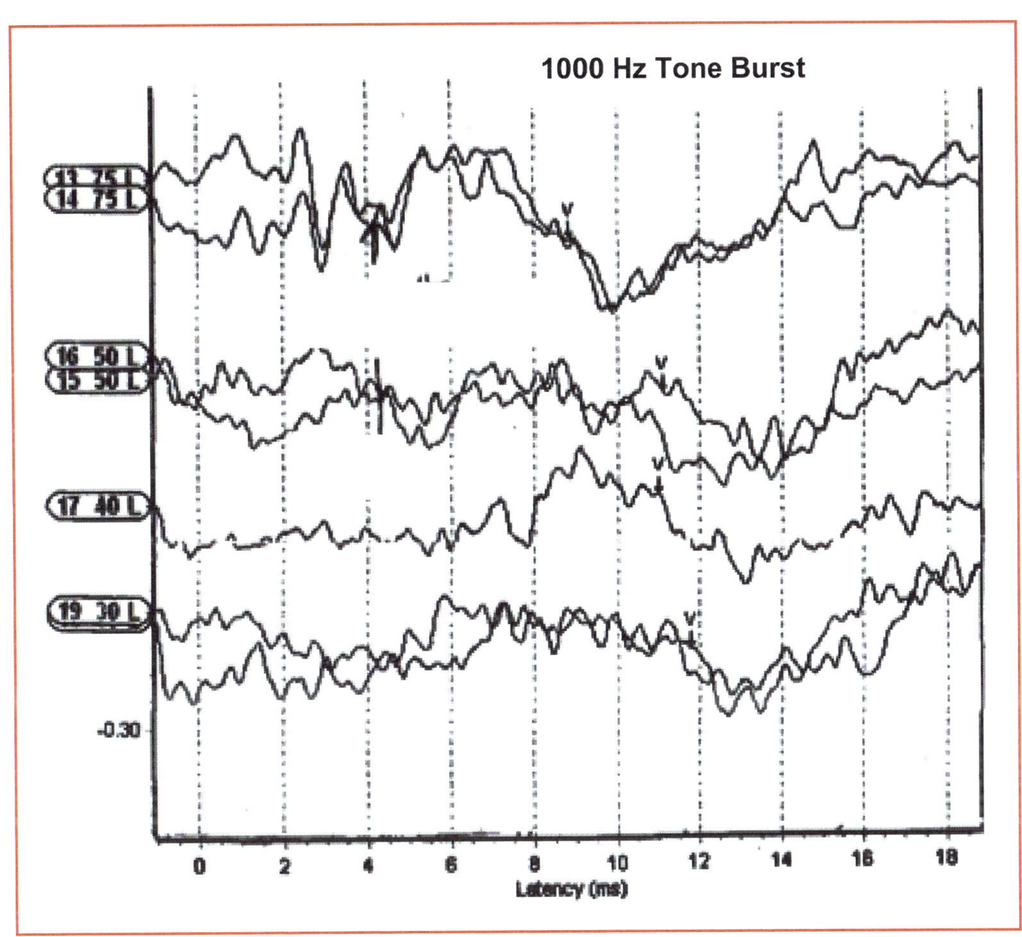

FIGURE 8–18. ABR recordings evoked with 1000 Hz tone burst stimulus presented to the left ear for AS with the Vivosonic Integrity device on the follow-up visit to the audiology clinic, confirming hearing within normal limits in the middle of the speech frequency region.

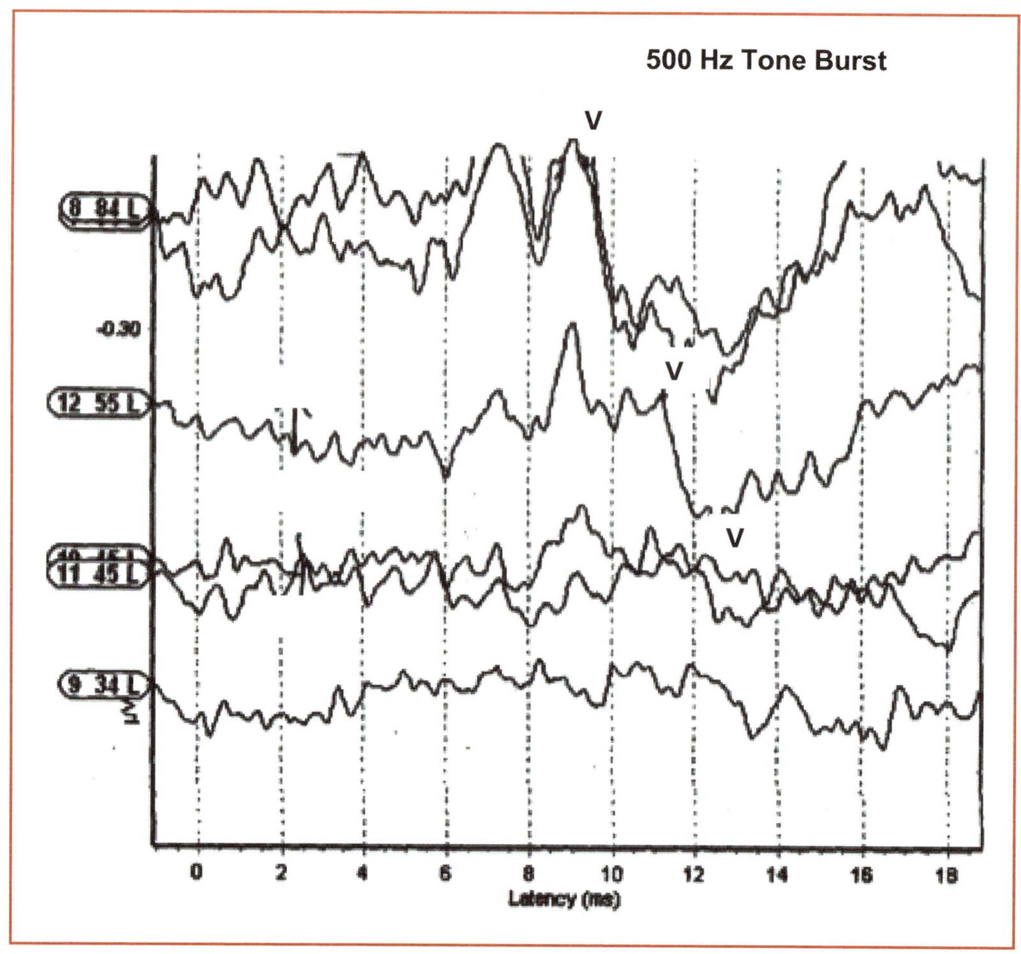

FIGURE 8–19. ABR recordings evoked with 500 Hz tone burst stimulus presented to the left ear for AS with the Vivosonic Integrity device on the follow-up visit to the audiology clinic, confirming hearing within normal limits in the low frequency region.

CASE: BILATERAL PROFOUND SENSORY HEARING LOSS

Patient

Case AT was a female who was 2 years 6 months of age at time of the audiologic assessment.

History

AT was born at term (40 weeks gestational age) with no obvious health problems. She reportedly did not pass a routine newborn hearing screening in the well baby nursery at another hospital. The mother, a speech pathologist, was confident that her child did not have a hearing loss. The child's primary care physician apparently was not convinced that the hearing screening findings warranted follow-up hearing assessment, and no audiology assessment was scheduled. The child had a history of ear infections during the first 2 years of life. Serious delay in speech and language development was attributed to middle ear dysfunction and hearing loss associated with the ear infections.

Sedation

An ABR assessment was performed in the operating room with AT anesthetized with light anesthesia.

Otoscopic Examination and Immittance Measurement

Otoscopic examination showed clear ear canals and normal tympanic membranes.

Immittance measurements made in the audiology clinic following the ABR evaluation showed type A tympanograms bilaterally. Acoustic reflexes for a BBN signal were not present in the ipsilateral condition for either ear.

DPOAE Measurement

DPOAEs were recorded in the audiology clinic following the ABR assessment. No DPOAEs were detected in either ear.

ABR Evaluation

There was no click-evoked ABR at maximum stimulus intensity level (95 dB nHL).

Given the absence of an ABR, ASSR measurement was immediately conducted while the child remained lightly anesthetized. As shown in Figure 8–20, there was no ASSR bilaterally for fast modulation rate stimulation for carrier frequencies of 500, 1000, 2000, and 4000 Hz, even for stimulus intensity levels up to 115 dB.

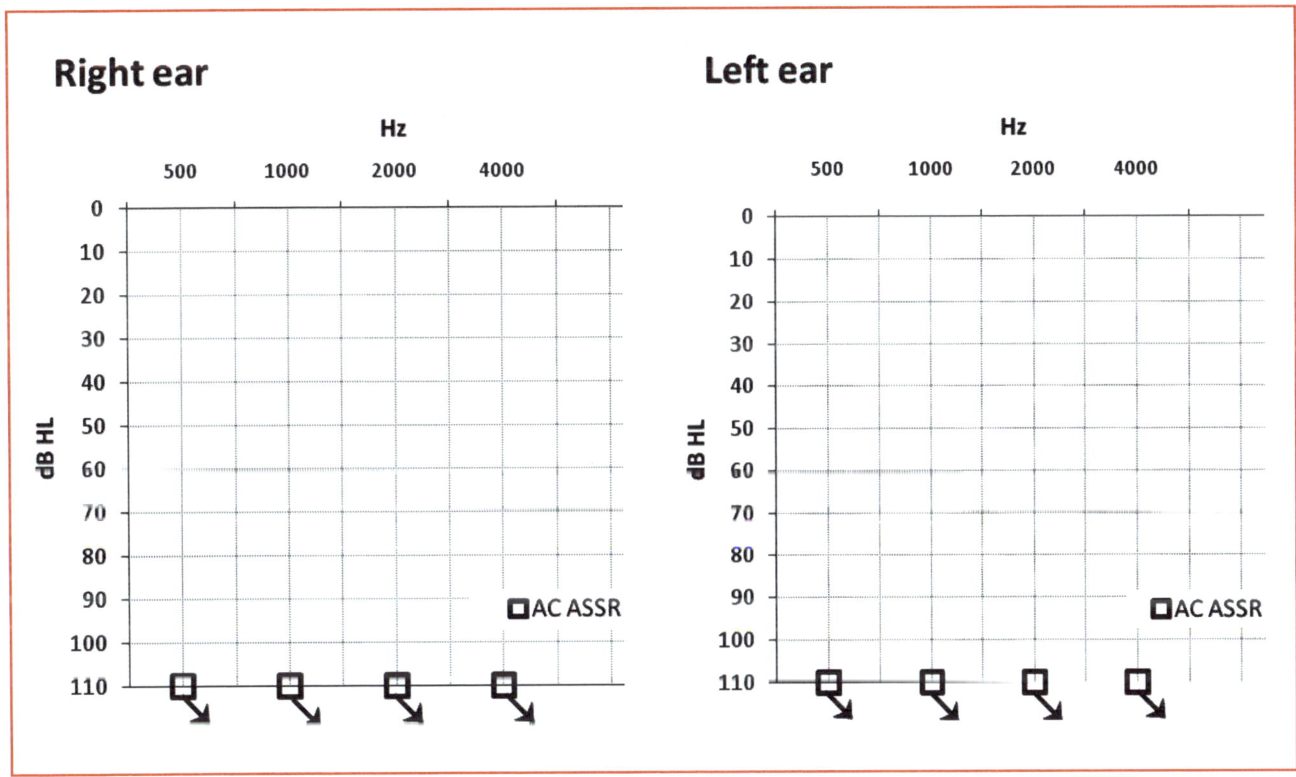

FIGURE 8–20. Auditory steady-state response (ASSR) findings for infant AT aged 2 months. There was no evidence of a reliable ABR at maximum click stimulus intensity levels (95 dB nHL). ASSR assessment yielded no response for intensity levels up to 110 dB HL, confirming a profound hearing loss in both ears.

Diagnosis and Recommendations

AT's extended family (mother and grandmother) were counseling extensively regarding the findings indicating a significant sensory hearing loss bilaterally. Despite the objective documentation of a bilateral severe-to-profound permanent hearing loss, and the child's marked speech and language delay, the family members questioned the accuracy of audiologic findings. The child was rescheduled for a follow-up assessment in the clinic 2 weeks later to verify the findings. Early intervention personnel contacted mother to enroll AT in a program for speech and language development. Meanwhile, with mother's approval ear mold impressions were made and a hearing aid fitting visit was scheduled. The patient was dispensed a powerful digital hearing aid on a temporary (3 to 4 month) basis while candidacy for cochlear implantation was evaluated by audiology and otolaryngology. Two years after the initial ABR assessment, and following a period of hearing aid use and then cochlear implantation, speech and language development is mildly delayed but the child is communicating effectively.

References

Aiken, S. J., & Picton, T. W. (2006). Envelope following responses to natural vowels. *Audiology and Neurotology, 11*, 213–232.

Allen, J. B. (1986). Measurement of eardrum acoustic impedance. In J. B. Allen, J. L. Hall, A. Hubbard, S. T. Neely, & A. Tubis (Eds.), *Peripheral auditory mechanisms* (pp. 44–51). New York: Springer-Verlag.

Allen, R. L., Stuart, A., Everett, D. & Elangovan, S. (2004). Preschool hearing screening. *American Journal of Audiology, 13*, 29–38.

American Academy of Pediatrics Task Force on Newborn and Infant Hearing. (1999). Newborn and infant hearing loss: Detection and intervention. *Pediatrics, 103*, 527–529.

American Speech-Language-Hearing Association. (1990). Guidelines for screening for hearing impairment and middle-ear disorders. *ASHA, 32*(Suppl. 2), 17–24.

American Speech–Language-Hearing Association (ASHA). (1997). *Guidelines for audiological screening*. Rockville Pike, MD: Author.

Aoyagi, M., Kiren, T., Furuse, H., Fuse, T., Suzuki, Y., Yokota, S., et al. (1994). Pure tone threshold prediction by 80 Hz amplitude modulation following response, *Acta Otolaryngologica*, (Suppl. 504), 7–14.

ASHA Audiologic Assessment Panel 1996. (1997). Guidelines for screening infants and children for outer and middle ear disorders, birth through 18 years. In *ASHA 2002 Desk Reference* (Vol. 4, pp. 342–349). Rockville, MD: American Speech-Language-Hearing Association.

Babac, S., Djeriç, D., & Ivankoviç, Z. (2007). Newborn hearing screening. [Article in Serbian]. *Srp Arh Celok Lek, 135*, 264–268.

Balkany, T. J., Berman, S. A., Simmons, M. A., & Jafek, B. (1978). Middle ear effusions in neonates. *Laryngoscope, 88*, 398–405.

Benito-Orejas, J. I., Ramírez, B., Morais, D., Almaraz, A., & Fernández-Calvo, J. L. (2008). Comparison of two-step transient evoked otoacoustic emissions (TEOAE) and automated auditory brainstem response (AABR) for universal newborn hearing screening programs. *International Journal of Pediatric Otorhinolaryngology, 72*, 1193–1201.

Berg, A. L., Papri, H., Ferdous, S., Khan, N. Z., & Durkin, M. S. (2006) Screening methods for childhood hearing impairment in rural Bangladesh. *International Journal of Pediatric Otorhinolaryngology, 70*, 107–114.

Boege, P., & Janssen, T. (2002). Pure-tone threshold estimation from extrapolated distortion product otoacoustic emission I/O-functions in normal and cochlear hearing loss ears. *Journal of the Acoustical Society of America, 111*, 1810–1818.

Brooks, D. N. (1968). An objective method of determining fluid in the middle ear. *International Audiology, 7*, 280–286.

Brzezinski, A. (1997). Melatonin in humans. *New England Journal of Medicine, 336*, 186–195

Burkard, R. F., Don, M. & Eggermont, J. J. (2007). *Auditory evoked potentials: basic principles and clinical application.* Baltimore: Lippincott Williams & Wilkins.

Calevo, M. G., Mezzano, P., Zullino, E., Padovani, P., Scopesi, F., & Serra, G. (2007). Neonatal hearing screening model: An Italian regional experience. *Journal of Maternal, Fetal & Neonatal Medicine, 20*, 441–448.

Cebulla, M., Stürzebecher, E., & Elberling, C. (2006). Objective detection of auditory steady-state responses:

Comparison of one-sample and q-sample tests. *Journal of the American Academy of Audiology*, *17*, 93–103.

Chiong, C., Ostrea, E., Jr., Reyes, A., Llanes, E. G., Uy, M. E., & Chan, A. (2007). Correlation of hearing screening with developmental outcomes in infants over a 2-year period. *Acta Otolaryngologica, 127*, 384–388.

Clarke, P., Iqbal, M., & Mitchell, S. (2003). A comparison of transient-evoked otoacoustic emissions and automated auditory brainstem responses for predischarge neonatal hearing screening. *International Journal of Audiology*, *42*, 443–447

Cohen, L. T., Rickards, F. W., & Clark, G. (1991). A comparison of steady-state evoked potentials to modulated tones in awake and sleeping humans. *Journal of the Acoustical Society of America*, *90*, 2467–2479.

Colletti, V. (1975). Methodologic observations on tympanometry with regard to the probe-tone frequency. *Acta Oto-Laryngologica*, *80*, 53–60.

Cone-Wesson, B. (2008). Subject variables in auditory steady-state response testing: State, anesthesia, age, and attention. In G. Rance (Ed.), *The auditory steady-state response* (pp. 109–117). San Diego, CA: Plural Publishing.

Cone-Wesson, B., Parker, J., Swiderski, N., & Rickards, F. (2002). The auditory steady state response: Full-term and premature neonates. *Journal of the Academy of Audiology*, *13*, 260–269.

Cone-Wesson, B., Rickards, F., Poulis, C., Parker, J., Tan, L., & Pollard, J. (2002b). The auditory steady-state response. III. Clinical observations and applications in infants and children. *Journal of the Academy of Audiology*, *13*, 270–282.

Cooper, J. C., Jr., Hearne, E. M., III, & Gates, G. A. (1982). Normal tympanometric shape. *Ear and Hearing*, *3*, 241–245.

de Jonge, R. (1986). Normal tympanometric gradient: A comparison of three methods. *Audiology*, *25*, 299–308.

Del Buono, Z. G., Mininni, F., Delvecchio, M., Pannacciulli, C. & Mininni, S. (2005). Neonatal hearing screening during the first and second day of life. *Minerva Pediatrica*, *57*, 167-172.

Dhar, S. & Hall, J. W. III. (In Press). *Otoacoustic Emissions: Principles, Procedures, and Protocols.* San Diego, CA: Plural Publishing.

Dille, M., Glattke, T. J., & Earl, B. R. (2007). Comparison of transient evoked otoacoustic emissions and distortion product otoacoustic emissions when screening hearing in preschool children in a community setting. *International Journal of Pediatric Otorhinolaryngology*, *71*, 1789–1795.

Dimitrijevic, A., & Ross, B. (2008). Neural generators of the auditory steady-state response. In G. Rance (Ed.), *The auditory steady-state response* (pp. 83–108). San Diego, CA: Plural Publishing.

Dimitrijevic, A., John, M. S., & Picton, T. W. (2004). Auditory steady-state responses and word recognition scores in normal hearing and hearing-impaired adults. *Ear and Hearing*, *25*, 68–84.

Dimitrijevic, A., John, M. S., van Roon, P., & Picton, T. W. (2001). Human auditory steady-state responses to tones independently modulated in both frequency and amplitude. *Ear and Hearing*, *22*, 100–111.

Dimitrijevic, A., John, M. S., Van Roon, P., Purcell, D. W., Adamonis, J., Ostroff, J., et al. (2002). Estimating the audiogram using multiple auditory steady-state responses. *Journal of the American Academy of Audiology*, *13*, 205–224.

Dobie, R. A., & Wilson, M. J. (1998). Low-level steady-state auditory evoked potentials: Effects of rate and sedation on detectability. *Journal of the Acoustical Society of America*, *104*, 3482–3488.

Dorn, P. A., Piskorski, P., Gorga, M. P., Neely, S. T., & Keefe, D. H. (1999). Predicting audiometric status from distortion product otoacoustic emissions using multivariate analysis. *Ear and Hearing*, *20*, 149–163.

Downs, M.P. 2000. The quest for early identification and intervention. *Seminars in Hearing*, *21*, 285–294.

Eiserman, W. D., Hartel, D. M., Shisler, L., Buhrmann, J., White, K. R., & Foust, T. (2008). Using otoacoustic emissions to screen for hearing loss in early childhood care settings. *International Journal of Pediatric Otorhinolaryngology*, *72*, 475–482.

Elberling, C., Don, M., Cebulla, M., & Stürzebecher, E. (2007). Auditory steady-state responses to chirp stimuli based on cochlear traveling wave delay. *Journal of the Acoustical Society of America*, *122*, 2772.

Galambos, R., Makeig, S., & Talmachoff, P. J. (1981). A 40-Hz auditory potential recorded from the human scalp. *Proceedings of the National Academy of Sciences*, *78*, 2643–2647.

Georgalas, C., Xenellis, J., Davilis, D., Tzangaroulakis, A., & Ferekidis, E. (2008). Screening for hearing loss and middle-ear effusion in school-age children, using transient evoked otoacoustic emissions: A feasibility study. *Journal of Laryngology & Otology*, *21*, 1–6.

Gilron, I., Plourde, G., Marcantoni, W., & Varin, F. (1998). 40 Hz auditory steady-state response and EEG spectral edge frequency during sufentanil anaesthesia. *Canadian Journal of Anaesthesia*, 45, 115–121.

Gorga, M. P., Neely, S. T., Dorn, P. A., & Hoover, B. M. (2003). Further efforts to predict pure-tone thresholds from distortion product otoacoustic emission input/output functions. *Journal of the Acoustical Society of America*, *113*, 3275–3284.

Gorga, M. P., Neely, S. T., Hoover, B. M., Dierking, D. M., Beauchaine, K. L., & Manning, C. (2004). Determining the upper limits of stimulation for auditory steady-state response measurements. *Ear and Hearing*, *25*, 302–307.

Granell, J., Gavilanes, J., Herrero, J., Sánchez-Jara, J. L., Velasco, M. J., & Martín, G. (2008). Is universal newborn hearing screening more efficient with auditory evoked potentials compared to otoacoustic emissions? [Article in Spanish]. *Acta Otorrinolaringologica Espania*, *59*, 170–175.

Gravel, J. S., White, K. R., Johnson, J. L., Widen, J. E., Vohr, B. R., James, M., et al. (2005). A multisite study to examine the efficacy of the otoacoustic emission/automated auditory brainstem response newborn hearing screening protocol: Recommendations for policy, practice, and research. *American Journal of Audiology*, *14*, S217–228.

Hall, J. W., III. (1978). Predicting hearing loss from the acoustic reflex: A comparison of three methods. *Archives of Otolaryngology*, *104*, 601–605.

Hall, J. W., III. (1992). *Handbook of auditory evoked responses*. Boston: Allyn & Bacon.

Hall, J. W., III. (1985). The acoustic reflex in central auditory dysfunction. In M. L. Pinheiro & F. E. Musiek (Eds.), *Assessment of central auditory dysfunction: Foundations and clinical correlates* (pp. 103–130). Baltimore: Williams & Wilkins.

Hall, J. W., III. (2000). *Handbook of otoacoustic emissions*. San Diego, CA: Singular Publishing Group.

Hall, J. W., III. (2006, April). *Hearing screening of kindergarten children: Increasing efficiency and accuracy*. Paper presented at the Convention of the American Academy of Audiology, Minneapolis, MN.

Hall, J. W., III (2007). *New handbook of auditory evoked responses*. Boston: Allyn & Bacon.

Hall, J. W., III, Berry, G. A., & Olson, K. (1982). Identification of serious hearing loss with acoustic reflex data. *Scandinavian Audiology*, *11*, 251–255.

Hall, J. W., III, Kileny, P. R., & Ruth, R. A. (1987). *Clinical trials for the ALGO-1 newborn hearing screening device*. Presented at the tenth biennial meeting of the International Electric Response Study Group, Charlottesville, VA.

Hall, J. W., III, & Chandler, D. (1994). Tympanometry in clinical audiology. In J. Katz (Ed.), *Handbook of clinical audiology* (4th ed., pp. 283–299). Baltimore: Williams & Wilkins.

Hall, J. W., III, & Johnston, K. N. (2007). Electroacoustic and electrophysiologic auditory measures in the assessment of (central) auditory processing disorder. In F. E. Musiek & G. D. Chermak (Eds.), *Handbook of (central) auditory processing Disorder: Vol. I. Auditory neuroscience and diagnosis* (pp. 287–315). San Diego, CA: Plural Publishing.

Hall, J. W., III, Smith, S. D., & Popelka, G. R. (2004). Newborn hearing screening with combined otoacoustic emissions and auditory brainstem responses. *Journal of the American Academy of Audiology*, *15*, 414–425.

Hanks, W. D., & Kinder, M. A. (March, 2007). *Tympanometry protocols used by early intervention Audiologists*. Paper presented at the 2007 EHDI Conference, Salt Lake City, Utah.

Helge, T., Werle, E., Barnick, M., Wegner, C., Rühe, B., Aust, G., et al. (2005). Two-tier screening process (TEOAE/AABR) reduces recall rates in newborn hearing screening. [Article in German]. *HNO*, *53*, 655–660.

Herdman, A. T., & Stapells, D. R. (2003). Auditory steady-state response thresholds of adults with sensorineural hearing impairments. *International Journal of Audiology*, *42*, 237–248.

Hergils, L. (2007). Analysis of measurements from the first Swedish universal neonatal hearing screening program. *International Journal of Audiology*, *46*, 680–685.

Hild, U., Hey, C., Baumann, U., Montgomery, J., Euler, H. A., & Neumann, K. (2008). High prevalence of hearing disorders at the Special Olympics indicate need to screen persons with intellectual disability. *Journal of Intellectual Disability Research*, *52*, 520–528.

Ho, V., Daly, K. A., Hunter, L. L., & Davey, C. (2002). Otoacoustic emissions and tympanometry screening among 0–5 year olds. *Laryngoscope*, *112*, 513–519.

Hof, J. R., Anteunis, L. J., Chenault, M. N., & van Dijk, P. (2005). Otoacoustic emissions at compensated middle ear pressure in children. *International Journal of Audiology*, 44, 317–320.

Holte, L., Margolis, R. H., & Cavanaugh, R. M., Jr. (1991). Developmental changes in multifrequency tympanograms. *Audiology*, *30*, 1–24

Hunter, L. L., Davey, C. S., Kohtz, A., & Daly, K. A. (2007). Hearing screening and middle ear measures in American Indian infants and toddlers. *International Journal of Pediatric Otorhinolaryngology*, *71*, 1429–1438.

Hunter, L. L., Tubaugh, L., Jackson, A., & Prospes, S. (2008). Wideband middle ear power measurements in infants and children. *Journal of the American Academy of Audiology*, *19*, 309–324.

Iley, K., & Addis, R. (2000). Impact of technology choice on service provision for universal newborn hearing screening within a busy district hospital. *Journal of Perinatology*, *20*, S122–S127.

Jeng, F.-C., Brown, C. J., Johnson, T. A., & Vander Werff, K. R. (2004). Estimating air-bone gaps using auditory steady-state responses. *Journal of the American Academy of Audiology, 15*, 67–78.

Jerger, J. (1970). Clinical experience with impedance audiometry. *Archives of Otolaryngology, 92*, 311–324.

Jerger, J., Anthony, A., Jerger, S., & Mauldin, L. (1974). Studies in impedance audiometry. III. Middle ear disorders. *Archives of Otolaryngology, 99*, 165–171.

Jerger, J., Burney, P., Mauldin, L., & Crump, B. (1974). Predicting hearing loss from the acoustic reflex. *Journal of Speech & Hearing Disorders, 39*, 11–22.

Jerger, J., & Hayes, D. (1976). The cross-check principle in pediatric audiology. *Archives of Otolaryngology, 102*, 614–620.

Jerger, J., & Jerger, S. (1974). Auditory findings in brain stem disorders. *Archives of Otolaryngology, 99*, 342–350.

Jerger, S., & Jerger, J. (1977). Diagnostic value of crossed versus uncrossed acoustic reflexes: Eighth nerve and brainstem disorders. *Archives of Otolaryngology, 103*, 445–453.

Jerger, J. F., Jerger, S., & Hall, J. W., III. (1979). A new acoustic reflex pattern. *Archives of Otolaryngology, 105*, 24–28.

Jerger, J., Jerger, S., & Mauldin, L. (1972). Studies in impedance audiometry. I. Normal and sensorineural ears. *Archives of Otolaryngology, 96*, 513–523.

Jerger, J., Jerger, S., Mauldin, L., & Segal, P. (1974). Studies in impedance audiometry. II. Children less than 6 years old. *Archives of Otolaryngology, 99*, 1–9.

John, M. S., Brown, D. K., Muir, P. J., & Picton, T. W. (2004). Recording steady-state responses in young infants. *Ear and Hearing, 25*, 539–553.

John, M. S., Dimitrijevic, A., & Picton, T. W. (2002). Auditory steady-state responses to exponential modulation envelopes. *Ear and Hearing, 23*, 106–117.

John, M. S., & Purcell, D. W. (2008). Introduction to technical principles of auditory steady-state response testing. In G. Rance (Ed.), *The auditory steady-state response* (pp. 11–54). San Diego, CA: Plural Publishing.

John, M. S., Purcell, D. W., Dimitrijevic, A., & Picton, T. W. (2002). Advantages and caveats when recording steady-state responses to multiple simultaneous stimuli. *Journal of the American Academy of Audiology, 13*, 246–259.

Johnson, B. W., Weinberg, H., Ribary, U., Cheyne, D. O., & Ancill, R. (1988). Topographic distribution of the 40 Hz auditory evoked-related potential in normal and aged subjects. *Brain Topography, 1*, 117–121.

Johnson, J. L., White, K. R., Widen, J. E., Gravel, J. S., & Meyer, S. (2005). A multi-center evaluation of how many infants with permanent hearing loss pass a two-stage otoacoustic emissions/automated auditory brainstem response newborn hearing screening protocol. *Pediatrics, 116*, 663– 672.

Joint Committee of Infant Hearing. (2007). *Year 2007 position statement: Principles and guidelines for early hearing detection and intervention programs. I, 120*(4), 898–921.

Keefe, D. H. (1992) Method to measure acoustic impedance and reflectance coefficient. *Journal of the Acoustical Society of America, 91*, 470–485.

Keefe, D. H., Folsom, R. C., Gorga, M. P., Vohr, B. R., Bulen, J .C., et al., 2000. Identification of neonatal hearing impairment: Ear-canal measurements of acoustic admittance and reflectance in neonates. *Ear and Hearing, 21*, 443–461.

Keefe, D. H., Gorga, M. P., Neely, S. T., Zhao, F., & Vohr, B. R. 2003. Ear-canal acoustic admittance and reflectance measurements in human neonates. II. Predictions of middle-ear in dysfunction and sensorineural hearing loss. *Journal of the Acoustical Society of America, 113*, 407–422.

Kei, J., Allison-Levick, J., Dockray, J., Harrys, R., Kirkegard, C., Wong, J. et al. (2003). High-frequency (1000 Hz) tympanometry in normal neonates. *Journal of the American Academy of Audiology, 14*, 20–28.

King, C., Warrier, C. M., Hayes, E., & Kraus, N. (2002). Deficits in auditory brainstem pathway encording of speech sounds in children with learning problems. *Neuroscience Letters, 319*, 111–115.

Koebsell, K. A., & Margolis, R. H. (1986). Tympanometric gradient measured from normal preschool children. *Audiology, 25*, 149–157.

Kok, M., van Zanten, G., Brocaar, M., & Jongejan, H. (1994). Click-evoked oto-acoustic emissions in very low birthweight infants: A cross-sectional data analysis. *Audiology, 33*, 152–164.

Korres, S. G., Balatsouras, D. G., Lyra, C., Kandiloros, D., & Ferekidis, E. (2006). A comparison of automated auditory brainstem responses and transiently evoked otoacoustic emissions for universal newborn hearing screening. *Medical Science Monitor, 12*, CR260–263.

Krumm, M., Huffman, T., Dick, K., & Klich, R. (2008). Telemedicine for audiology screening of infants. *Journal of Telemedicine & Telecare, 14*, 102–104.

Levi, E. C., Folsom, R. C., & Dobie, R. A. (1993). Amplitude-modulation following response (AMFR): Effects of modulation rate, carrier frequency, age and state. *Hearing Research, 68*, 42–52.

Lilly, D. (2005, April 12). The evolution of aural acoustic-immittance measurements. *The ASHA Leader, 6*, 24.

Lilly, D. J. (1977, November). *Prediction of points on the audiogram from acoustic reflex data.* Paper presented to the American Speech and Hearing Association Convention, Chicago.

Lin, H. C., Shu, M. T., Lee, K. S., Lin, H. Y., & Lin, G. (2007). Reducing false positives in newborn hearing screening program: How and why. *Otology and Neurotology, 28*, 788–792.

Lins, O. G., Picton, T. W., Boucher, B. L., Durieux-Smith, A., Champagne, S. C., Moran, L. M., et al. (1996). Frequency-specific audiometry using steady-state responses. *Ear and Hearing, 17*, 81–96.

Lu, Y., Zhang, Q., Wen, Y., Ji, F., Chen, A., Xi, X., & Li, X. (2008). The SP-AP compound wave in patients with auditory neuropathy. *Acta Otolaryngologica, 128*, 896–900.

Luo, R. Z., Wen, R. J., Huang, Z. Y., Zhou, J. L., & Chen, Q. (2007). Hearing evaluation of infants failed in hearing screening. [Article in Chinese]. *Zhonghua Er Bi Yan Hou Tou Jing Wai Ke Za Zhi, 42*, 33–37.

Luts, H., Desloovere, C., & Wouters, J. (2006). Clinical application of dichotic multiple-stimulus auditory steady-state responses in high-risk newborns and young children. *Audiology and Neuro-otology, 11*, 24–37.

Luts, H., Van Dun, B., Alaerts, J., & Wouters, J. (2008). The influence of the detection paradigm in recording auditory steady-state responses. *Ear and Hearing, 29*, 638–650.

Lyons, A., Kei, J., & Driscoll, C. (2004). DPOAEs in children at school entry: A comparison with pure-tone screening and tympanometry results. *Journal of the American Academy of Audiology, 15*, 702–715.

Makeig, S., & Galambos, R. (1989). The CERP: Event-related perturbations in steady-state responses. In E. Basar (Ed.), *Brain dynamics: Progress and perspectives* (pp. 373–400). Berlin/Heidelberg: Springer.

Margolis, R. H., Bass-Ringdahl, S., Hanks, W. D., Holte, K. & Zapala, D. A. (2003). Tympanometry in newborn infants—1K Hz norms. *Journal of the American Academy of Audiology, 14*, 383–392.

Margolis, R. H., & Popelka, G. (1975). Status and dynamic acoustic impedance measurements in infant ears. *Journal of Speech and Hearing Research, 18*, 435–453.

Marques, T. R., Mendes, P. C., Bochnia, C. F., Jacob, L. C., Roggia, S. M., & Marques, J. M. (2008). Newborn hearing screening: The relation between bathing and the retesting rate. [Article in Portuguese]. *Review of Brasilian Otorrinolaringology, 74*(Engl. Ed.), 375–381.

Martin, G. K., Ohms, L. A., Franklin, D. J., Harris, F. P., & Lonsbury-Martin, B. L. (1990). Distortion product emissions in humans: III. Influence of sensorineural hearing loss. *Annals of Otology, Rhinology, and Laryngology, 147*(Suppl.), 30–42.

McMahon, C. M., Patuzzi, R. B., Gibson, W. P. R., & Sanli, H. (2008). Frequency-specific electrocochleography indicates that presynaptic and postsynaptic mechanisms of auditory neuropathy exist. *Ear and Hearing, 29*, 314–325.

Metz, O. (1946). The acoustic impedance measured on normal and pathological ears. *Acta Otolaryngologica, 63*(Suppl.), 1–254.

Meier, S., Narabayashi, O., Probst, R., & Schmuziger, N. (2004). Comparison of currently available devices designed for newborn hearing screening using automated auditory brainstem and/or otoacoustic emission measurements. *International Journal of Pediatric Otorhinolaryngology, 68*, S39–S43.

Mesner, A., Price, M., Kwast, K., Gallagher, K., & Forte, J. (2001). Volunteer-based newborn universal newborn hearing screening program. *International Journal of Pediatric Otorhinolaryngology, 60*, 123–130.

Murray, G., Ormson, M., Loh, M., Ninan, B., Ninan, D., Dockery, L., & Fanaroff, A. (2004). Evaluation of Natus ALGO 3 newborn hearing screener. *Journal of Obstetric, Gynecologic, & Neonatal Nursing, 33*, 183–190.

Neumann, K., Dettmer, G., Euler, H. A., Giebel, A., Gross, M., Herer, G., et al. (2006). Auditory status of persons with intellectual disability at the German Special Olympic Games. *International Journal of Audiology, 45*, 83–90.

Niemeyer, W., & Sesterhenn, G. (1972, October). *Calculating the hearing threshold from the stapedial reflex threshold for different sound stimuli.* Paper presented at the Eleventh International Congress of Audiology, Budapest, Hungary.

Niemeyer, W., & Sesterhenn, G. (1974). Calculating the hearing threshold from the stapedial reflex threshold for different sound stimuli. *Audiology, 13*, 421–427.

Norton, S. J., Gorga, M. P., Widen, J. E., Folsom, R. C., Sininger, Y., Cone-Wesson, B., et al. (2000). Identification of neonatal hearing impairment: Evaluation of transient evoked otoacoustic emissions, distortion product otoacoustic emissions, and auditory brainstem response test performance. *Ear and Hearing, 21*, 508–528.

Nozza, R. J., Bluestone, C. D., Kardatzke, D., & Bachman, R. (1992). Towards the validation of aural acoustic immittance measures for diagnosis of middle ear effusion in children. *Ear and Hearing, 13*, 442–453.

Nozza, R. J., Bluestone, C. D., Kardatzke, D., & Bachman, R. (1994). Identification of middle ear effusion by aural acoustic admittance and otoscopy. *Ear and Hearing, 15*, 310–323.

Nozza, R. J., Sabo, D. L., & Mandel, E. M. (1997). A role for otoacoustic emissions in screening for hearing impairment and middle ear disorders in school-age children. *Ear and Hearing, 18*, 227–239.

Ohio Department of Health, Bureau of Child & Family Health Services. (2007). *Hearing screening guidelines & requirements for school age children.* Retrieved October, 20, 2009, from http://www.odh.ohio.gov

Ohwatari, R., Fukuda, S., Chida, E., Matsumura, M., Kuroda, T., Kashiwamura, M., et. al. (2001). Preserved otoacoustic emission in a child with profound unilateral sensorineural hearing loss. *Auris Nasus Larynx, 28*(Suppl.), 117–120.

Paradise, J. L., Smith, C. G., & Bluestone, C. D. (1976). Tympanometric detection of middle ear effusion in infants and young children. *Pediatrics, 58*, 198–210.

Pedersen, L., Møller, T. R., Wetke, R., & Ovesen, T. (2008). Neonatal hearing screening. A comparison of automatic auditory brainstem audiometry and otoacoustic emissions. [Article in Danish]. *Ugeskr Laeger, 170*, 642–646.

Pethe, J., von Specht, H., Muhler, R., & Hocke, T. (2001). Amplitude modulation following response in awake and sleeping humans—A comparison for the 40 Hz and 80 Hz modulation frequency. *Scandinavian Audiology, 52*(Suppl.), 152–155.

Picton, T. W., Dimitrijevic, A., John, M. S., & van Roon, P. (2001). The use of phase in the detection of auditory steady-state responses. *Clinical Neurophysiology, 112*, 1692–1711.

Picton, T. W., Dimitrijevic, A., van Roon, P., John, M. S., Reed, M., & Finkelstein, H. (2002). Possible roles for the auditory steady-state responses in fitting hearing aids. In R. C. Seewald & J. S. Gravel (Eds.), *A sound foundation through early amplification: Proceedings of the Second International Conference* (pp. 63–73). Stäfa, Switzerland.

Picton, T. W., Durieux-Smith, A., Champagne, S. C., Whittingham, J., Moran, L. M., Giguere, C., et al. (1998). Objective evaluation of aided thresholds using auditory steady-state responses. *Journal of the American Academy of Audiology, 9*, 315–331.

Picton, T. W., & John, M. S. (2004). Avoiding electromagnetic artifacts when recording auditory steady-state responses. *Journal of the American Academy of Audiology, 15*, 541–554.

Picton, T. W., John, M. S., & Dimitrijevic, A. (2002). Possible roles for the auditory steady state responses in identification, evaluation and management of hearing loss in infancy. *Audiology Today, 14*, 29–34.

Picton, T. W., John, M. S., Dimitrijevic, A., & Purcell, D. (2003). Auditory steady-state responses. *International Journal of Audiology, 42*, 177–219.

Plourde, G. (1996). The effects of propofol on the 40-Hz auditory steady-state response and on the electroencephalogram in humans. *Anesthesia and Analgesia, 82*, 1015–1022.

Plourde, G., Baribeau, J., & Bonhomme, V. (1997). Ketamine increases the amplitude of the 40-Hz auditory steady-state response in humans. *British Journal of Anaesthesia, 78*, 524–529.

Plourde, G., & Picton, T. W. (1990). Human auditory steady state responses during general anesthesia. *Anesthesia and Analgesia, 71*, 460–468.

Plourde, G., & Villemure, C. (1996). Comparison of the effects of enflurane/N2O on the 40-Hz auditory steady-state response versus the auditory middle-latency response. *Anesthesia and Analgesia, 82*, 75–83.

Popelka, G. R., Margolis, R. H., & Wiley, T. L. (1976). Effect of activating signal bandwidth on acoustic reflex thresholds. *Journal of the Acoustical Society of America, 59*, 153–159.

Prieve, B. A., Calandruccio, L., Fitzgerald, T., Mazevski, A., & Georgantas, L. M. (2008). Changes in transient-evoked otoacoustic emission levels with negative tympanometric peak pressure in infants and toddlers. *Ear and Hearing, 29*, 533–542.

Psarommatis, I., Valsamakis, T., Raptaki, M., Kontrogiani, A., & Douniadakis, D. (2007). Audiologic evaluation of infants and preschoolers: A practical approach. *American Journal of Otolaryngology, 28*, 392–396.

Psillas, G., Psifidis, A., Antoniadou-Hitoglou, M., & Kouloulas, A. (2006). Hearing assessment in preschool children with speech delay. *Auris Nasus Larynx, 33*, 259–263.

Rance, G. (2005). Auditory neuropathy/dys-synchrony and its perceptual consequences. *Trends in Amplification, 9*, 1–43.

Rance, G. (2008). Auditory steady-state responses in neonates and infants. In G. Rance (Ed.), *The auditory steady-state response* (pp. 161–184). San Diego, CA: Plural Publishing.

Rance, G., Beer, D. E., Cone-Wesson, B., Shepherd, R. K., Dowell, R. C., King, A. M., et al. (1999). Clinical findings for a group of infants and young children with auditory neuropathy. *Ear and Hearing, 20*, 238–252.

Rance, G., & Briggs, R. J. S. (2002). Assessment of hearing in infants with moderate to profound impairment: The Melbourne experience with auditory steady-state evoked potential testing. *Annals of Otology, Rhinology, and Laryngology, 111*(Suppl. 189), 22–28.

Rance, G., Luts, H., Cone-Wesson, B., Van Maanen, A., & King, A. (2008). Case studies in application of auditory steady-state response testing. In G. Rance (Ed.), *The auditory steady-state response* (pp. 161–184). San Diego, CA: Plural Publishing.

Rance, G., & Rickards, F. (2002). Prediction of hearing threshold in infants using auditory steady-state evoked potentials. *Journal of the American Academy of Audiology, 13*, 236–245.

Rance, G., Rickards, F. W., Cohen, L. T., De Vidi, S., & Clark, G. M. (1995). The automated prediction of hearing thresholds in sleeping subjects using auditory steady-state evoked potentials. *Ear and Hearing, 16*, 499–507.

Rance, G., Roper, R., Symonds, L., Moody, L. J., Poulis, C., Dourlay, M., et al. (2005). Hearing threshold estimation in infants using auditory steady state responses. *Journal of the American Academy of Audiology, 16*, 293–302.

Rance, G., & Tomlin, D. (2006). Maturation of auditory steady-state response in normal babies. *Ear and Hearing, 27*, 20–29.

Rance, G., Tomlin, D., & Rickards, F. W. (2006). Comparison of auditory steady-state responses and tone-burst auditory brainstem responses in normal babies. *Ear and Hearing, 27*, 751–762.

Rapin, I., & Gravel, J. S. (2006). Auditory neuropathy: A biologically inappropriate label unless acoustic nerve involvement is documented. *Journal of the American Academy of Audiology, 17*, 147–150.

Rickards, F. W., Tan, L. E., Cohen, L. T., Wilson, O. J., Drew, J. H., & Clark, G. M. (1994). Auditory steady state evoked potentials in newborns. *British Journal of Audiology, 28*, 327–337.

Rizzo, S. Jr. & Greenberg, H. J. (1979). Influence of ear canal air pressure on acoustic reflex threshold. *Journal of the American Auditory Society, 5*, 21–24.

Robinette, M. S., & Glattke, T. J. (Eds.). (2007). *Otoacoustic emissions: Clinical applications*. New York: Thieme.

Ross, B., Picton, T. W., Herdman, A. T., Hillyard, S. A., & Pantev, C. (2004). The effect of attention on the auditory steady-state response. *Neurology and Clinical Neurophysiology, 22*, 1–4.

Roush, J., Bryant, K., Mundy, M., Zeisel, S., & Roberts, J. (1995). Developmental changes in static admittance and tympanometric width in infants and toddlers. *Journal of the American Academy of Audiology, 6*, 334–338

Sadri, M., Thornton, A. R., & Kennedy, C. R. (2007). Effects of maturation on parameters used for pass/fail criteria in neonatal hearing screening programs using evoked otoacoustic emissions. *Audiology and Neurotology, 12*, 226–233.

Santarelli, R., Starr, A., Michalewski, H. J., & Arlsan, E. (2008). Neural and receptor cochlear potentials obtained by transtympanic electrocochleography in auditory neuropathy. *Clinical Neurophysiology, 119*, 1028–1041.

Sauter, T. B. (2007). Initial audiologic assessment of infants: Comments on Karzon and Lieu (2006). *American Journal of Audiology, 16*(1), 75–76 [author reply 77–78].

Schmidt, C.-M., Knief, A., Deuster, D., Matulat, P., & am Zehnhoff-Dinnesen, A. G. (2007). Melatonin is a useful alternative to sedation in children undergoing brainstem audiometry with an age dependent success rate: A field report of 250 investigations. *Neuropediatrics 38*, 2–4.

Schmuziger, N., Lodwig, A., & Probst, R. (2006). Influence of artifacts and pass/refer criteria on otoacoustic emission hearing screening. *International Journal of Audiology, 45*, 67–73.

Schoonhoven, R., Lamore, P. J., de Laat, J. S., & Grote, J. J. (1999). The prognostic value of electrococheography in severely hearing-impaired infants. *Audiology, 38*, 141–154.

Sideris, I., & Glattke, T. J. (2006). A comparison of two methods of hearing screening in preschool population. *Journal of Communication Disorders, 39*, 391–401.

Sininger, Y. S., Cone-Wesson, B., Folsom, R. C., Gorga, M. P., Vohr, B., & Widen, J., et al. (2000). Identification of neonatal hearing impairment: Auditory brainstem response in the perinatal period. *Ear and Hearing, 21*, 383–399.

Sininger, Y. S. (2002) Identification of auditory neuropathy in infants and children. *Seminars in Hearing, 23*(3), 193–200.

Small, S. A., Hatton, J. L., & Stapells, D. R. (2007). Effects of bone oscillator coupling method, placement location, and occlusion on bone-conduction auditory steady-state responses in infants. *Ear and Hearing, 28*, 83–98.

Small, S. A., & Stapells, D. R. (2004). Artifactual responses when recording auditory steady-state responses. *Ear and Hearing, 25*, 611–623.

Small, S. A., & Stapells, D. R. (2005). Multiple auditory steady-state responses to bone-conduction stimuli in adults with normal hearing. *Journal of the American Academy of Audiology, 16*, 172–183.

Small, S. A., & Stapells, D. R. (2006). Multiple auditory steady state response thresholds to bone-conduction stimuli in young infants with normal hearing. *Ear and Hearing, 27*, 219–228.

Small, S. A., & Stapells, D. R. (2008). Bone conduction auditory steady-state responses. In G. Rance (Ed.), *The auditory steady-state response* (pp. 201–228). San Diego, CA: Plural Publishing.

Small, S. A., & Stapells, D. R. (2008). Normal ipsilateral/contralateral asymmetries in infant multiple auditory steady-state responses to air- and bone-conduction stimuli. *Ear and Hearing, 29*, 185–198.

Small, S. A., & Stapells, D. R. (2008). Maturation of bone-conduction multiple auditory steady-state responses. *International Journal of Audiology, 47*, 476–488.

Smith, C. G., Paradise, J. L., Sabo, D. L., Rockette, H. E., Kurs-Lasky, M., Bernard, B. S., et al. (2006). Tympanometric findings and the probability of middle-ear effusion in 3686 infants and young children. *Pediatrics, 118*, 1–13.

Spektor, Z., Leonard, G., Kim, D. O., Jung, M. D., & Smurzynski, J. (1991). Otoacoustic emissions in normal and hearing impaired children and adults. *Laryngoscope, 101*, 965–976.

Srisuparp, P., Gleebbur, R., Ngerncham, S., Chonpracha, J., & Singkampong, J. (2005). High-risk neonatal hearing screening program using automated screening device performed by trained nursing personnel at Siriraj Hospital: Yield and feasibility. *Journal of the Medical Association of Thailand, 88*(Suppl. 8), S176–182.

Stapells, D. R. (2000). Threshold estimation by the tone-evoked auditory brainstem response: A literature meta-analysis. *Journal of Speech-Language Pathology and Audiology, 24*, 74–83.

Stapells, D. R. (2008). The 80-Hz auditory steady-state response compared with other auditory evoked potentials. In G. Rance (Ed.), *The auditory steady-state response* (pp. 149–160). San Diego, CA: Plural Publishing.

Stapells, D. R., Galambos, R., Costello, J. A., & Makeig, S. (1988). Inconsistency of auditory middle latency and steady-state responses in infants. *Electroencephalography Clinical Neurophysiology, 71*, 289–295.

Starr, A., Picton, T., Sininger, Y., Hood, L., & Berlin, C. (1996). Auditory neuropathy. *Brain, 119*, 741–753.

Stewart, D., Mehl, A., Hall, J. W., III, Thompson, V., Carrol, M., & Hamlett, J. (2000). Universal newborn hearing screening with automated auditory brainstem response. *Journal of Perinatalogy, 20*, S128–S131.

Stroebel, D., Swanepoel, D., & Groenewald, E. (2007). Aided auditory steady-state responses in infants. *International Journal of Audiology, 46*, 287–292.

Stürzebecher, E., Cebulla, M., Elberling, C., & Berger, T. (2006). New efficient stimuli for evoking frequency specific auditory steady-state responses. *Journal of the American Academy of Audiology, 17*, 448–461.

Suppiej, A., Rizzardi, E., Zanardo, V., Franzoi, M., Ermani, M., & Orzan, E. (2007). Reliability of hearing screening in high-risk neonates: Comparative study of otoacoustic emission, automated and conventional auditory brainstem response. *Clinical Neurophysiology, 118*, 869–876.

Swanepoel, D., Ebrahim, S., Friedland, P., Pottas, L., & Swanepoel, A. (2008). Auditory steady-state responses to bone conduction stimuli in children with hearing loss. *International Journal of Pediatric Otorhinolaryngology, 72*, 1861–1871.

Swanepoel, D., Werner, S., Hugo, R., Louw, B., Owen, R., & Swanepoel, A. (2007). High frequency immittance for neonates: a normative study. *Acta Otolaryngologica, 127*, 49–56.

Tatli, M. M., Bulent Serbetcioglu, M., Duman, N., Kumral, A., Kirkim, G., Ogun, B., et al. (2007). Feasibility of neonatal hearing screening program with two-stage transient otoacoustic emissions in Turkey. *Pediatrics International, 49*, 161–166.

Taylor, C. L., & Brooks, R. P. (2000). Screening for hearing loss and middle ear disorders in children using TEOAEs. *American Journal of Audiology, 9*, 50–55.

Tompkins, S. M. & Hall, J. W., III. (1990). Comparison of two gradient methods in normal ears versus otitis media [abstract]. *Journal of the American Academy of Audiology, 1*, 49–50.

Uchida, Y., Ando, F., Nakata, S., Ueda, H., Nakashima, T., Niino, N., et al. (2006). Distortion product otoacoustic emissions and tympanometric measurements in an adult population-based study. *Auris Nasus Larynx, 33*, 97–401.

Valdes, J. L., Perez-Abalo, M. C., Martin, V., Savio, G., Sierra, C., Rodriguéz, E., et al. (1997). Comparison of statistical indicators for the automatic detection of 80 Hz auditory steady state responses. *Ear and Hearing*, 18, 420–429.

Van Strääten, H. L., Tibosch, C. H., Dorrepaal, C., Dekker, F. W., & Kok, J. H. (2001). Efficacy of automated auditory brainstem response hearing screening in very preterm newborns. *Journal of Pediatrics, 138*, 674–678.

Vander Werff, K., Johnson, T., & Brown, C. (2008). Behavioural threshold estimation for auditory steady-state response testing. In G. Rance (Ed.), *The auditory steady-state response* (pp. 125–148). San Diego, CA: Plural Publishing.

Vanhuyse, V. J., Creten, W. L., & Van Camp, K. J. (1975). On the W-notching of tympanograms. *Scandinavian Audiology, 4*, 45–50.

Vohr, B. R., Oh, W., Stewart, E. J., Bentkover, J. D., Gabbard, S., Lemons, J., et al. (2001). Comparison of costs and referral rates of 3 universal newborn hearing screening protocols. *Journal of Pediatrics, 139*, 239–244.

Wever, E. G., & Bray, C. W. (1930). Auditory nerve impulses. *Science, 71*, 215.

White, K. R., Vohr, B. R., Meyer, S., Widen, J. E., Johnson, J. L., Gravel, J. S., et al. (2005). A multisite study to examine the efficacy of the otoacoustic emission/automated auditory brainstem response newborn hearing screening protocol: Research design and results of the study. *American Journal of Audiology, 14*, S186–199.

Wong, S. H.-W., Gibson, W. P. R., & Sanli, H. (1997). Use of transtympanic round window electrocochleography for threshold estimation in children. *The American Journal of Otology, 18*, 632–636.

Xu, Z. M., Li, J., Hu, T. Z., Sun, J. H., & Shen, X. M. (2003). Sensitivity of distortion product otoacoustic emissions and auditory brain-stem response in neonatal hearing screening, a comparative study. [Article in Chinese]. *Zhonghua Yi Xue Za Zhi, 25*, 278–280.

Zenker-Castro, F., & Barajas, J. J. (2008). Auditory steady-state responses and hearing device fitting: Part A. The role of auditory steady-state response in fitting hearing aids. In G. Rance (Ed.), *The auditory steady-state response* (pp. 241–258). San Diego, CA: Plural Publishing.

Index

Note: Numbers in **bold** reference non-text material.

B

C

D

E